Atlas of **Cardiovascular Magnetic Resonance** *Imaging*

An Imaging Companion to Braunwald's Heart Disease

Atlas of Cardiovascular Magnetic Resonance Imaging
An Imaging Companion to Braunwald's Heart Disease

Christopher M. Kramer, MD
Professor, Departments of Medicine and Radiology
Director, Cardiovascular Imaging Center
University of Virginia Health System
Charlottesville, Virginia

W. Gregory Hundley, MD
Professor, Departments of Internal Medicine
(Section on Cardiology) and Radiology
Wake Forest University School of Medicine
Winston-Salem, North Carolina

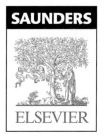

SAUNDERS

ELSEVIER

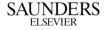

SAUNDERS
ELSEVIER

1600 John F. Kennedy Blvd.
Ste 1800
Philadelphia, PA 19103-2899

ISBN: 978-1-416-06135-9

Executive Publisher: Natasha Andjelkovic
Senior Art Manager: Ceil Nuyianes
Publishing Services Manager: Julie Eddy
Project Manager: Marquita Parker
Design Manager: Steven Stave
Marketing Manager: Courtney Ingram

Working together to grow
libraries in developing countries

www.elsevier.com | www.bookaid.org | www.sabre.org

ELSEVIER | BOOK AID International | Sabre Foundation

Printed in Canada

Last digit is the print number: 9 8 7 6 5 4 3 2 1

Contributors

Rajiv Agarwal, MD
Cardiovascular Association PLLC, Houston, Texas

Rahul Aggarwal, MD
Department of Internal Medicine, Section of Cardiology, Wake Forest University School of Medicine, Winston-Salem, North Carolina

Andrew E. Arai, MD
National Heart, Lung, and Blood Institute, National Institutes of Health, Bethesda, Maryland

Niranjan Balu, PhD
Vascular Imaging Laboratory, Department of Radiology, University of Washington, Seattle, Washington

Rebecca S. Beroukhim, MD
Instructor in Pediatrics, Harvard Medical School, Assistant in Cardiology, Children's Hospital Boston, Boston, Massachusetts

David A. Bluemke, MD, PhD, MsB
Director of Radiology and Imaging Sciences, Clinical Center, National Institutes of Health, Bethesda, Maryland

Ugur Bozlar, MD
Department of Radiology, Gulhane Military Medical Academy, Etlik, Ankara, Turkey

Hugh Calkins, MD
Professor, Department of Medicine, Division of Cardiology, Johns Hopkins University School of Medicine, Baltimore, Maryland

Marcus Y. Chen, MD
National Heart, Lung, and Blood Institute, National Institutes of Health, Bethesda, Maryland

Amedeo Chiribiri, MD
Clinical Research Fellow, King's College London, Division of Imaging Sciences, St Thomas' Hospital, London, UK

Robin P. Choudhury, MA, DM, MRCP
Wellcome Trust Clinical Research Fellow, Department of Cardiovascular Medicine, University of Oxford, Honorary Consultant Cardiologist, John Radcliffe Hospital, Oxford, UK

Baocheng Chu, MD, PhD
Biomolecular Imaging Center, Department of Radiology, University of Washington, Seattle, Washington

Jennifer A. Dickerson, MD
Assistant Professor of Clinical Internal Medicine, Ohio State University College of Medicine, Columbus, Ohio

Frederick H. Epstein, PhD
Associate Professor of Radiology and Biomedical Engineering, University of Virginia, Charlottesville, Virginia

Marina Ferguson, MT
Vascular Imaging Laboratory, Department of Radiology, University of Washington, Seattle, Washington

Scott D. Flamm, MD
Section of Cardiovascular Imaging, Department of Radiology, Cleveland Clinic, Cleveland, Ohio

Andrew S. Flett, MBBS, MRCP
Department of Cardiology, The Heart Hospital, University College London Hospitals NHS Trust, London, UK

Mark A. Fogel, MD, FACC, FAHA, FAAP
Associate Professor of Pediatrics, Cardiology and Radiology, University of Pennsylvania School of Medicine, Director of Cardiac MR, Children's Hospital of Philadelphia, Philadelphia, Pennsylvania

Christopher J. François, MD
Department of Radiology, University of Wisconsin School of Medicine and Public Health, Madison, Wisconsin

Matthias G. Friedrich, MD, FESC
Associate Professor, University of Calgary, Stephenson CMR Centre, Foothills Medical Centre,
Calgary, Alberta, Canada

Tal Geva, MD
Professor of Pediatrics, Harvard Medical School, Chief, Division of Noninvasive Cardiac Imaging, Department of Cardiology, Children's Hospital Boston, Boston, Massachusetts

Nilesh R. Ghugre, PhD
Division of Cardiology, Children's Hospital Los Angeles, Keck School of Medicine, University of Southern California, Los Angeles, California

Thomas M. Grist, MD
Department of Radiology, University of Wisconsin School of Medicine and Public Health, Madison, Wisconsin

Dipti Gupta, MD, MPH
Division of Cardiology, Department of Medicine, SUNY at Stony Brook, Stony Brook, New York

Henry R. Halperin, MD
Professor, Department of Medicine, Division of Cardiology, Johns Hopkins University School of Medicine, Baltimore, Maryland

Klaus D. Hagspiel, MD
Professor, Department of Radiology, University of Virginia Health System, Charlottesville, Virginia

Thomas S. Hatsukami, MD
Professor of Surgery, Co-Director, Vascular Imaging Laboratory, University of Washington; Surgical Service, Veterans AA Puget Sound Health Care System, Seattle, Washington

Shahriar Heidary, MD
Adjunct Clinical Instructor, Division of Cardiovascular Medicine, Stanford University School of Medicine, Stanford, California

Charles B. Higgins, MD
Professor, Department of Radiology, University of California, San Francisco School of Medicine, San Francisco, California

Ahmed M. Housseini, MD
Department of Radiology, Suez Canal University, Ismailia, Egypt

W. Gregory Hundley, MD, FACC
Professor, Departments of Internal Medicine (Section on Cardiology) and Radiology, Wake Forest University School of Medicine, Winston-Salem, North Carolina

Yasutaka Ichikawa, MD
Department of Radiology, Mie University Hospital, Mie, Japan

Alexander B. Jehle, MD
Cardiovascular Division, Department of Medicine, University of Virginia Health System, Charlottesville, Virginia

Raymond J. Kim, MD
Duke Cardiovascular Magnetic Resonance Imaging Center, Duke University Medical Center, Durham, North Carolina

Simon C. Koestner, MD
Department of Cardiology, VU University Medical Center, Amsterdam, The Netherlands

Christopher M. Kramer, MD
Professor, Departments of Medicine and Radiology, Director, Cardiovascular Imaging Center, University of Virginia Health System, Charlottesville, Virginia

Raymond Y. Kwong, MD, MPH, FACC
Co-Director, Cardiac Magnetic Resonance Imaging, Cardiovascular Division, Department of Medicine, Brigham and Women's Hospital, Instructor, Harvard Medical School, Boston, Massachusetts

Ilias Kylintireas, MD
Department of Cardiovascular Medicine, John Radcliffe Hospital, University of Oxford, Oxford, UK

Mark A. Lawson, MD, FACC
Assistant Professor of Medicine and Radiology, Vanderbilt University School of Medicine; Director, Cardiovascular MRI, Vanderbilt University Medical Center, Nashville, Tennessee

Justin M. Lee, MA, MRCP
Department of Cardiovascular Medicine, John Radcliffe Hospital, University of Oxford, Oxford, UK

Alistair C. Lindsay, MBChB, MRCP
Clinical Research Fellow, Department of Cardiovascular Medicine, University of Oxford, Honorary Specialist Registrar in Cardiology, John Radcliffe Hospital, Oxford, UK

Michael V. McConnell, MD
Associate Professor, Division of Cardiovascular Medicine, Stanford University School of Medicine, Stanford, California

James Moon, MD, MRCP
Department of Cardiology, The Heart Hospital, University College London Hospitals

Saul G. Myerson, MB ChB, MRCP, MD, FESC
Department of Cardiovascular Medicine, University of Oxford, John Radcliffe Hospital, Oxford, UK

Saman Nazarian, MD
Assistant Professor, Department of Medicine, Division of Cardiology, Johns Hopkins University School of Medicine, Baltimore, Maryland

Stefan Neubauer, MD, FRCP, FACC, FMedSci
Department of Cardiovascular Medicine, University of
Oxford, John Radcliffe Hospital, Oxford, UK

Eike Nagel, MD
Professor of Clinical Cardiovascular Imaging, King's College
London, Division of Imaging Sciences, St. Thomas' Hospital,
London, UK

Partick T. Norton, MD
Assistant Professor, Department of Radiology, University of
Virginia Health System, Charlottesville, Virginia

William O. Ntim, MB, ChB, FACC, FACP
Assistant Professor, Department of Internal Medicine, Section
of Cardiology, Wake Forest University School of Medicine,
Winston-Salem, North Carolina

Karen G. Ordovas, MD
Assistant Professor, Department of Radiology, University of
California, San Francisco School of Medicine, San Francisco,
California

Nael F. Osman, PhD
Associate Professor of Radiology, Medicine, and Electrical
and Computer Engineering,
Johns Hopkins University, Baltimore, Maryland

Rajan A.G. Patel, MD
Cardiovascular Division, Department of Medicine, University
of Virginia Health System, Charlottesville, Virginia

Sven Plein, MD, PhD
Senior Lecturer, Academic Unit of Cardiovascular Research,
University of Leeds, Leeds General Infirmary, Leeds, UK

Chirapa Puntawangkoon, MD
Department of Internal Medicine, Section of Cardiology,
Wake Forest University School of Medicine, Winston-Salem,
North Carolina

Subha V. Raman, MD, MSEE, FACC
Assistant Professor, Departments of Internal Medicine and
Biomedical Informatics, Ohio State University College of
Medicine, Columbus, Ohio

Nathaniel Reichek, MD, FACC, FAHA
Professor of Medicine and Biomedical Engineering, SUNY at
Stony Brook, Stony Brook, New York

Matthew D. Robson, PhD
Department of Cardiovascular Medicine, John Radcliffe
Hospital, University of Oxford Centre for Clinical Magnetic
Resonance Research, Oxford, UK

Hajime Sakuma, MD
Department of Radiology, Mie University Hospital, Mie,
Japan

Annamalai Senthilkumar, MD
Duke Cardiovascular Magnetic Resonance Imaging Center,
Duke University Medical Center,
Durham, North Carolina

Chetan Shenoy, MBBS
Duke Cardiovascular Magnetic Resonance Imaging Center,
Duke University Medical Center,
Durham, North Carolina

Oliver Strohm, MD, FESC
Associate Professor, University of Calgary, Stephenson CMR
Centre, Foothills Medical Centre, Calgary, Alberta, Canada

Nikolaos Tzemos, MD, MRCP
Cardiovascular Division, Department of Medicine, Brigham
and Women's Hospital, Boston, Massachusetts

Albert C. van Rossum, MD, PhD
Department of Cardiology, VU University Medical Center,
Amsterdam, The Netherlands

Gabriel Vorobiof, MD
Cardiovascular Division, Department of Medicine, Brigham
and Women's Hospital, Boston, Massachusetts

John C. Wood, MD, PhD
Division of Cardiology, Children's Hospital Los Angeles,
Keck School of Medicine, University of Southern California,
Los Angeles, California

Chun Yuan, PhD
Professor of Radiology, Co-Director, Vascular Imaging
Laboratory, University of Washington, Seattle, Washington

Foreword

The rapid advances in cardiology during the first half of the twentieth century may be fairly ascribed to the introduction of new techniques.

Paul Wood, 1951
Diseases of the Heart and Circulation

These prophetic words of Dr. Paul Wood, the preeminent London cardiologist of the 1950s, clearly have even a more meaningful relevance as we near the end of the first decade of the twenty-first century. Dr. Wood died prematurely from coronary artery disease at the age of 55, 11 years after publishing his textbook *Diseases of the Heart and Circulation*, and thus was not witness to the explosive growth of cardiovascular technology over the second half of the last century. In that same period of time, coronary heart disease deaths were cut in half.

It is unclear what role imaging has played in these improved outcomes. But it is clear that diagnostic imaging has increased more rapidly than any other component of medical care.

Cardiovascular magnetic resonance (CMR) is among the most exciting and most advanced of the imaging modalities, and its ability to visualize cardiac structures dynamically represents a true breakthrough in imaging technology. CMR has important real and potential applications for assessing vascular anatomy, the structure and function of the cardiac chambers (including ventricular mass and volume), myocardial perfusion, and myocardial scar.

Many of the applications of CMR are those that can be performed using more readily available and less expensive technology. For example, evaluation of left ventricular mass, shape, volume, and both region and global systolic function are obtained with echocardiography on a routine basis, and radionuclide imaging is in a strong leadership position for myocardial perfusion imaging. CMR is useful for these purposes when either echocardiography or nuclear perfusion imaging is unable to obtain adequate image quality or provides equivocal findings. However, CMR is not relegated to this second-tier position for many other indications in which CMR has been established as the gold standard. Most notably, the ability to visualize myocardial necrosis and fibrosis using late gadolinium hyperenhancement is an attribute that is unique to CMR. Contrast-enhanced CMR accurately identifies the location, transmural and circumferential extent, and mass of infarcted myocardium, in both acute and chronic settings. The detection of even small infarct zones detects previous myocardial infarction in patients in whom this diagnosis cannot be made by other methods. Infarct mass measured shortly after treatment for myocardial infarction predicts the degree of subsequent left ventricular remodeling and thus has important prognostic implications. As a marker of non-viable myocardium, contrast-enhanced CMR is an excellent method for determining the presence or absence of viable myocardium, which predicts the likelihood of reversal of regional and global dysfunction after revascularization.

Another means to assess myocardial viability is imaging regional left ventricular function during low-dose dobutamine administration to demonstrate contractile reserve, and studies have demonstrated that the combination of low-dose dobutamine CMR and contrast-enhanced CMR provides diagnostic accuracy in identifying viable myocardium that is greater than either method alone.

Contrast hyperenhancement has also been observed in a number of other conditions beyond coronary artery disease, including myocarditits, dilated cardiomyopathy, hypertrophic cardiomyopathy, and infiltrative conditions such as amyloidosis and sarcoidosis, which reflect pathophysiologic processes affecting the myocardial extracellular space. In some disorders, detection of these processes has prognostic as well as diagnostic value.

Unlike perfusion imaging with single photon or positron emitting radionuclides, which has limited spatial resolution, CMR perfusion imaging with pharmacologic stress provides information regarding the transmural extent of myocardial ischemia. CMR is thus able to visualize small areas of ischemia (usually present in the subendocardial zone) and also detects subendocardial ischemia in patients with multivessel coronary artery disease who might be misdiagnosed as normal by nuclear imaging because of a uniform, balanced reduction in flow. Similar methods have detected diffuse subendocardial hypoperfusion during vasodilator stress in patients with microvascular abnormalities such as those with syndrome X. New methods have evolved for quantification of regional myocardial blood flow distribution from endocardium to epicardium. Such quantitative methods will be valuable for assessing therapies, such as those stimulating angiogenesis, that result in small increases in endocardial perfusion within the ischemic zones.

CMR has become established as the most accurate noninvasive method for measuring left ventricular mass and volume, and thus ejection fraction measurements also have a high degree of accuracy and reproducibility. Strain imaging using tagging techniques offer exciting possibilities to further the understanding of regional systolic and diastolic function in a variety of cardiac diseases.

Coronary magnetic resonance angiography (MRA) remains an elusive target as a procedure that can yield images of diagnostic quality on a uniform, reproducible basis. The small caliber and tortuosity of the vessels, combined with cardiac and respiratory motion, have presented hurdles that are yet to be surmounted. Nonetheless, progress is being made. In contrast, MRA of the larger and relatively stationary non-coronary vessels is now commonplace in clinical practice, providing excellent visualization of the vessel wall and lumen, with and without the use of contrast media. Arterial remodeling is readily apparent in atherosclerotic vessels with large plaque volumes before there is significant encroachment of the vascular lumen, and important progress has been made in tissue characterization of the atherosclerotic plaques. There is promise that, with further technical advances, similar inroads will be made in coronary MRA and coronary plaque characterization.

One of the major advantages of CMR is the ability to obtain images of such excellent spatial resolution without ionizing radiation. Thus, when future research ultimately achieves the goal of routine, high quality coronary artery imaging, coronary MRA will undoubtedly compete very favorably with coronary CT angiography as the preferred tool for noninvasive assessment of coronary atherosclerotic burden and severity of coronary stenosis.

Other unresolved issues still linger: Who should be studied? Who should interpret the study? Who will pay for the study? Who will train whom? How will guidelines be affected? How will quality be determined and maintained? Hopefully, these are not unresolvable, and the cardiovascular societies are collectively addressing these complex and inter-related questions. Measuring performance in cardiac imaging is inherently difficult as it is not possible to connect the results of an imaging test to health-related outcomes. Patient selection is a key variable as it impacts importantly on downstream management decisions including further testing, interventions and costs.

On the other hand, cardiovascular imaging has transformed, and will continue to transform, cardiovascular care. CMR in particular represents a revolutionary imaging modality that creates a unique opportunity to improve diagnosis and streamline clinical management strategies but also creates challenges in patient selection, clinical training, resource utilization and cost effectiveness. That will be our challenge going forward.

The editorial team of *Braunwald's Heart Disease* is delighted to launch a series of four imaging companions, each dedicated to one of the key cardiac imaging modalities. This companion on cardiovascular magnetic resonance, expertly edited by Drs. Kramer and

Hundley, covers all of the important technical and clinical aspects of this exciting field and provides a unique case-based perspective into the tremendous potential for magnetic resonance imaging to enhance patient diagnosis and management. We believe that this companion will be a highly valuable resource for clinicians, imaging subspecialists and cardiovascular trainees and that it will contribute in a significant manner to the care of the patients they serve.

ROBERT O. BONOW, MD, MACC
Goldberg Distinguished Professor
Northwestern University Feinberg School of Medicine
Chief, Division of Cardiology
Northwestern Memorial Hospital
Chicago, Illinois

Contents

Abbreviations

A = atrium
AA = aortic arch
ACC = American College of Cardiology
ACE = angiotension converting enzyme
AHA = American Heart Association
AL = anterolateral
AO = aorta
Ao S = aortic sinus
ARVC = arrhythmogenic right ventricular cardiomyopathy
ARVC/D = arrhythmogenic right ventricular cardiomyopathy/dysplasia
Asc Ao = ascending aorta
ASD = atrial septal defect
AV = atrioventricular valves
AVS = antrioventricular septum
Az V = azygous vein
BMI = body mass index
BP = blood pressure
BSA = body surface area
CA = conus arteriosus
CABG = coronary artery bypass graft
CAD = coronary artery disease
Circ = Circumflex
CMR = Cardiovascular magnetic resonance
COPD = Chronic Obstructive Pulmonary Disease
CRT = cardiac resynchronization therapy
CS = coronary sinus
CT = computed tomography
DE = delayed enhancement
DE-CMR = delayed enhancement cardiovascular magnetic resonance
Desc Ao = descending aorta
DSCMR = dobutamine stress cardiovascular magnetic resonance
ECG = electrocardiogram
EDV = end-diastolic volume
EEST = electrocardiogram exercise stress testing
Eso = esophagus

ESRD = end-stage renal disease
ESV = end-systolic volume
F = Fontan conduit
FDG – PET = fludeoxyglucose positron emission tomography
FO = foramen ovale
FOV = field of view
Gd = gadolinium
Gd-DTPA = gadolinium diethyltriaminepentaacetic acid
HASTE = half-Fourier acquisition single-shot turbo spin echo
HCM = hypertrophic cardiomyopathy
Hep V = hepatic vein
HLA = horizontal long axis
HR = heart rate
i = index
IB = inferior baffle
IDCM = idiopathic dilated cardiomyopathy
IF = inflow tract
ILB = inferior limbic band
Inf = infundibulum
innom = innominate / brachiocephalic artery
IVC = inferior vena cava
LA = left atrium
LAA = left atrial appendage
LAD = left anterior descending
LCC = left common carotid artery
LCX = left coronary artery
LGE = late gadolinium enhancement
LLPV = left lower pulmonary vein
LM = left main coronary artery
LMB = left main bronchi
LPA = left pulmonary artery
LPV = left pulmonary vein
LSA = left subclavian artery
LUPV = left upper pulmonary
LV = left ventricular
LVA = left ventricular inferior wall aneurysm

LVEF = left ventricular ejection fraction
LVIDD = left ventricular internal diameter in diastole
LVM = left ventricular mass
LVOT = left ventricular outflow tract
LVV = left ventricular volume
MACE = major adverse cardiac events
MET = metabolic equivalent
MI = myocardial infarction
MIP = maximum intensity projection
MPA = main pulmonary artery
MPHRR = maximum predicted heart rate response
MPR = multi-planar reformatted
MSCT = multislice spical computed tomography
NYHA = New York Heart Association
OM = obtuse marginal
PA = pulmonary artery
PAPVC = partially anomalous pulmonary venous connection
PCI = percutaneous intervention
PDA = patent ductus arterious
PDA = posterior descending artery
PeriC = pericardium
PET = positron emission tomography
PFO = patent foramen ovale
PM = posteromedial
PV = pulmonary valve
PVA = pulmonary venous atrium
Qp = pulmonary blood flow
Qs = systemic blood flow
RA = right atrium
RAO = right anterior oblique
RCA = right coronary artery
Res = respiration
RF = radio frequency
RLPV = right lower pulmonary vein
RMB = right main bronchi
RPA = right pulmonary artery

RPV = right pulmonary vein
RUPV = right upper pulmonary vein
RV = right ventricular
RVOT = right ventricular outflow
SA = short axis
SA = sinoatrial
SB = superior baffle
SCD = sudden cardiac death
SE = spin echo
SLB = superior limbic band
SP = saturation pulse
SNR = signal-to-noise ratio
SPECT = single photon emission computed tomography
SSFP = steady-state free procession
ST = systolic wall thickening
STIR = short tau inversion recovery
SV = stroke volume
SVA = systemic venous atrium
SVC = superior vena cava
SVD = sinus venous defect
TD = trigger delay
TE = echo time
TGA = transposition of great arteries
TGrE = turbo-gradient echo imaging
TI = inversion time
TR = repetition time
Tr = trachea
TSE = turbo spin echo
TTC = triphenyl tetrazolium chloride
TV = tricuspid valve
VEC-CMR = velocity encoded CMR
VLA = vertical long axis
VSD = ventricular septal defect
VT = ventricular tachycardia
WMSI = wall motion score index

Chapter 1

Normal Cardiac Anatomy

Saul G. Myerson and Stefan Neubauer

KEY POINTS

- Knowledge of the anatomy of the heart and in particular the three-dimensional (3D) relationships of the various normal structures is essential.

- The heart lies at an oblique and variable angle within the chest, and standard cardiovascular magnetic resonance (CMR) imaging planes are relative to the long axis of the heart rather than the body. Standard image planes relative to body position (e.g., coronal, transaxial) can provide useful anatomic information, but it should be made clear how the image plane was positioned to avoid confusion.

- Three-dimensional spatial awareness is important in appreciating normal cardiac anatomy. Because of the oblique nature of many cardiac structures and the two-dimensional plane of a single CMR image slice, it is possible to "slice" through a structure at an oblique angle, which may appear abnormal. Further imaging in different planes (often perpendicular to the one with the apparent abnormality) is recommended to fully appreciate the nature of the anatomy and determine whether it is normal or abnormal.

- Modification of the image position may be required if the initial image is not ideal. Do not be afraid of repeating the sequence, having moved the image plane slightly or obtained other image slices to better position the image slice.

- Optimization of the sequence to each patient is important for obtaining the highest-quality images (e.g., the trade-off between spatial and temporal resolution may have to be adjusted individually). If the initial image is of poor quality, repeat with better parameters as necessary.

- For many images, cine imaging is recommended because of the continuously moving heart, because this provides a better appreciation of the anatomy in motion.

- Spin-echo images provide good contrast between tissues containing adipose tissue (e.g., pericardial fat) and tissues with high water content (e.g., myocardium) or fibrous tissue (e.g., pericardium).

- Beware of partial volume effects. The relatively thick slice thickness of CMR images (5 to 8 mm) can include parts of two structures combined in one image plane.

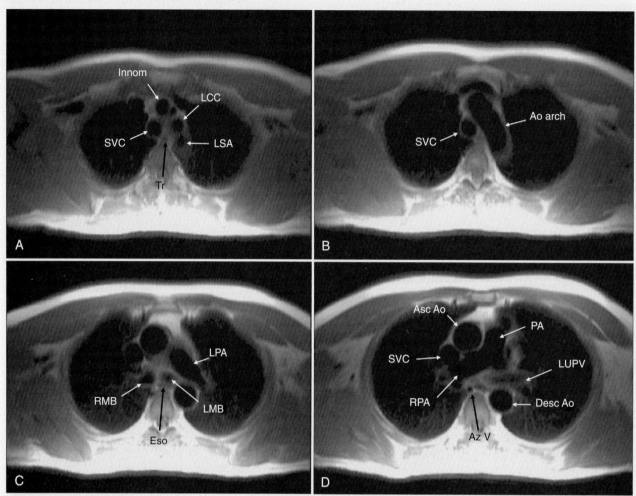

■ **Figure 1-1** Transverse views from HASTE sequence in upper thorax, from superior (**A**) to inferior (**D**). Black-blood sequence, with adipose tissue appearing bright (high signal), air and flowing blood appearing dark (low signal), and most other tissues of mid-gray intensity (intermediate signal); slice thickness = 7 mm. In (**A**), the great vessel origins can be seen—innominate/brachiocephalic artery (innom), left common carotid artery (LCC), left subclavian artery (LSA), and superior vena cava (SVC), in addition to the trachea (Tr). The esophagus (Eso) is located posterior to the Tr, but is normally compressed when lying flat, and is difficult to visualize; it can be seen lower down in (**C**). The aortic arch (Ao arch) and SVC appear in (**B**). Just below the aortic arch in (**C**), the left pulmonary artery (LPA) can be seen along with the right (RMB) and left (LMB) main bronchi, highlighted against the mediastinal fat. Lower still in (**D**), the main pulmonary artery/trunk (PA) and right pulmonary artery (RPA) and left upper pulmonary vein (LUPV) are visible between the ascending and descending (Desc Ao) limbs of the thoracic aorta. The pulmonary veins are often better visualized on coronal imaging because of their thin wall and angulated course but ideally imaged with magnetic resonance (MR) contrast angiography. The azygous vein (Az V) can also be seen just anterior to the spine on the right side.

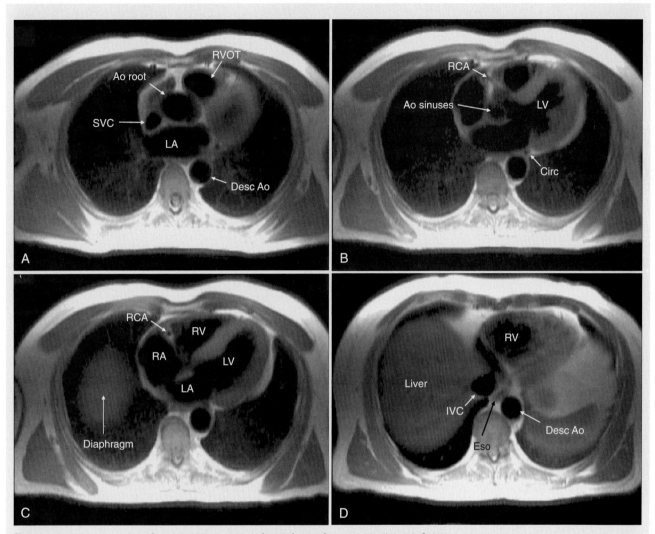

■ **Figure 1-2** Transverse views from HASTE sequence in lower thorax, from superior (**A**) to inferior (**D**). The sequence characteristics are as for Figure 1-1. **A**, The superior aspects of the heart are now in plane, aortic root (Ao root), right ventricular outflow tract (RVOT) and left atrium (LA) visible, along with the SVC. The very top of the left ventricle (LV) can also be seen adjacent to the RVOT, although is better appreciated in the slightly lower slices. **B**, The aortic sinuses (Ao sinuses) and LV are visible, and the circumflex artery (Circ) is highlighted as a small circular black void within the fat in the left atrioventricular groove. The origin of the right coronary artery (RCA) can be seen arising from the right coronary cusp. **C**, The RCA is further seen, highlighted in a similar fashion to the circumflex, within the right atrioventricular groove. The main cardiac chambers are also seen—LA, LV, right atrium (RA), right ventricle (RV), and the dome of the diaphragm. At the lowest thoracic level (**D**), the liver can be seen because of the more superior position of the right diaphragm, along with the inferior vena cava (IVC). The Eso can be seen again adjacent to the descending aorta (Desc Ao), because both penetrate the diaphragm on entering the abdomen.

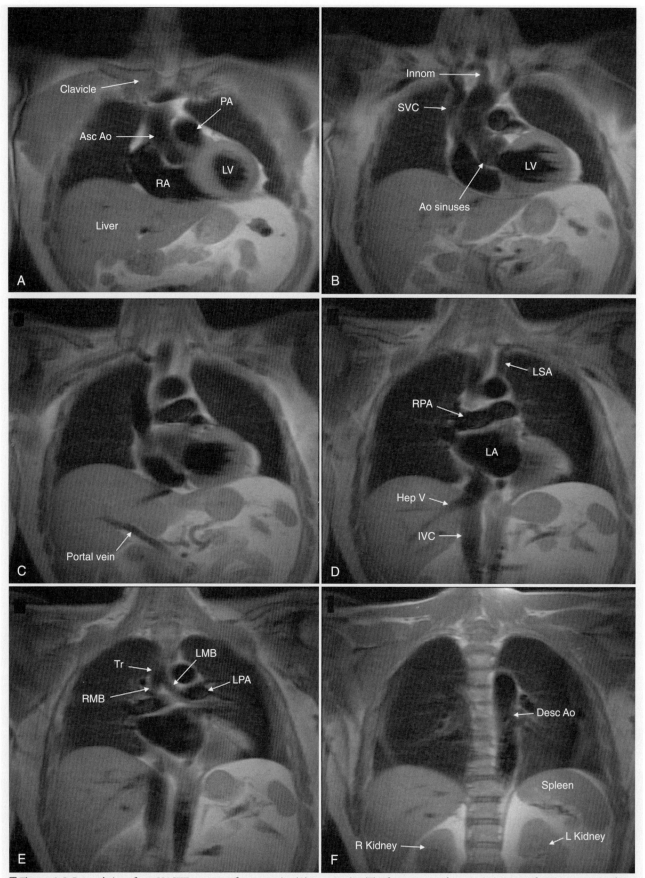

■ **Figure 1-3** Coronal views from HASTE sequence, from anterior (**A**) to posterior (**F**). The sequence characteristics are as for Figure 1-1. **A,** Slice through the clavicles, with the ascending aorta (Asc Ao), PA, RA, and LV visible. **B,** The SVC and the innominate artery (innom) arising from the AO arch can be seen. **D,** In the mid-mediastinum, the RPA, LA, and LSA can be seen (Hep V, hepatic vein; IVC, IVC). **E,** The bifurcation of the Tr into the left main bronchus (LMB) and right main bronchus (RMB) can be seen, crossing the left pulmonary artery (LPA). **F,** The most posterior slice shows the Desc Ao and the retroperitoneal abdominal organs.

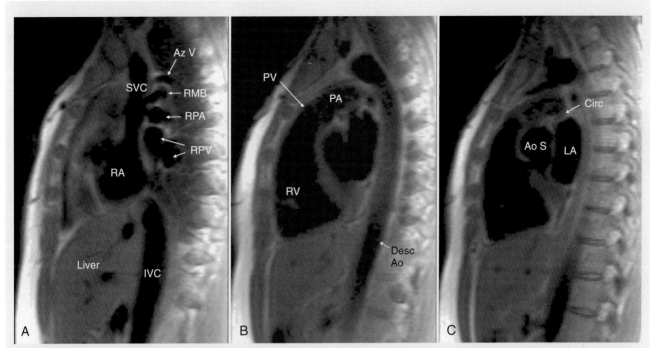

■ **Figure 1-4** Sagittal views through the right ventricular outflow tract from right (**A**) to left (**C**), HASTE sequence. The sequence characteristics are as follows for Figure: 1-1. **A,** The RA can be seen with the major veins draining into it, the superior vena cava (SVC) and inferior vena cava (IVC) (the insertion of which is just out of plane). The Az V can be seen inserting into the posterior aspect of the SVC, just above the right main bronchus (RMB) cut obliquely. The RPA is below that, with the right pulmonary veins (RPV) inferiorly. **B,** More medially, the right ventrical (RV) and main pulmonary artery (PA) can be seen. The pulmonary valve (PV) is difficult to visualize on HASTE imaging because of its thin structure with little signal, but the position is shown just at the base of the pulmonary sinuses. **C,** The Ao S are seen, with the first section of the Circ coursing in the atrioventricular groove, adjacent to the LA.

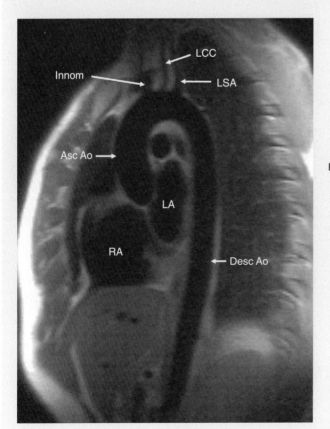

■ **Figure 1-5** Oblique sagittal view through the thoracic aorta, HASTE sequence. The characteristics are as follows for Figure 1-1: The ascending (Asc Ao) and descending (Desc Ao) limbs of the aorta can be seen in the same plane. The three great vessels arising from the arch can also be seen—the innominate/brachiocephalic (innom), left common carotid (LCC), and left subclavian (LSA) arteries. The craniocaudal relationship of the atria can also be appreciated, with the LA in a more superior location relative to the RA.

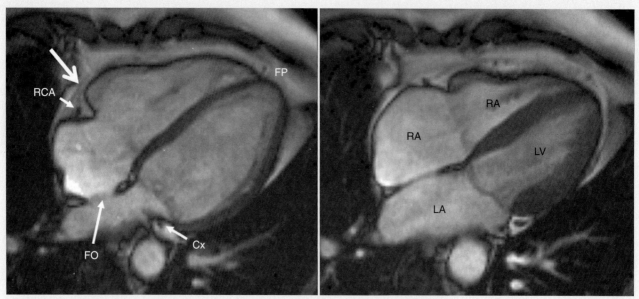

■ **Figure 1-6** Horizontal long axis view at end-diastole (*left*) and end-systole (*right*); still frame from SSFP movie sequence; TE = 1.54 msec; TR = 3.1 msec; slice thickness = 7 mm; flip angle 60°. Both blood and adipose tissue appear bright (high signal), myocardium is mid-dark gray and air almost black. Note the small atria at end-diastole, the normal-sized ventricles with normal wall thickness, and the absence of the LV outflow tract in this view. The apex is formed by the LV and there is mild bowing of the mitral leaflets. The RCA and circumflex coronary artery (Cx) can be seen in cross-section surrounded by fat in the atrioventricular groove. The pericardium can just be seen (*arrow*) and there is a moderate cardiac fat pad (FP). The atrial septum (apart from the foramen ovale; FO) is slightly thickened (6 mm) with high signal in the center and very low signal between this and the blood, characteristic of the chemical shift artifact at a fat/water interface. This patient is likely to have mild lipomatous hypertrophy of the atrial septum, a relatively common and mostly benign finding in later life, in which adipose cells infiltrate the atrial septum. This view is analogous to the apical four-chamber view in echocardiography.

■ **Figure 1-7** Turbo spin echo (black-blood) image in the HLA view (TE = 34 msec; TR = 750 msec; slice thickness = 7 mm). Note the high signal from adipose tissue, almost absent signal from blood, and the mid-gray signal from the myocardium, skeletal muscle, and vessel walls. The pericardium (PeriC) and RCA are easily seen among the adipose tissue.

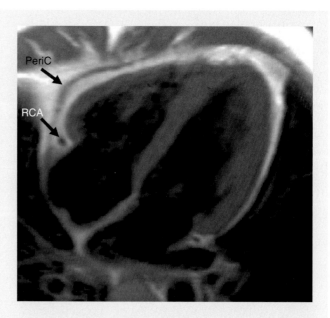

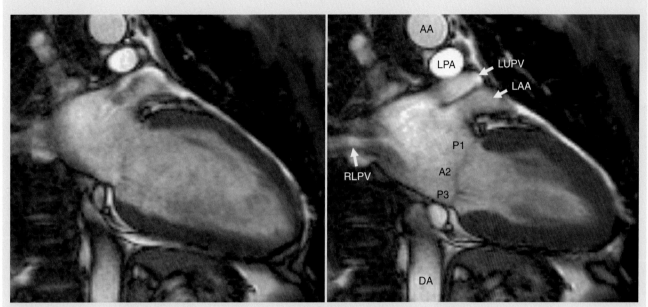

■ **Figure 1-8** Vertical long axis view of the LV at end-diastole (*left*) and end-systole (*right*). The slice passes through the LV apex and the commissure of the mitral valve, with the A2, P1, and P3 segments of the mitral valve visible in systole along with the papillary muscles. The left atrial appendage (LAA), LUPV, and right lower pulmonary vein (RLPV) can often be seen. The aortic arch (AA), Desc Ao, and LPA are also visible. This view is analogous to the two-chamber view in echocardiography.

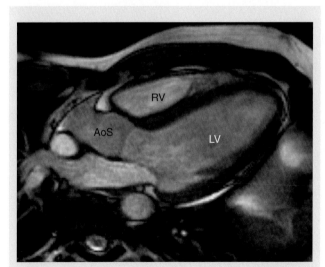

■ **Figure 1-9** Standard left ventricular outflow tract view (SSFP sequence at end-diastole). Note the good view of the LV outflow tract, the aortic valve, and the Ao S. The RV appears smaller compared with Figure 1-1 because of the rotated position of the image plane. Both aortic and mitral valves are closed because this image was taken immediately after the R-wave of the EKG, during isovolumetric contraction just prior to aortic valve opening. This view is analogous to the three-chamber view in echocardiography.

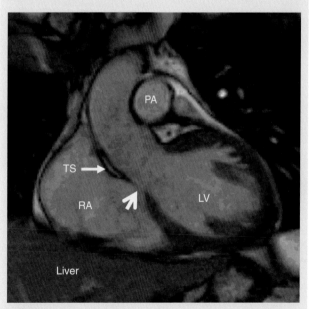

■ **Figure 1-10** Coronal left ventricular outflow tract view, acquired by placing a slice through the left ventricular outflow tract and aortic sinuses in Figure 1-4. The LV is foreshortened, but the ascending aorta is now visible passing around the main PA. The transverse sinus of the PeriC (TS) can be seen between the aortic root and the RA, which can resemble an aortic dissection to the uninitiated. The membranous portion of the ventricular septum is also seen (*arrowhead*), which separates the left ventricular outflow tract from the RA, because of the slightly more apical insertion of the tricuspid valve on the septum. The proximity of the liver to the RA can be appreciated.

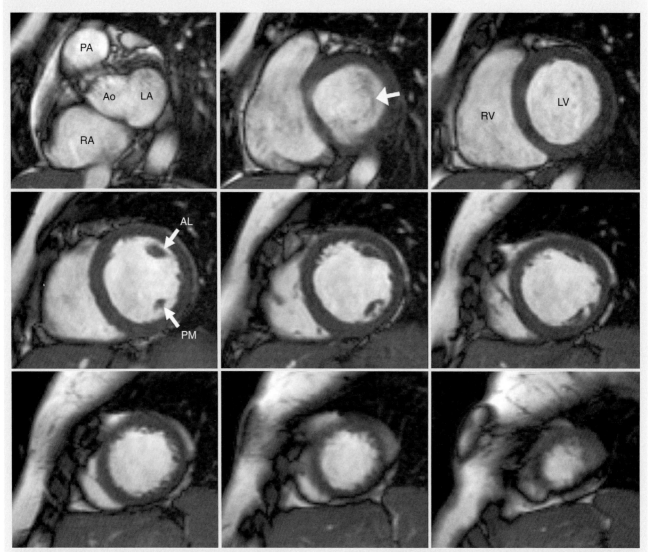

■ **Figure 1-11** Stack of short axis images of the LV and RV from base to apex at end-diastole. The first slice (*top left*) is through the atria, just basal to the mitral/tricuspid annulus. The posterior mitral valve leaflet is easily seen (*arrow*; center of top row), as are the anterolateral (AL) and posteromedial (PM) papillary muscles.

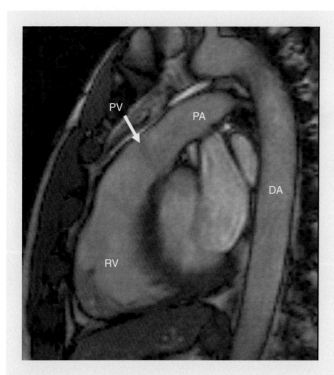

■ **Figure 1-12** RVOT in diastole. This is an oblique sagittal view through the RV infundibulum, PV, and proximal PA. The anatomy and contraction of the outflow tract can be visualized and any turbulence from PV disease noted. The RV is very foreshortened and the Desc AO is often seen in this view.

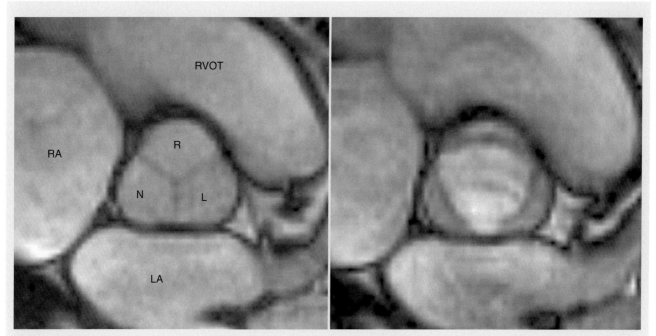

■ **Figure 1-13** Transverse view through the aortic valve in diastole (*left*) and systole (*right*). The leaflet tips can be clearly seen and the tricuspid anatomy of the valve noted (*R*, right coronary cusp; *L*, left coronary cusp; *N*, noncoronary cusp).

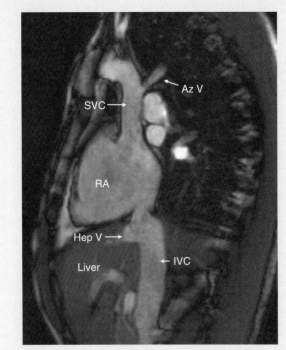

■ **Figure 1-14** Oblique sagittal view through the systemic venous return to the heart.

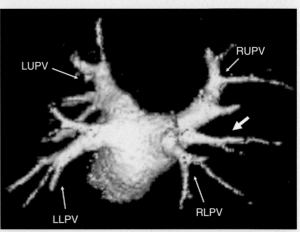

■ **Figure 1-15** Contrast magnetic resonance angiogram of the LA, viewed from posterior. A 20-ml bolus of gadolinium contrast is delivered via a power injector and imaging is timed to contrast arrival in the LA. The 3D data set is processed to remove voxels below a set intensity threshold, leaving only the high signal voxels from the contrast, which are then surface rendered, creating a "cast" of the LA and pulmonary veins. These data are commonly used for locating the pulmonary vein ostia during radiofrequency left atrial circumferential ablation for atrial fibrillation. It may also be used to fuse the anatomic images from CMR with the electrical maps acquired during invasive catheterization using proprietary software, and significantly shortens the procedure time. Care should be taken to ensure precise timing of the imaging as the contrast bolus travels through the LA, and either test sequences or bolus tracking are required. In this case, normal insertion of the four pulmonary veins can be seen, along with a common variant—a right middle accessory vein (*thick arrow*), draining the right middle lobe. As a result of this, the RLPV is smaller than the others, as in other cases, the middle lobe drains into a branch of the RLPV instead of directly into the LA.

SUGGESTED READING

Agur AMR, Dalley AF (eds): Grant's Atlas of Anatomy, 11th Edition. Philadelphia, Lippincott Williams & Wilkins, 2005.

Netter FH (ed): Atlas of Human Anatomy, 4th Edition. ICON learning systems. Philadelphia, Elsevier, 2006.

Standring S (ed): Gray's Anatomy, 40th Edition. Philadelphia, Elsevier, 2009.

Chapter 2

Normal Vessel Anatomy

Housseini M. Ahmed, Ugur Bozlar, Patrick T. Norton, and Klaus D. Hagspiel

KEY POINTS

- Optimal visualization of normal vascular anatomy with magnetic resonance angiography can be achieved with gadolinium-enhanced three-dimensional (3D) techniques, phased array surface coils, and parallel imaging.

- Three-dimensional reconstruction techniques are typically used and consist of multiplanar reformatted images and full or subvolume maximum intensity projection images in various planes.

This chapter reviews the normal arterial and venous anatomy as well as some of the more common normal variants for the extracranial circulation in the form of an anatomic atlas. All images were obtained on state-of-the-art 1.5T and 3T whole-body scanners. Gadolinium-enhanced 3D techniques were used for all cases using phased array surface coils and parallel imaging. To optimally visualize the individual vascular territories, the most appropriate 3D reconstruction techniques were used. These consist of multiplanar reformatted images and full or subvolume maximum intensity projection images in various planes, in addition to source images.

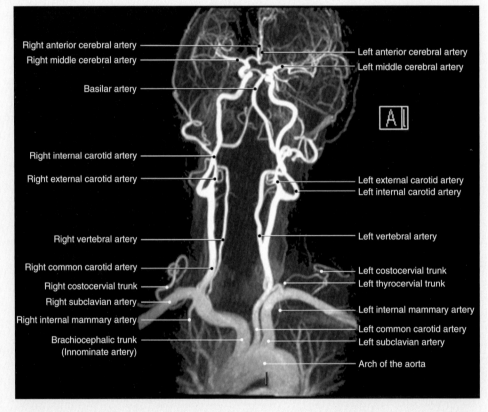

■ **Figure 2-1** Coronal maximum intensity projection (MIP) image of contrast-enhanced magnetic resonance angiogram at 3 Tesla (3T contrast-enhanced MRA) of the supraaortic arteries in a 78-year-old man. The three main supraaortic branches include the brachiocephalic, left common carotid, and left subclavian arteries, which supply the head and upper extremities.

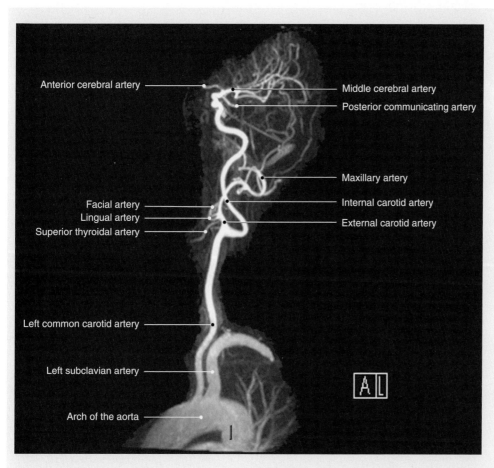

■ Figure 2-2 Oblique sagittal MIP image of 3T contrast-enhanced MRA of the left carotid artery in a 78-year-old man. The internal carotid artery has a more posterior and lateral course as compared with the external carotid artery. There are no branches of the internal carotid artery below the skull base (cervical portion).

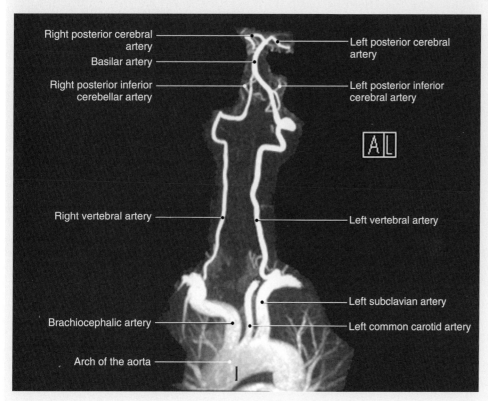

■ Figure 2-3 Coronal MIP image of 3T contrast-enhanced MRA of the vertebral arteries in a 78-year-old man. In the majority of patients, there is a dominant vertebral artery that is larger than its contralateral counterpart. In this case, the left vertebral artery is dominant.

■ **Figure 2-4** Coronal MIP image of 1.5T contrast-enhanced MRA of the upper extremity arterial tree in a 74-year-old man. The right subclavian artery originates at the bifurcation of the brachiocephalic artery and right common carotid artery, extending to the point where it crosses the outer border of the first rib, where it becomes the axillary artery. The axillary artery continues to the lower border of the tendon of the teres major muscle, where it becomes the brachial artery.

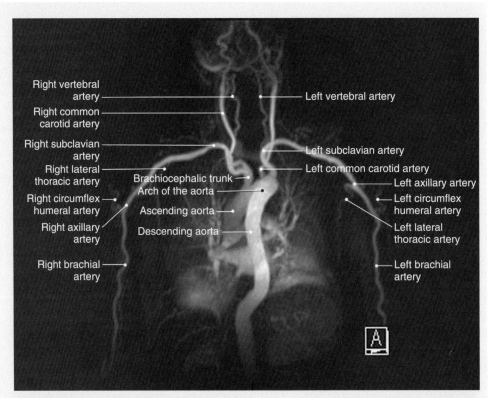

■ **Figure 2-5** Left anterior oblique MIP image of 1.5T contrast-enhanced MRA of the upper extremity arterial tree in a 74-year-old man. The ascending aorta is comprised of the aortic root (sinuses of Valsalva) and the tubular portion. The aortic arch gives rise to the supraaortic branches (see Fig. 2-1). The descending aorta begins in the region of the ligamentum arteriosum (remnant of the ductus arteriosus).

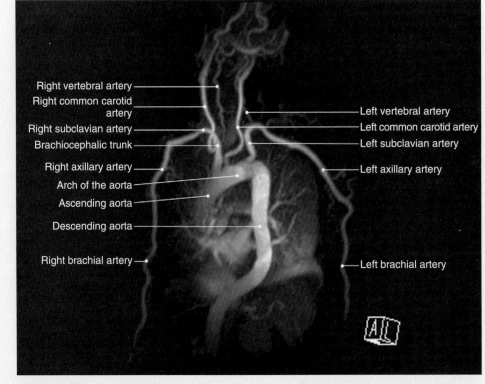

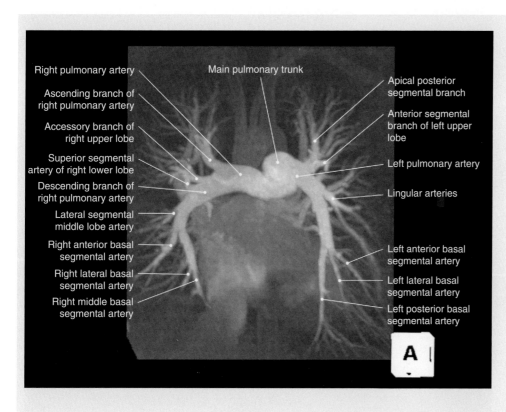

Right pulmonary artery

Ascending branch of
right pulmonary artery

Accessory branch of
right upper lobe

Superior segmental
artery of right lower lobe

Descending branch of
right pulmonary artery

Lateral segmental
middle lobe artery

Right anterior basal
segmental artery

Right lateral basal
segmental artery

Right middle basal
segmental artery

Main pulmonary trunk

Apical posterior
segmental branch

Anterior segmental
branch of left upper
lobe

Left pulmonary artery

Lingular arteries

Left anterior basal
segmental artery

Left lateral basal
segmental artery

Left posterior basal
segmental artery

A

■ **Figure 2-6** Coronal MIP image of 1.5T contrast-enhanced MRA of the pulmonary arteries in a 25-year-old woman. The main pulmonary artery bifurcates into left and right pulmonary arteries. The right pulmonary artery courses to the right, whereas the left pulmonary artery continues posteriorly.

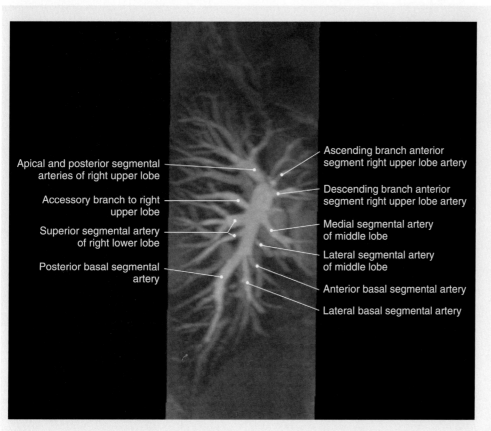

Apical and posterior segmental
arteries of right upper lobe

Accessory branch to right
upper lobe

Superior segmental artery
of right lower lobe

Posterior basal segmental
artery

Ascending branch anterior
segment right upper lobe artery

Descending branch anterior
segment right upper lobe artery

Medial segmental artery
of middle lobe

Lateral segmental artery
of middle lobe

Anterior basal segmental artery

Lateral basal segmental artery

■ **Figure 2-7** Sagittal subvolume MIP image of 1.5T contrast-enhanced MRA of the right pulmonary artery (RPA) in a 25-year-old woman. The RPA gives rise to ascending and descending branches, with the ascending branch supplying the segmental arteries of the upper lobe. An accessory branch to the right upper lobe is present in approximately 90% of individuals. The descending branch gives rise to the segmental branches of the right middle and lower lobes.

Figure 2-8 Sagittal subvolume MIP image of 1.5T contrast-enhanced MRA of the left pulmonary artery in a 25-year-old woman. The left pulmonary artery (LPA) is a little shorter and smaller than the RPA. It runs horizontally in front of the descending aorta and left bronchus to the root of the left lung, where is divides into two branches: one for upper lobe (gives off apical, posterior, anterior descending, anterior descending, and lingular arteries) and one for lower lobe (gives off superior "apical," medial basal, anterior basal, lateral basal, and posterior basal arteries).

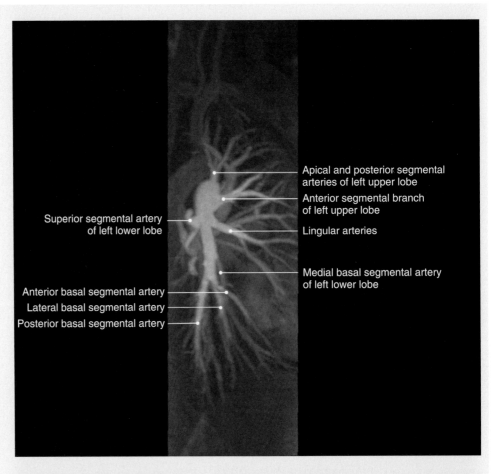

Superior segmental artery of left lower lobe

Apical and posterior segmental arteries of left upper lobe

Anterior segmental branch of left upper lobe

Lingular arteries

Medial basal segmental artery of left lower lobe

Anterior basal segmental artery
Lateral basal segmental artery
Posterior basal segmental artery

Figure 2-9 Sagittal subvolume MIP image of 1.5T contrast-enhanced MRA of the thoracic aorta in a 29-year-old woman. The bronchial arteries are quite variable, and can arise directly from the aorta or a common trunk with posterior intercostal arteries. The most superior posterior intercostal arteries arise either from the costocervical trunk (branch of the subclavian artery) or common trunks arising from the proximal descending aorta. The more inferior posterior intercostal arteries arise in left and right pairs from the descending aorta at each level.

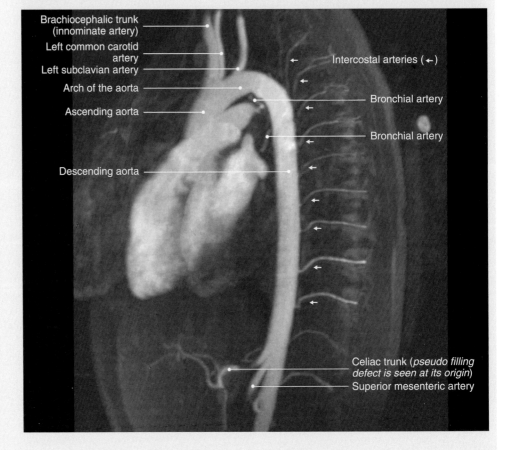

Brachiocephalic trunk (innominate artery)

Left common carotid artery

Left subclavian artery

Arch of the aorta

Ascending aorta

Descending aorta

Intercostal arteries (←)

Bronchial artery

Bronchial artery

Celiac trunk (*pseudo filling defect is seen at its origin*)
Superior mesenteric artery

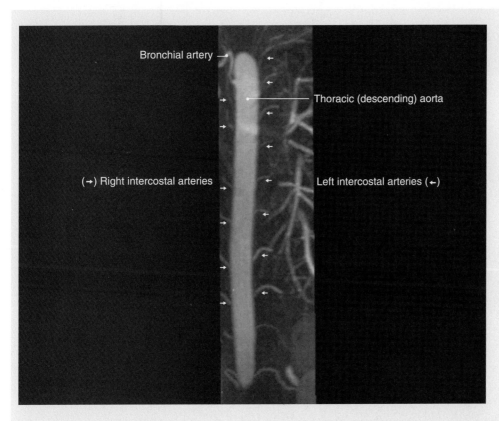

Bronchial artery

Thoracic (descending) aorta

(→) Right intercostal arteries

Left intercostal arteries (←)

■ Figure 2-10 Coronal subvolume MIP image of 1.5T contrast-enhanced MRA of descending thoracic aorta in a 29-year-old woman. Three types of intercostal arteries are present: superior intercostal arteries (from the costocervical trunk and supplying the first and second posterior intercostal spaces), anterior intercostal arteries (six pairs arising from the internal thoracic artery and supplying the upper six intercostal spaces), and posterior intercostal arteries (nine pairs arising from the thoracic aorta and supplying the lower nine intercostal spaces). The intercostal arteries originate separately, one on each side, from the descending thoracic aorta (80% of individuals), or from a common trunk. A unilateral trunk is present in 10% to 15% of individuals.

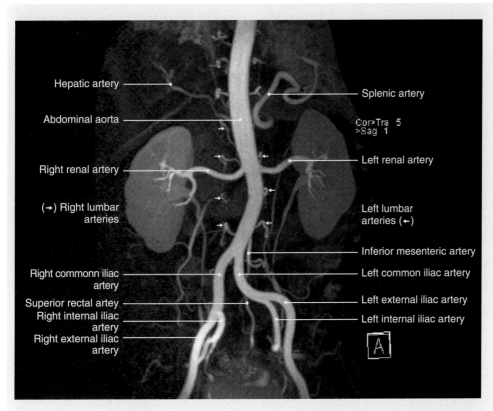

Hepatic artery

Abdominal aorta

Right renal artery

(→) Right lumbar arteries

Right commonn iliac artery

Superior rectal artey

Right internal iliac artery

Right external iliac artery

Splenic artery

Cor>Tra 5
>Sag 1

Left renal artery

Left lumbar arteries (←)

Inferior mesenteric artery

Left common iliac artery

Left external iliac artery

Left internal iliac artery

■ Figure 2-11 Coronal MIP image of 3T contrast-enhanced MRA of abdominal aorta in a 24-year-old woman. The abdominal aorta begins at the aortic hiatus of the diaphragm and ends normally at the level of the body of the fourth lumbar vertebra by dividing into the two common iliac arteries. (Occasionally, the aortic bifurcation is higher or lower.) Its branches may be divided into four sets: dorsal (supplying the body wall), ventral and lateral (supplying the viscera), and terminal (supplying pelvis and lower limbs).

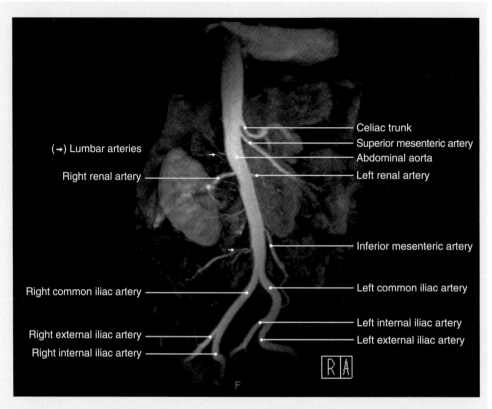

■ **Figure 2-12** Right anterior oblique MIP image of 3T contrast-enhanced MRA of abdominal aorta in a 34-year-old woman. The ventral branches of the abdominal aorta include celiac, superior mesenteric, and inferior mesenteric arteries. The dorsal branches include lumbar and median sacral arteries. The common iliac arteries are the terminal branches of the abdominal aorta. (Absent or very short common iliac arteries are rare.)

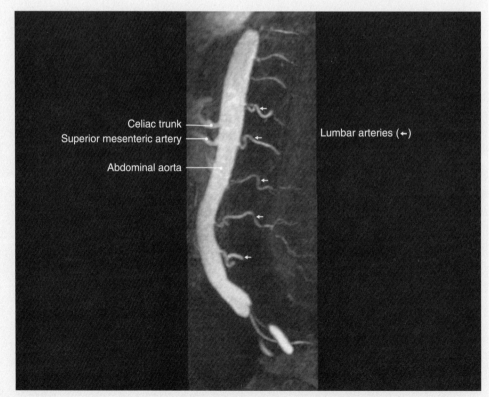

■ **Figure 2-13** Sagittal subvolume MIP image of 3T contrast-enhanced MRA of abdominal aorta in a 62-year-old woman. Lumbar arteries (usually four on each side) arise from the back of the aorta opposite the bodies of the upper four lumbar vertebrae. A fifth pair, smaller in size, occasionally arises from the median sacral artery, but the lumbar branches of iliolumbar arteries usually take their place.

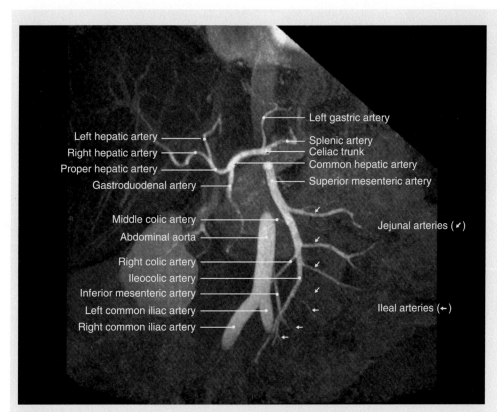

Left gastric artery
Left hepatic artery
Right hepatic artery
Proper hepatic artery
Gastroduodenal artery
Splenic artery
Celiac trunk
Common hepatic artery
Superior mesenteric artery

Middle colic artery
Abdominal aorta
Right colic artery
Ileocolic artery
Inferior mesenteric artery
Left common iliac artery
Right common iliac artery

Jejunal arteries (✔)

Ileal arteries (←)

■ **Figure 2-14** Coronal subvolume MIP image of 3T contrast-enhanced MRA of celiac and mesenteric arteries in a 47-year-old woman. The celiac trunk arises at the T12-L1 level and is usually directed inferiorly but can be horizontal or craniad. Classically, (in 65% to 75% of individuals) it divides into left gastric (usually the first branch), common hepatic, and splenic arteries. The superior mesenteric artery (SMA) origin is located around L1, slightly below the celiac artery (range, 2 mm to 2 cm). It supplies the whole of the small intestine (except the superior part of the duodenum), cecum, the ascending colon and most of the transverse colon. The SMA gives off inferior pancreaticoduodenal, ileocolic, right colic, middle colic, jejunal, and ileal branches.

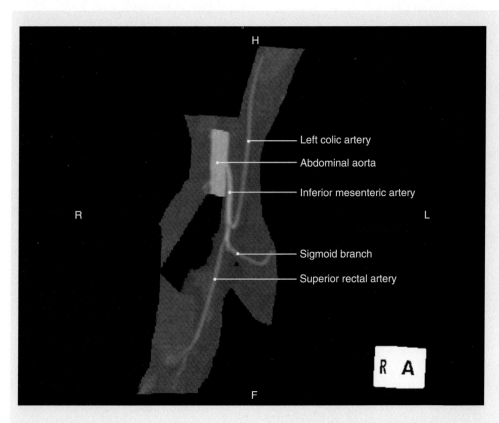

H

Left colic artery

Abdominal aorta

Inferior mesenteric artery

R

L

Sigmoid branch

Superior rectal artery

R A

F

■ **Figure 2-15** Right anterior oblique subvolume MIP image of 3T contrast-enhanced MRA of inferior mesenteric artery (IMA) in a 47-year-old woman. The IMA arises 3 or 4 cm above the aortic bifurcation (just above the lower border of the horizontal part of the duodenum). It supplies the left third of the transverse colon, the whole of the descending colon, the sigmoid colon, and parts of the rectum. The IMA gives off left colic, sigmoid, and superior rectal branches.

■ **Figure 2-16** Coronal subvolume MIP image of 3T contrast-enhanced MRA of renal arteries in a 24-year-old woman. Two renal arteries arise nearly at right angles from the sides of the aorta immediately below the SMA at L1-L2 level in around 75% of individuals. The renal artery divides at the renal hilum (in 60% of individuals) into anterior and posterior branches. In a typical case, the anterior division supplies the anterior, upper, middle, and lower segments of the kidney, whereas the posterior division (which courses behind the renal pelvis) supplies the posterior segment.

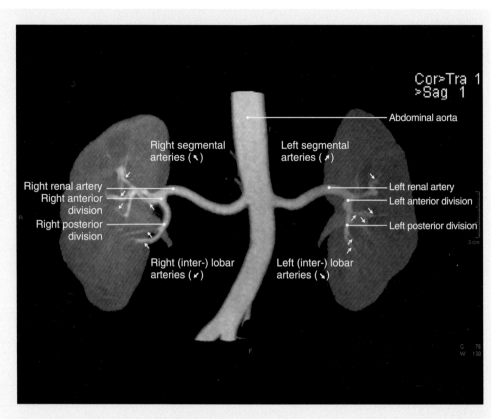

■ **Figure 2-17** Sagittal subvolume MIP image of 1.5 T contrast-enhanced MRA of the penile artery in a 33-year-old man. The blood supply of the penis is via the internal pudendal artery, which is the smaller of the two terminal branches of the anterior trunk of the internal iliac artery. After giving off the perineal artery to the perineum and scrotum, it continues as the penile artery. In the classic pattern, the penile artery gives off the dorsal penile, bulbourethral, and cavernosal arteries.

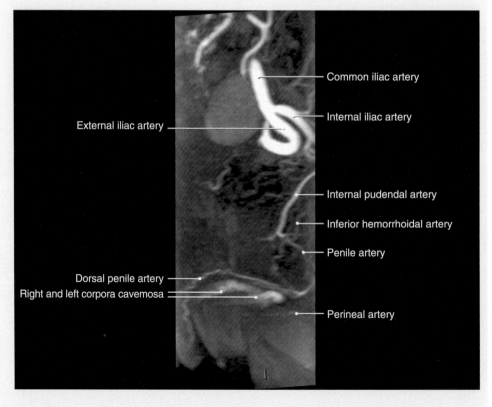

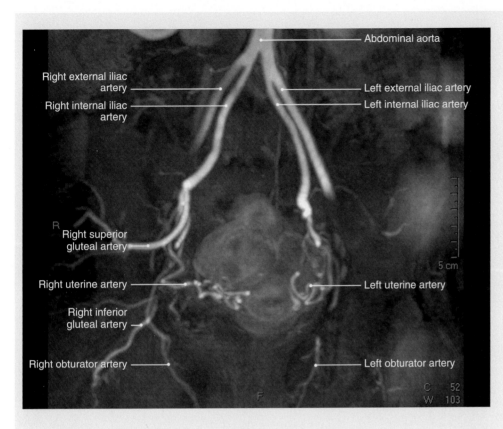

Abdominal aorta

Right external iliac artery

Left external iliac artery

Right internal iliac artery

Left internal iliac artery

Right superior gluteal artery

Right uterine artery

Left uterine artery

Right inferior gluteal artery

Right obturator artery

Left obturator artery

■ **Figure 2-18** Coronal subvolume MIP image of 1.5T contrast-enhanced MRA of uterine arteries in a 30-year-old woman. The uterine artery is a branch of the anterior trunk of the internal iliac artery. It gives off the fundal branch to the fundus of the uterus, and cervicovaginal, ovarian, and tubal arteries in addition to a small branch to the distal ureter. The terminal branches in the uterine muscle are exceedingly tortuous (helicine arteries).

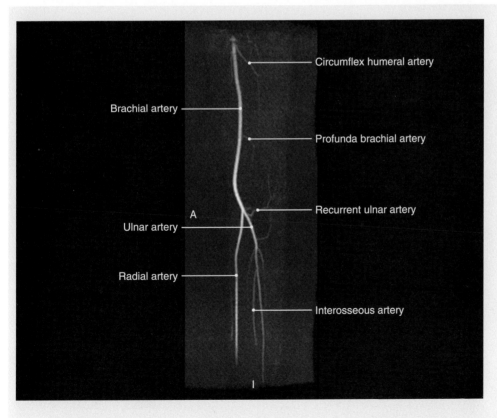

Circumflex humeral artery

Brachial artery

Profunda brachial artery

Recurrent ulnar artery

Ulnar artery

Radial artery

Interosseous artery

■ **Figure 2-19** Coronal MIP image of 3T contrast-enhanced MRA of upper extremity arteries in a 26-year-old man. The axillary artery becomes the brachial artery at the lateral margin of the teres major muscle. It ends about a centimeter or so below the elbow joint by dividing into radial and ulnar arteries. The brachial artery is superficial throughout its course; it is covered only by skin and superficial and deep fasciae. Major branches of the brachial artery include deep brachial, superior ulnar collateral, inferior ulnar collateral (supratrochlear), muscular, and nutrient arteries.

Figure 2-20 Coronal MIP image of 3T contrast-enhanced MRA hand arteries in a 26-year-old man. At the level of radial styloid process, the radial artery divides into a superficial palmar branch (anastomoses with superficial palmar arch) and a deep palmar branch (continues to form the deep palmar arch that gives off four palmar metacarpal arteries). At the pisiform bone, the ulnar artery gives off a deep palmar branch (anastomoses with deep palmar arch) and superficial palmar branch (forms the superficial palmar arch). The latter gives rise to four common palmar digital arteries to join the palmar metacarpal arteries from the deep palmar arch.

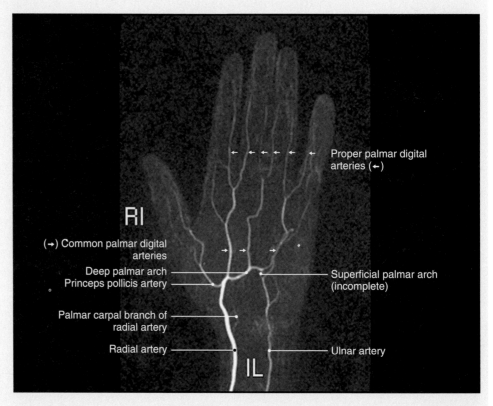

Figure 2-21 Coronal MIP image of 3T contrast-enhanced MRA of pelvic arteries in a 36-year-old man. Distal to the inguinal ligament, the external iliac artery (EIA) continues as the common femoral artery (CFA), which in turn bifurcates into the superficial femoral artery (SFA) and profunda femoris artery (PFA). Rarely, the CFA is absent and both SFA and PFA originate directly from the EIA. More commonly, the CFA is very short, giving rise to a high bifurcation. In around 60% of individuals, the PFA exists as a single trunk. Branches of the CFA include superficial epigastric, superficial circumflex iliac, superficial external pudendal, and deep external pudendal arteries in addition to muscular branches. Branches of the PFA include lateral femoral circumflex, medial femoral circumflex, and descending genicular arteries in addition to perforating and muscular branches.

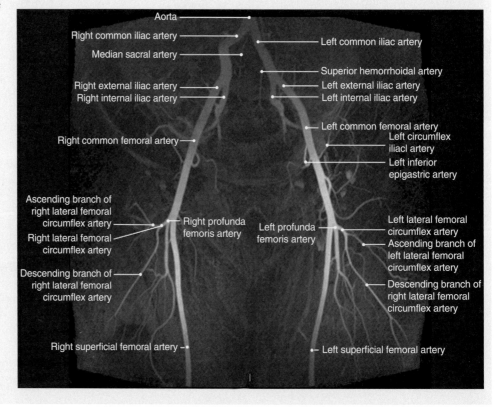

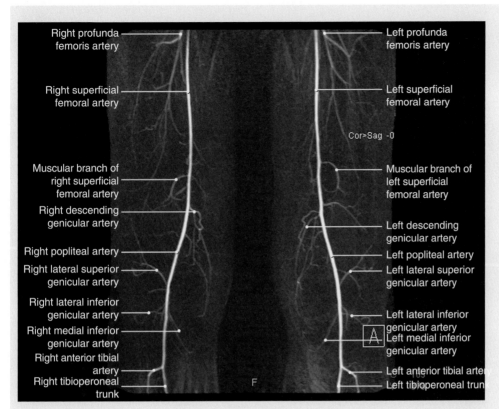

Right profunda femoris artery
Left profunda femoris artery
Right superficial femoral artery
Left superficial femoral artery
Cor>Sag -0
Muscular branch of right superficial femoral artery
Muscular branch of left superficial femoral artery
Right descending genicular artery
Left descending genicular artery
Right popliteal artery
Left popliteal artery
Right lateral superior genicular artery
Left lateral superior genicular artery
Right lateral inferior genicular artery
Left lateral inferior genicular artery
Right medial inferior genicular artery
Left medial inferior genicular artery
Right anterior tibial artery
Left anterior tibial arte
Right tibioperoneal trunk
Left tibioperoneal trun
F

■ **Figure 2-22** Coronal MIP image of 3T contrast-enhanced MRA of thigh arteries in a 36-year-old man. The popliteal artery is the continuation of the superficial femoral artery where it passes through the opening in the adductor magnus muscle (at the junction of middle and distal thirds of the thigh-adductor canal). It divides at the lower border of popliteus muscle into anterior tibial artery and tibioperoneal trunk in 95% of individuals. Branches of the popliteal artery include superior genicular, middle genicular, inferior genicular, and sural arteries in addition to cutaneous and superior muscular branches.

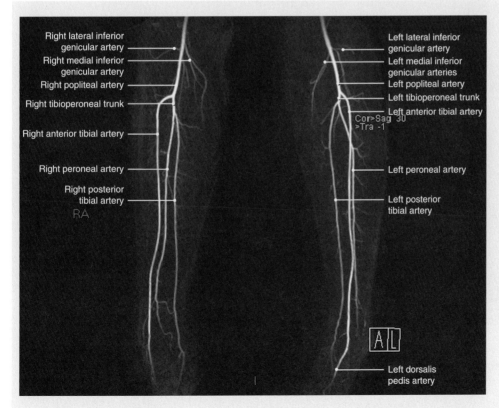

Right lateral inferior genicular artery
Left lateral inferior genicular artery
Right medial inferior genicular artery
Left medial inferior genicular arteries
Right popliteal artery
Left popliteal artery
Right tibioperoneal trunk
Left tibioperoneal trunk
Cor>Sag 30
>Tra -1
Left anterior tibial artery
Right anterior tibial artery
Right peroneal artery
Left peroneal artery
Right posterior tibial artery
Left posterior tibial artery
RA
Left dorsalis pedis artery

■ **Figure 2-23** Coronal MIP image of 3T contrast-enhanced MRA of runoff arteries in a 22-year-old woman. The anterior and posterior tibial arteries arise at the lower border of popliteus muscle. Branches of anterior tibial artery are posterior tibial recurrent a., anterior tibial recurrent a., anterior medial malleolar a., anterior lateral malleolar a., arcuate a., tarsal a., and dorsalis pedis a. in addition to numerous unnamed muscular branches. Branches of the posterior tibial artery are circumflex fibular and peroneal arteries. Branches of the peroneal artery are nutrient a., medial plantar a., and lateral plantar a. in addition to muscular, communicating, medial malleolar, and calcanean branches.

■ **Figure 2-24** Coronal MIP image of 1.5T contrast-enhanced MRA of neck veins in a 48-year-old man. The superior vena cava (SVC) is formed by the junction of the two brachiocephalic veins at the lower margin of the first right costal cartilage. The lower half of the SVC lies within the pericardium. Its major tributaries include the brachiocephalic, azygos, and small veins from the pericardium and mediastinum. The major SVC variants include duplicated SVC (observed in 0.3% of the general population), and single left superior vena cava. The brachiocephalic veins are formed by the junction of the internal jugular and subclavian veins at the base of the neck and upper thorax. Their major tributaries include vertebral, internal thoracic, inferior thyroid, superior and first posterior intercostal veins, and occasionally thymic and pericardial veins.

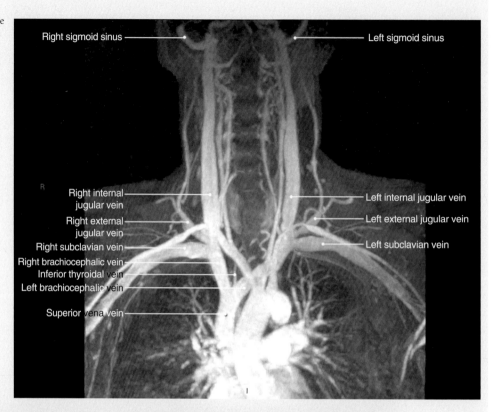

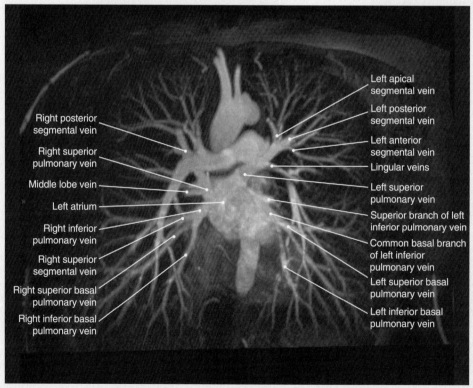

■ **Figure 2-25** Coronal subvolume MIP image of 1.5T contrast-enhanced MRA of pulmonary veins in a 55-year-old woman. Each lung is drained by its own superior and inferior pulmonary vein (SPV and IPV). The right SPV is usually formed by the junction of four veins: the apical, anterior, and posterior segmental veins and the middle lobe vein (formed by the junction of lateral and medial segmental veins). The right IPV is formed by the junction of the superior and common basal pulmonary veins. The latter has two tributaries, the superior and inferior basal pulmonary veins. The left SPV is usually formed by the junction of three veins: the apical-posterior, anterior segmental, and lingular veins. The latter has two tributaries, the superior and inferior lingular veins. The left IPV is formed by the superior and common basal pulmonary veins. The latter is formed by the junction of superior and inferior basal pulmonary veins. The SPV and IPV drain separately into the left atrium but may form a single confluence on one or both sides (common trunk).

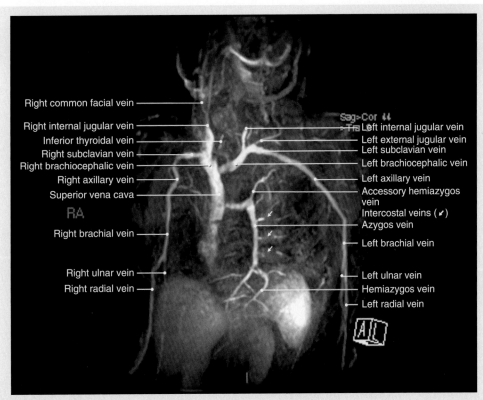

Right common facial vein
Right internal jugular vein
Inferior thyroidal vein
Right subclavian vein
Right brachiocephalic vein
Right axillary vein
Superior vena cava
RA
Right brachial vein
Right ulnar vein
Right radial vein

Sag>Cor
Left internal jugular vein
Left external jugular vein
Left subclavian vein
Left brachiocephalic vein
Left axillary vein
Accessory hemiazygos vein
Intercostal veins (✔)
Azygos vein
Left brachial vein
Left ulnar vein
Hemiazygos vein
Left radial vein

■ **Figure 2-26** Left anterior oblique subvolume MIP image of 1.5T contrast-enhanced MRA of central veins in a 74-year-old man. The azygos vein is inconstant in origin. It most frequently forms at the L1-L2 level but occasionally forms below the renal veins (lumbar azygos vein). It is joined by the right ascending lumbar and right subcostal (12th intercostal) veins at the T12 level. Major tributaries to the azygos vein include hemiazygos, right superior intercostal vein (second to fourth intercostal veins), and right posterior fifth to 11th intercostal veins. In addition, the azygos veins also receive esophageal, mediastinal, pericardial, and right bronchial veins. The hemiazygos vein also forms at L1-L2 level. It is joined at the T12 level by the left subcostal and ascending lumbar veins. Major tributaries to the hemiazygos vein include esophageal, mediastinal, left bronchial, left eighth to 12th posterior intercostal veins, and occasionally the upper lumbar veins.

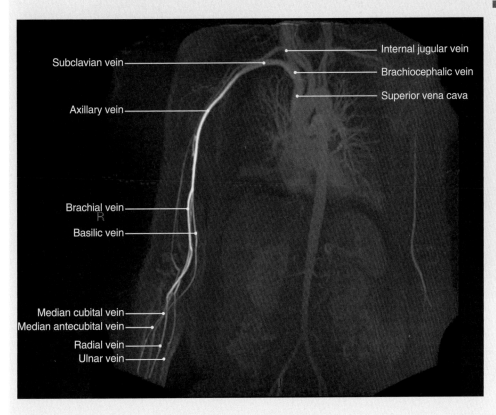

Subclavian vein
Axillary vein
Brachial vein
R
Basilic vein
Median cubital vein
Median antecubital vein
Radial vein
Ulnar vein

Internal jugular vein
Brachiocephalic vein
Superior vena cava

■ **Figure 2-27** Coronal MIP image of 1.5T contrast-enhanced MRA of upper extremity veins in a 36-year-old woman. (The technique used was direct MR venography, in which dilute contrast is injected into a vein at the dorsum of the right hand.) The superficial system of the upper extremity veins is composed of the dorsal venous network of the hand, superficial veins of the palm, median cubital and antecubital veins, in addition to basilic and cephalic veins; however, a great variation is present in the superficial veins of the forearm. The basilic or cephalic vein can be dominant or one may be absent. The deep veins are usually paired and follow their respective arteries, and include deep palmar venous arch, radial, ulnar, interosseous, brachial, and axillary veins. The deep veins of the forearm and upper arm are usually relatively small because the superficial veins provide the predominant venous return to the upper extremities.

■ **Figure 2-28** Coronal subvolume MIP image of 3T contrast-enhanced MRA of inferior vena cava (IVC) in a 49-year-old woman. The IVC is formed at the L5 level by the junction of the common iliac veins and drains the lower half of the body. It enters the thorax through the tendinous portion of the diaphragm and enters the inferior aspect of the right atrium at approximately the T9 level. The IVC is considerably distensible, with an average diameter of about 2.5 cm. Major tributaries to the IVC, in addition to common iliac veins, include the ascending lumbar, renal, adrenal, gonadal, inferior phrenic, and hepatic veins. Major IVC variants include duplicated infrarenal IVC (occurs in 2% of individuals), left-sided IVC (observed in 0.5% of individuals), and absent hepatic segment of IVC with azygos continuation.

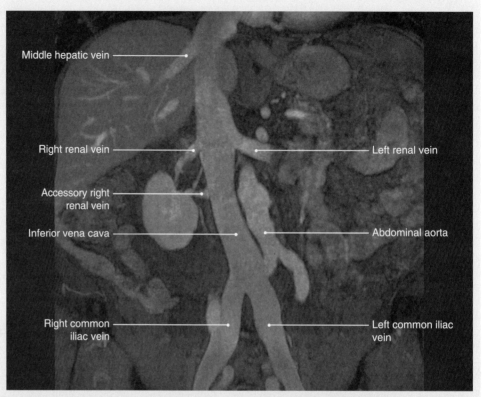

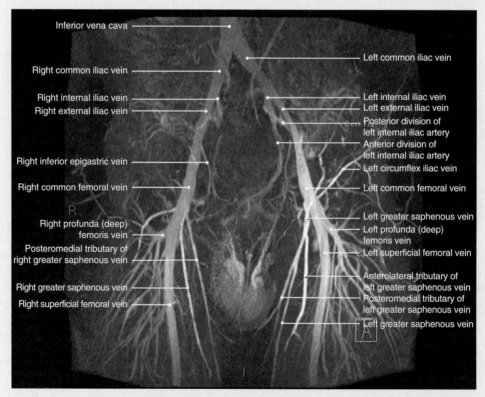

■ **Figure 2-29** Coronal subvolume MIP image of 3T contrast-enhanced MRA of pelvic veins in a 36-year-old man. (The arterial phase images were subtracted from the venous phase images resulting in a subtraction MRV.) The common femoral vein (CFV) is formed just below the inguinal ligament by the junction of the superficial and deep femoral veins (SFV and DFV). It is about 4 to 10 cm in length and continues as the external iliac vein (EIV) above the inguinal ligament. Major tributaries of the CFV include the greater saphenous vein (GSV) and lateral and medial circumflex femoral veins in about 86% of individuals. Major tributaries of the EIV include the inferior epigastric, deep circumflex iliac, and pubic veins. Tributaries of the internal iliac vein are numerous and include superior and inferior gluteal, internal pudendal, obturator, inferior and middle hemorrhoidal, vesical, prostatic, uterine, vaginal, and posterior pelvic veins.

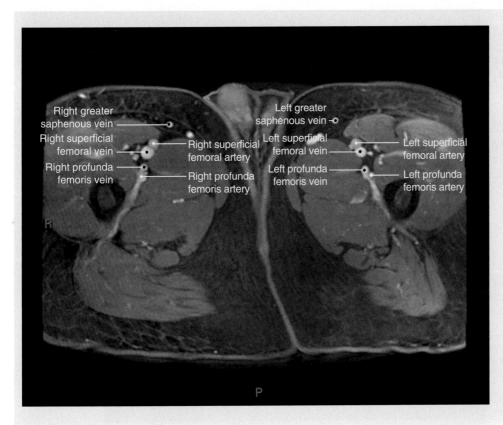

■ **Figure 2-30** Axial 3T contrast-enhanced fat-suppressed images of the pelvic veins in a 34-year-old man. The DFV (profunda femoris) lies in the proximal two thirds of the thigh and originates from the muscular tributaries in the posterior thigh. It courses anterior to the deep femoral artery and terminates in SFV. In around 50% of individuals, the DFV has a large connection inferiorly with the popliteal vein or SFV at the adductor canal. Major tributaries of the DFV include perforating veins of the posterior thigh and occasionally the medial and lateral circumflex femoral veins.

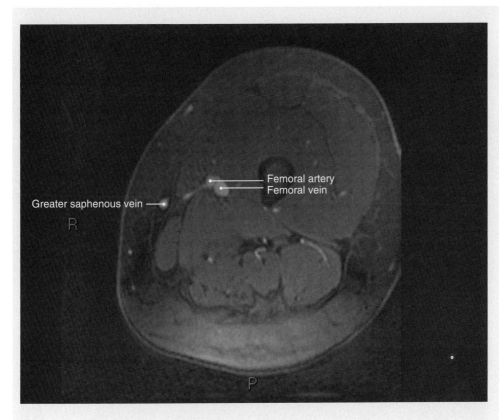

■ **Figure 2-31** Axial 3T contrast-enhanced fat-suppressed images of the thigh veins in a 22-year-old woman. The SFV begins at the adductor hiatus as a continuation of the popliteal vein. It courses posterolateral to the superficial femoral artery in the lower adductor canal and medial to the SFA in the upper adductor canal. It is most often single but may be paired or partially duplicated in 25% of individuals. The only major tributary of the SVF is the DFV. The femoral vein has several valves; the most constant sites are the SFV just below the DFV insertion and the CFV just below the inguinal ligament.

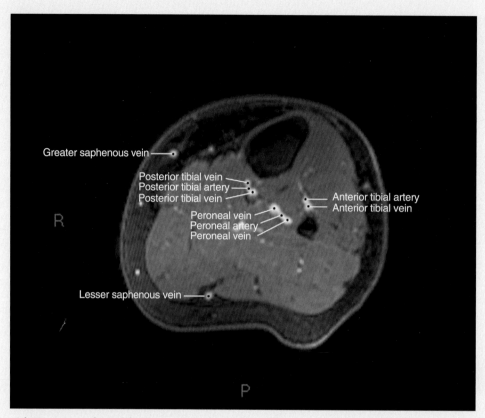

■ **Figure 2-32** Axial 3T contrast-enhanced fat-suppressed images of the calf veins in a 22-year-old woman. The GSV and lesser saphenous vein (LSV) are the direct continuation of the medial and lateral marginal veins of the foot, respectively, and they are considered the major superficial veins of the legs. The GSV is the longest vein in the body; it courses just anterior to the medial malleolus and drains anteriorly into the CFV about 3 cm below the inguinal ligament. It usually has three large tributaries: (1) at the ankle joint (joined by perforating veins from the posterior tibial veins), (2) at the calf (communicates with LSV), and (3) just below the knee joint (has two or three large tributaries). The LSV begins posterior to the lateral malleolus and ascends in the middle of the back of the calf to join the popliteal vein about 3 to 7 cm above the level of the knee joint. Less frequently it terminates in the GSV in the proximal thigh. It receives numerous cutaneous branches from the posterior aspect of the leg.

■ **Figure 2-33** Right coronal oblique MIP image of 3T contrast-enhanced MRA of the celiac artery in a 30-year-old woman showing absent proper hepatic artery (normal variant). The normal pattern of the common hepatic artery is to form the gastroduodenal and proper hepatic artery, which then divides distally into right and left hepatic branches. This pattern is present in only 54% to 75% of the population, the remainder having aberrant hepatic branches from the left gastric artery or SMA. Division of the hepatic artery into its right and left hepatic branches may take place at any point between the proper hepatic artery and the aortic origin of the main hepatic trunk. The right hepatic artery may arise from the gastroduodenal artery (absent proper hepatic artery), common hepatic artery, or celiac trunk.

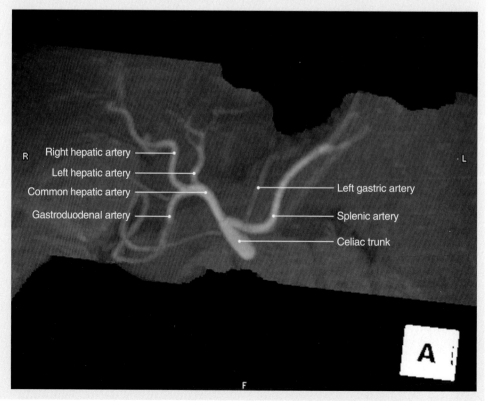

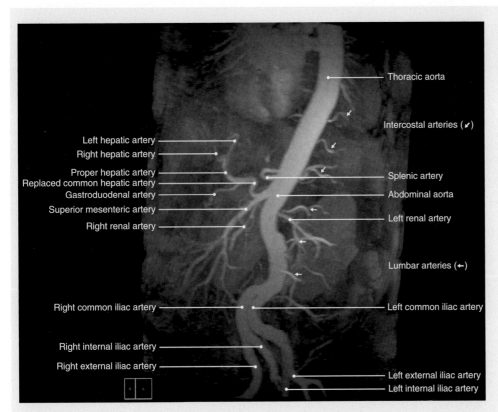

Left hepatic artery
Right hepatic artery
Proper hepatic artery
Replaced common hepatic artery
Gastroduodenal artery
Superior mesenteric artery
Right renal artery

Right common iliac artery

Right internal iliac artery
Right external iliac artery

Thoracic aorta
Intercostal arteries (↙)
Splenic artery
Abdominal aorta
Left renal artery
Lumbar arteries (←)
Left common iliac artery
Left external iliac artery
Left internal iliac artery

■ **Figure 2-34** Left anterior oblique MIP image of 3T contrast-enhanced MRA of abdominal aorta in a 70-year-old man showing a replaced common hepatic artery off the superior mesenteric artery (normal variant). Variations in the arrangement of the hepatic artery and its branches are common and of surgical importance. (1) The common hepatic artery may arise from the SMA or less commonly from the abdominal aorta (2.5% and 2%, respectively). (2) An accessory left hepatic artery arises most frequently from the left gastric artery. (3) An accessory right hepatic artery arises most commonly from the SMA.

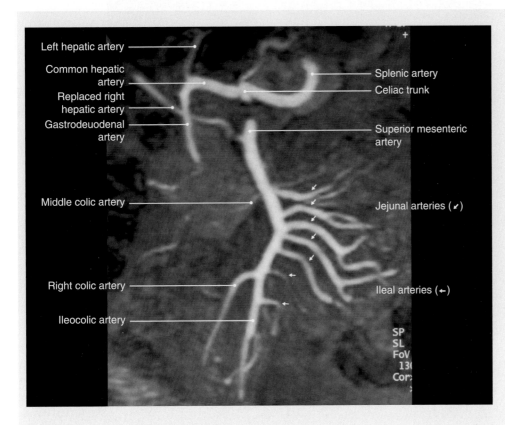

Left hepatic artery
Common hepatic artery
Replaced right hepatic artery
Gastrodeuodenal artery

Middle colic artery

Right colic artery

Ileocolic artery

Splenic artery
Celiac trunk
Superior mesenteric artery
Jejunal arteries (↙)
Ileal arteries (←)

SP
SL
FoV
13
Cor

■ **Figure 2-35** Coronal subvolume MIP image of 1.5T contrast-enhanced MRA of the superior mesenteric artery in a 41-year-old man showing replaced right hepatic artery (normal variant). Accessory right and left hepatic arteries may also arise from gastroduodenal artery or the aorta. They may exist in conjunction with normal branches of the hepatic artery and constitute additional sources of blood supply to the liver. On the other hand, they may replace the normal branches in 41% of individuals and constitute the sole supply to the corresponding segments of the liver; they are then called replaced hepatic arteries. Replaced right hepatic arteries off the SMA are seen in 10% to 12% of individuals.

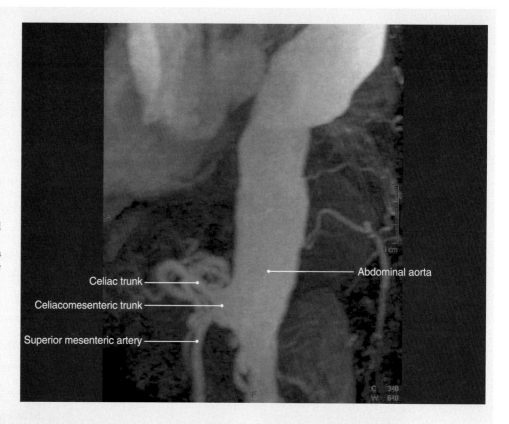

■ **Figure 2-36** Sagittal MIP image of 1.5T contrast-enhanced MRA of the abdominal aorta in a 66-year-old man with a thoracoabdominal aortic aneurysm showing a celiacomesenteric trunk (normal variant). Variations in the branching pattern of the celiac trunk are observed in around 25% to 35% of individuals. In 25% there is a true trifurcation of the three branches. The celiac and superior mesenteric arteries form a common trunk (celiacomesenteric trunk) in less than 1% of individuals.

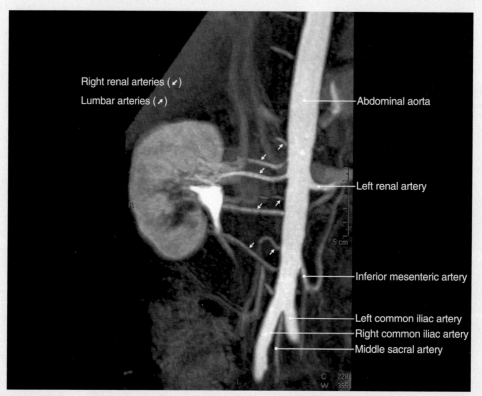

■ **Figure 2-37** Coronal subvolume MIP image of 1.5T contrast-enhanced MRA of the abdominal aorta in a 60-year-old man showing four right renal arteries (normal variant). Variant arterial anatomy of the kidney, including multiple arteries and early division, occurs in around 40% of individuals. In 30% of individuals, there are multiple (two to four) renal arteries. Multiple renal arteries are unilateral in 32% and bilateral in 12% of individuals. Approximately 10% are accessory vessels (supernumerary vessels that enter the kidney independently at the hilum and originate from the abdominal aorta in 98% of cases) and 20% are aberrant arteries (enter the kidney outside the hilum). Accessory and aberrant arteries have been observed to originate from iliac, superior mesenteric, inferior mesenteric, median sacral, intercostal, lumbar, adrenal, inferior phrenic, right hepatic, or right colic arteries in addition to abdominal aorta.

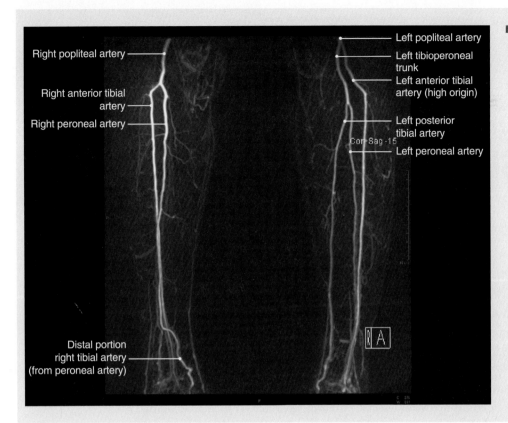

Right popliteal artery

Right anterior tibial artery

Right peroneal artery

Distal portion right tibial artery (from peroneal artery)

Left popliteal artery

Left tibioperoneal trunk

Left anterior tibial artery (high origin)

Left posterior tibial artery

Left peroneal artery

Cor-Sag-15

■ **Figure 2-38** Coronal MIP image of 3T contrast-enhanced MRA of the runoff vessels in a 42-year-old woman shows high origin of left anterior tibial artery and absent right anterior tibial artery (normal variants). The right distal posterior tibial artery comes off the peroneal artery. Variations in the branching pattern of the popliteal artery are observed in up to 12% of the population. It may divide into terminal branches above the level of popliteus muscle, so the anterior tibial artery descends anterior to it in around 5% of individuals. In 7% of individuals the peroneal artery is the major source of blood supply to the foot. The anterior and posterior tibial arteries are absent or terminate early in 2% and 5%, respectively. The perforating branch of the peroneal artery may continue as the dorsalis pedis artery. The popliteal artery is congenitally absent in less than 0.1% of individuals.

SUGGESTED READING

Agur AMR, Dalley AF (eds): Grant's Atlas of Anatomy, 11th Edition. Philadelphia, Lippincott Williams and Wilkins, 2005.

Khadir S (ed): Atlas of Normal and Variant Angiographic Anatomy. Philadelphia, Elsevier, 1991.

Netter FH (ed): Atlas of Human Anatomy, 4th Edition. ICON learning systems. Philadelphia, Elsevier, 2006.

Standring S (ed): Gray's Anatomy, 40th Edition. Philadelphia, Elsevier, 2009.

Chapter 3

Left Ventricular Volumes, Ejection Fraction, Mass, and Shape

Nathaniel Reichek and Dipti Gupta

KEY POINTS

- Cardiovascular magnetic resonance (CMR) is the most accurate and comprehensive method available for assessment of left ventricular structure and function. It provides high spatial and temporal resolution and volumetric quantitation throughout the cardiac cycle without any geometric assumptions.

- CMR is a powerful method for serial follow-up of ventricular remodeling of any cause. High test-retest reproducibility permits accurate detection of changes in left ventricular volumes, mass, and ejection fraction.

- CMR achieves statistical power in research protocols and clinical trials, while reducing sample sizes required compared with other imaging methods.

- Normal CMR values for left ventricular volumes, mass, and ejection fraction have been defined and can be adjusted for age and gender. Variations in methods may require development of laboratory-specific normal values.

- Using CMR LV mass and mass/volume ratio, left ventricular remodeling in hypertensive heart disease can be classified as concentric left ventricular hypertrophy, concentric remodeling without hypertrophy, or eccentric hypertrophy. Regression of hypertrophy with treatment, which reduces cardiovascular risk, is readily documented with CMR.

- CMR can depict complex patterns of interrelated changes in left ventricular volumes, systolic function, and mass that may be seen with treatment in hypertension, valvular regurgitation, and ischemic and idiopathic dilated cardiomyopathies.

- CMR is highly effective in quantitation of the left ventricular response to volume overload and resultant changes in left ventricular volumes and ejection fraction. Regurgitant volume and fraction are easily determined.

- CMR is a preferred method for assessment of left ventricular size and global and segmental myocardial function in ischemic heart disease. Combined with CMR viability imaging, it is a powerful tool for clinical decision making.

- CMR can detect patients regarded as having nonischemic cardiomyopathy who in fact have ischemic cardiomyopathy.

Accurate and reproducible quantitative assessment of left ventricular (LV) structure and function is an essential prerequisite in the diagnosis and management of almost all forms of adult cardiovascular disease. CMR is an extremely powerful noninvasive imaging modality that provides comprehensive anatomic and physiologic assessment of the left ventricle, including chamber volume, ejection fraction, myocardial mass, and shape. It offers three-dimensional (3D) visualization of the left ventricle through the cardiac cycle with high spatial and temporal resolution without use of ionizing radiation or contrast agents. CMR is especially useful in patients deemed technically difficult for echocardiography but is also more reliable than two-dimensional (2D) echocardiography when LV size and function are abnormal, particularly in ischemic heart disease. In addition, CMR permits assessment of regional structure and function parameters in correct spatial registration with powerful imaging methods for tissue characterization, such as delayed enhancement imaging of myocardial infarction.

CMR determinations of ejection fraction (EF), end-diastolic and end-systolic volumes (EDV, ESV), and left ventricular mass (LVM) have shown high levels of agreement with existing alternative invasive and noninvasive reference methods, including biplane invasive ventriculography, thermodilution and Fick stroke volumes, cardiac CT, and 3D echocardiography. These measurements also have shown excellent intraobserver, interobserver, and test-retest reproducibility. CMR reproducibility is superior to that of 2D echocardiography (Table 3-1).

Because the confidence limits of an image-based measurement are a function of the variability of the measurement, including the sum of intraobserver or interobserver variability and imaging variability (expressed as standard deviation), this enables CMR to reliably detect abnormalities and changes in ventricular structure and function that conventional 2D echocardiography cannot (Table 3-2). The smallest changes in left ventricular structure and function detectable in an individual patient are two times the test-test standard deviation in either direction. The smallest changes reliably detected by echocardiography are, in fact, rather large, perhaps larger than those likely to be seen in most patients with chronic cardiac disease.

METHODS AND NORMAL VALUES

CMR LV evaluation is typically performed using ECG-gated segmented breath-held cine imaging with a steady-state free procession (SSFP) sequence. A study is initiated by obtaining scout images in the axial, sagittal, and coronal planes. An iterative process is then used to define and confirm the LV long and short-axis planes as follows. The axial scouts are used to prescribe a scout two-chamber single-phase image. By imaging orthogonal to the two-chamber scout, an LV four chamber scout image is obtained. Prescription of a stack of short-axis scout images perpendicular to the long-axis on the four-chamber plane is then performed. A four-chamber cine image loop showing the left ventricular septal and lateral walls is then prescribed from the short-axis scout stack. Rotation of the imaging plane counterclockwise relative to the short-axis plane provides both a long-axis three-chamber plane extending from the aortic root to the LV apex showing the LV anteroseptal and posterolateral walls and a two-chamber cine showing the LV anterior and inferior walls. The four-chamber cine plane is then used to prescribe the stack of adjacent short-axis cine loops from the LV apex through the aortic and mitral valve planes. Although in normally shaped ventricles with uniform regional function, biplane long-axis analyses assuming rotational uniformity of the LV may provide clinically useful results, most laboratories use full analysis of the LV short-axis stack for quantitative assessments because they are independent of any geometric assumptions and integrate much more 3D data, and hence are more reproducible (Figs. 3-1 and 3-2).

By adding the LV cavity areas on all the slices at end-diastole and multiplying by the slice thickness, EDV is obtained by the analytic software. End-systolic volume is determined in a similar manner and EF calculated. A summation of all end-diastolic LV myocardial areas, multiplied by slice thickness and the specific gravity of the myocardium (1.055) provides LV mass.

CMR LV imaging and analysis is not entirely standardized at present, so local laboratory normal values are extremely valuable. Among variations in methods that can differ among CMR laboratories and may affect normal values and results in abnormal hearts are temporal and spatial resolution of CMR images, use of retrospective versus prospective gating, inclusion of papillary

TABLE 3-1 Test-Retest Reproducibility

VARIABLE	2D ECHO SD	CMR SD
LVEDV (ml)	24	7.4
LVESV (ml)	16	6.5
LVEF (%)	6.6	2.5
LVM (g)	36	6.4

LVEDV, left ventricular end-diastolic volume; LVEF, left ventricular ejection fraction; LVESV, left ventricular end-systolic volume; LVM, left ventricular mass; SD, standard deviation.
From Rajappan K, Bellenger NG, Anderson L, Pennell DJ: The role of cardiovascular magnetic resonance in heart failure. Eur J Heart Fail 2000;2:241-252, with permission.

TABLE 3-2 Smallest Detectable Changes in a Single Patient

VARIABLE	2D ECHO SD	CMR SD
LVEDV (ml)	48	14.8
LVESV (ml)	32	13
LVEF (%)	13.2	5
LVM (g)	72	12.8

LVEDV, left ventricular end-diastolic volume; LVEF, left ventricular ejection fraction; LVESV, left ventricular end-systolic volume; LVM, left ventricular mass; SD, standard deviation.

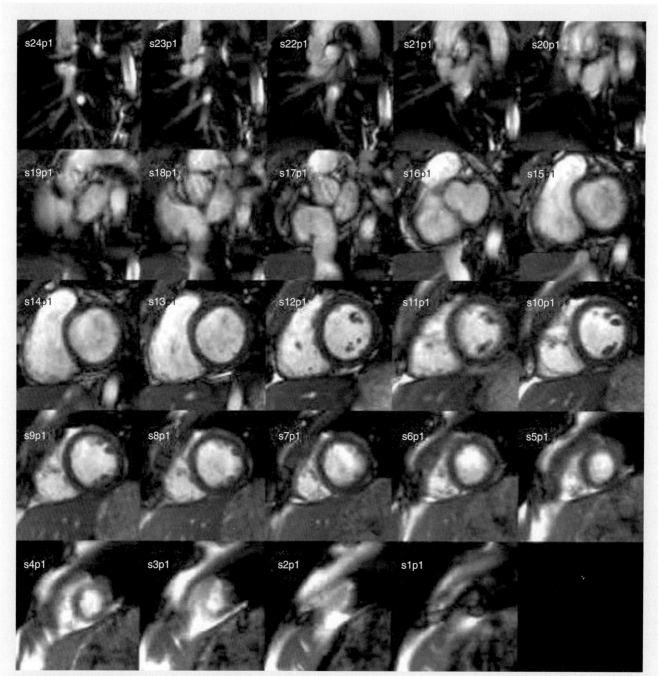

■ **Figure 3-1** Representative contiguous end-diastolic 8-mm short-axis slices of the left heart from the
dome of the left atrium (*upper left*) to the apex of the left ventricle (*lower right*).

muscles and trabeculae in the LV cavity or myocardial
mass, method of determining end-systole, analytic software package used, and intra observer and interobserver
variability.

Our laboratory developed a reference set of normal
LV values in an extensively screened normal cohort of
over 200 normotensive, nondiabetic, nonobese (body
mass index [BMI] < 28) volunteers without history of
cardiovascular disease or symptoms thereof, additionally screened with 2D echocardiography (Table 3-3).
We used maximal available temporal and spatial resolution in each subject, which are functions of heart rate and
body size. CMR was performed using prospectively gated

SSFP cine imaging with contiguous 8-mm slices in the
LV short-axis plane. LV end-diastolic and end-systolic
volumes, ejection fraction, and mass were determined using MASS software (Medis, New York, NY), including
papillary muscles and trabeculae in LV cavity and defining end-systole as the time of aortic valve closure. Results
were indexed (i) to body surface area.

Note that women have higher EF and lower EDVi,
ESVi, and LVMi compared with men, despite correction for body size. This finding also has been described in
several large population studies. In addition, even within
the normal range, systolic blood pressures are some-
what higher in men than women, which accounts for the

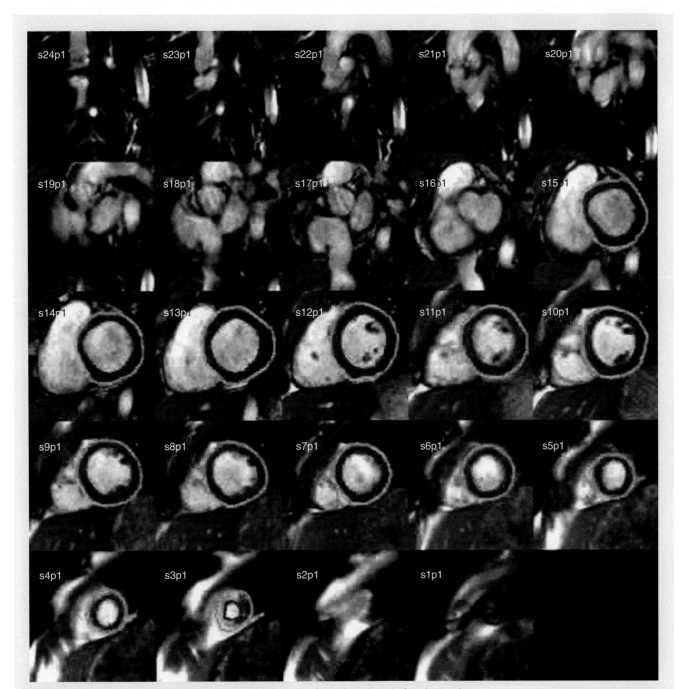

■ **Figure 3-2** Short-axis images from Figure 3-1 with left ventricular endocardium (*red*) and epicardium and right septal border (*green*) demarcated manually.

TABLE 3-3 LV Parameters Indexed to Body Surface Area in Normal Volunteers

VARIABLE	MALE	FEMALE
LVEDVi (ml/m^2)	74 ± 14	67 ± 11
LVESVi (ml/m^2)	32 ± 8	26 ± 7
LVEF (%)	57 ± 6	61 ± 6
LVMi (g/m^2)	67 ± 11	54 ± 9
LVM/EDV (g/ml)	0.9 ± 0.2	0.8 ± 0.2

LVEDVi, left ventricular end-diastolic volume index; LVEF, left ventricular ejection fraction; LVESVi, left ventricular end-systolic volume index; LVM/EDV, left ventricular mass:end-diastolic volume ratio; LVMi, left ventricular mass index.

higher LV mass/volume ratio in men than women. We and others have also noted that chamber volumes diminish with age, but development of age-specific laboratory normal values is hampered by the very large sample sizes required to cover the age range needed. Steady-state free procession cine left ventricular volume indices are higher and mass lower than those obtained using echocardiography or using older CMR gradient echo cine methods. The different results between gradient echo and SSFP CMR are likely caused by higher contrast between blood pool and myocardium found with SSFP and resultant differences in partial volume effects at the endocardium.

Case 1   Normal Left Ventricle

Figures 3-3 and 3-4 were taken in a normotensive, nonobese, nondiabetic, healthy 48-year-old female volunteer without any history of cardiovascular disease or symptoms thereof. Quantitative results: BP 118/70 mm Hg; BSA 1.42 m²; EDV 109 ml; EDVi 77 ml/m²; ESV 38 ml; ESVi 27 ml/m²; LVM 78 g; LVMi 55 g/m²; LVEF 65%.

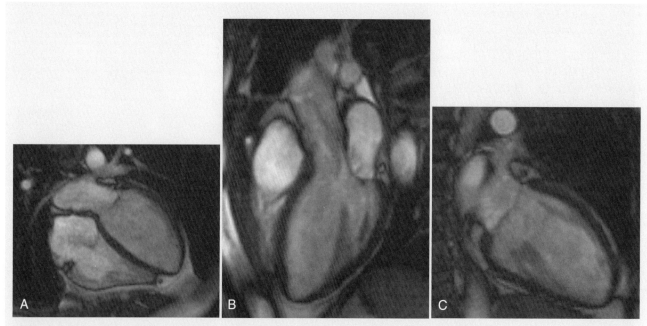

■ **Figure 3-3** After definition of the LV long-axis on scout images, CMR was performed using steady-state free procession (SSFP) cine imaging, obtaining LV four-chamber, three-chamber, and two-chamber cine loops (shown: LV four-chamber, three-chamber, and two-chamber images at end-diastole). Biplane estimation of LV volume, mass, and ejection fraction can be performed from such images but sacrifices the accuracy of volumetric imaging and works acceptably only if LV shape is normal.

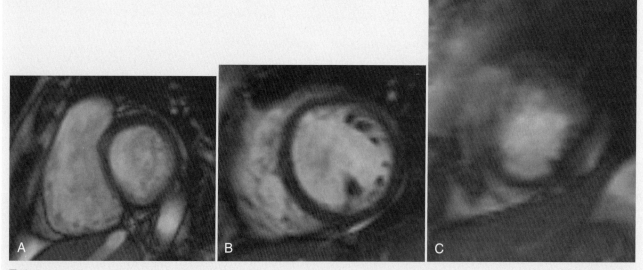

■ **Figure 3-4** Selected LV short-axis basal, mid-ventricular, and apical images at end-diastole are shown from a contiguous stack of short-axis cine loops from LV apex through the LV base in this normal volunteer. To quantitate LV end-diastolic and -systolic volumes, ejection fraction, mass, and shape, the LV epicardial and endocardial borders on each slice in the stack must be assessed with FDA-approved software using either manual planimetry or one of several available semiautomated methods that can incorporate the location of the mitral and aortic valve planes on the long-axis images into the analysis.

Comment

Although absolute values for volumes and mass are relatively low in this individual, the subject's body size is relatively small and EDVi is actually higher than the mean for normal women. All indexed results are within the normal range.

Case 2   Hypertension

This 59-year-old man with long-standing hypertension and EKG LVH, a risk factor connoting up to a tenfold increase in cardiovascular events is enrolled in a research treatment protocol combining an ACE inhibitor and an aldosterone antagonist. CMR was performed at intake and at 3.5 months of treatment (Figs. 3-5 to 3-7). At intake, BP is 185/104 mm Hg. Posttreatment BP is 147/94 mm Hg. Quantitative results before treatment: EDVi: 109 ml/m^2;* ESVi: 58 ml/m^2;* LV EF: 47%; LVM: 330 g; LVMi: 145 g/m^2;* mass/volume ratio: 1.34. [*, significantly abnormal, $p < 0.05$].

Quantitative results after 3.5 months treatment: EDVi: 87 ml/m^2;** ESVi: 39 ml/m^2;** LV EF: 56%;*,** LVM: 309 g;*,** LVMi: 136 g/m^2;*,** mass/volume ratio: 1.55.*,**

---

*, Significantly abnormal; **, significant change from pretreatment, $p < 0.05$.

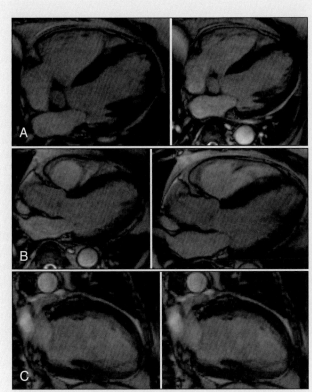

■ **Figure 3-5** Intake (*left*) and posttreatment (*right*) LV long-axis four-chamber, LVOT, and two-chamber end-diastolic images are shown.

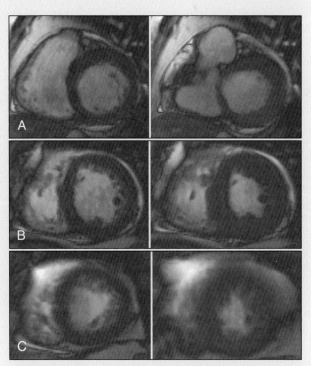

■ **Figure 3-6** Pretreatment short-axis end-diastolic (*left*) and -systolic (*right*) CMR images in this hypertensive man.

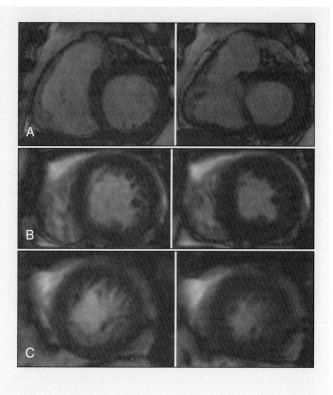

■ **Figure 3-7** Posttreatment short-axis end-diastolic and -systolic images in this hypertensive man treated for 3.5 months with a combination of an ACE inhibitor and aldosterone antagonist.

Discussion of Results

The baseline data demonstrate moderate concentric LVH with borderline LV systolic function. Despite the short period of follow-up, results demonstrate clear-cut significant LVH regression and reduction in chamber volumes associated with a significant increase in ejection fraction. Because of the large change in EDVi, the mass/volume ratio actually increases. Thus, because of multiple effects (change in BP, reduction in LV volume, increase in mass/volume ratio), the effective afterload per unit cross-sectional area of myocardium, or wall stress, is diminished, which may play an important role in the improvement of systolic function. Comparison of the pretreatment and posttreatment long-axis images in Figure 3-5 demonstrates that LV chamber shape also changed with treatment, becoming more elliptical in all three planes shown. The association of increasingly spherical LV shape with worse LV systolic function has long been noted but is not incorporated into conventional clinical quantitative analyses at this point in time. Comparison of the paired end-diastolic and end-systolic pretreatment short-axis images in Figure 3-6 and the posttreatment images in Figure 3-7 readily demonstrates the improvement in LV systolic function noted on quantitative analysis. The most apical slice shown is less crisp than the others because of the smaller radius of curvature of the ventricle near the apex, which increases partial volume effects with a constant slice thickness.

Comments

Left ventricular hypertrophy (LVH) is a powerful marker of end-organ damage in hypertension, is associated with more severe vascular disease, and identifies individuals with a marked increase in cardiovascular risk. The hypertrophic response to hypertension includes three subgroups with different patterns of LV remodeling (Table 3-4).

Each of these patterns is associated with increased cardiovascular risk. In addition, regression of LVH with blood pressure lowering has been shown to reduce cardiovascular risk, including death, stroke, and myocardial infarction. Although echocardiographic determination of LV mass is useful in identifying patients with severe LVH and for research studies with large sample sizes, its high measurement variability impairs its value in patients with milder concentric and/or eccentric LVH, in those with concentric remodeling, and serial evaluation of individual hypertensive patients. Because of its low measurement variability and ability to clearly define gender-adjusted normal values, CMR is more effective in these settings. Thus, in this patient, CMR could demonstrate parallel reductions in LV mass and chamber volume with normalization of LV ejection fraction during a relatively brief period of improved blood pressure control with multiple agents that interrupt hypertrophic stimuli from the renin-angiotensin-aldosterone system. Particularly notable is the short duration of treatment

TABLE 3-4 Patterns of LV Remodeling in Hypertension

	LVMI	EDVI	MASS/VOLUME RATIO
Concentric hypertrophy	↑	⇔/↓	↑
Concentric remodeling	⇔	↓	↑
Eccentric hypertrophy	↑	↑	⇔

EDVi, end-diastolic volume index; LVMi, left ventricular mass index.

required to detect such changes using a highly reproducible method such as CMR. Echocardiographic studies of LVH regression have typically required longer treatment periods to demonstrate LVH regression and require much larger sample sizes than similar studies based on CMR.

Case 3   Aortic Regurgitation

This patient is a 41-year-old white woman with a bicuspid aortic valve. On physical exam, the BP is 109/66 mm Hg. There are brisk aortic pulse upstrokes, and the LV apex impulse is enlarged. There is an aortic ejection sound and the second sound split, with a loud S2A. There is a medium-length grade 2 to 3 mid-systolic murmur at the second right intercostal space and left sternal border and a grade 3/6 early diastolic murmur at the left sternal border. Despite severe aortic regurgitation and moderate aortic root dilatation, she is asymptomatic and has been followed using serial 2D echocardiograms. The most recent echocardiogram showed a decrease in global EF from 65% to the 55% to 60% range and an increase in LV internal diameter in diastole (LVIDD) from 4.9 cm to 5.5 cm over a 6-month period. A stress echo was read as normal and revealed excellent exercise tolerance. The patient is referred for CMR to further evaluate severity of aortic regurgitation and related progressive LV dilatation and decline in LVEF (Figs. 3-8 and 3-9). Quantitative results: EDVi: 129 ml/m^2; ESVi: 51 ml/m^2; LVMi: 63 g/m^2; LV EF: 60%; LV mass/volume ratio: 0.5; regurgitant fraction: 38%.

Discussion of Results

The CMR results in this patient demonstrate moderate end-diastolic left ventricular dilation with a proportional increase in end-systolic volume index. Thus, the LV ejection fraction remains normal. Note that LV shape remains elliptical, as is commonly true when ejection fraction remains normal in the setting of significant left ventricular dilation. As in the previous patient, the apical short-axis slice is less distinct than the more basal slices because of a smaller radius of curvature and partial volume effects. CMR results show greater severity of LV dilation than did echocardiography, with better preservation of LV function. In addition, the regurgitant fraction is toward the high end of the moderate range. The mass/volume ratio is reduced, reflecting inadequate hypertrophy to match chamber dilation. This results in afterload excess, by the law of Laplace, because the force developed per unit cross-sectional area of myocardium in systole must equal the product of the intracavitary pressure and the cross-sectional area of the chamber. Afterload excess may be an important stimulus to progressive dilation and ventricular dysfunction. This may be the converse of the changes seen in Case 2. In the LVOT plane, an aortic regurgitant jet is shown. The aortic root is moderately dilated with a maximal diameter of 4.7 cm at the level of sinuses and a maximal aortic root diameter of 4.3 cm just above the sinuses. The ascending aorta tapers to normal diameter before the arch and the arch and descending aorta are normal in caliber. Additional evaluation of aortic regurgitation is performed using phase contrast imaging. Steady-state free processing (SSFP) cine imaging can depict regurgitant and stenotic jets and related turbulence but is less sensitive to these effects than pulsed or color echo-doppler, or even CMR gradient echo cine imaging. Thus, SSFP cines

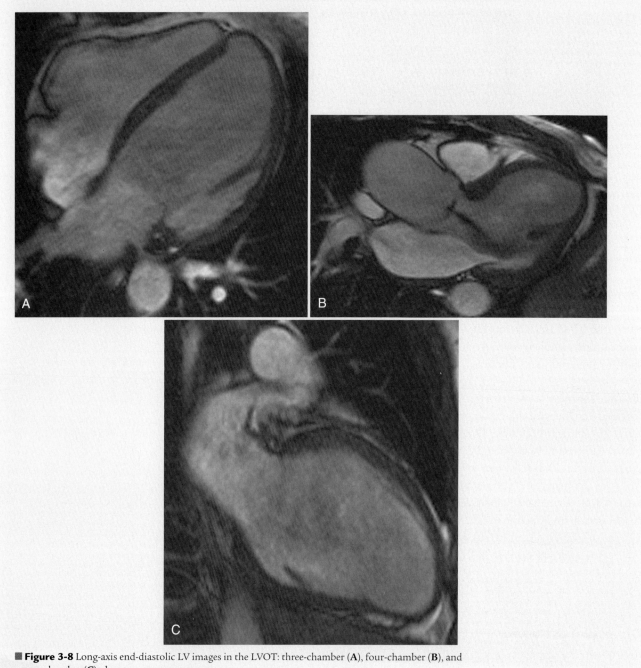

■ **Figure 3-8** Long-axis end-diastolic LV images in the LVOT: three-chamber (**A**), four-chamber (**B**), and two-chamber (**C**) planes.

should not be used for sensitive detection of regurgitation or even semiquantitative quantitation of regurgitation. For these purposes, phase contrast imaging and even gradient echo cine imaging, which shows the dephasing from regurgitant jets more readily than SSFP, are superior. Quantitation of isolated aortic regurgitation in the absence of other regurgitant lesions can be performed by comparison of right and left ventricular anatomic

stroke volumes but CMR phase contrast velocimetry methods are preferred by most laboratories. Using phase velocimetry either comparisons of through plane volumetric aortic and main pulmonary artery flow or the ratio of aortic root forward to backward flow, or both, can be used.

Although aortic contrast MRA is the standard method for assessment of thoracic aortic dilation, dissection, and

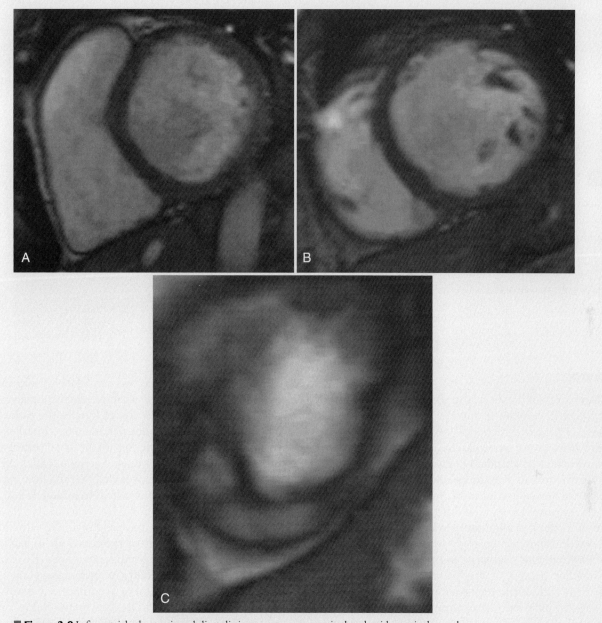

■ **Figure 3-9** Left ventricle short-axis end-diastolic images at representative basal, mid-ventricular, and apical planes from the short-axis SSFP stack obtained in the same patient as in Figure 3-8.

aneurysm, because aortic abnormalities in this patient on scout imaging appear limited to the aortic root, noncontrast SSFP cine imaging of the aortic root and ascending aorta in "candy cane" and short-axis planes is used instead. This approach deals more effectively with aortic sinus and root motion than MRA, which often shows blurring of the aortic root and sinuses, and may be preferable when abnormalities of the aorta are limited to the root. Multiple short-axis planes of the aortic valve are also obtained to directly visualize the regurgitant orifice (not shown).

Comments

Current guidelines for assessment and management of aortic regurgitation rely on echo-doppler indices of regurgitation for initial classification of severity and the combination of symptomatic status and either ejection fraction by any method or linear echo LV minor axis size at end-diastole and end-systole to guide management. Either symptoms or LV end-systolic diameter = 5.5 cm or 5.0 to 5.5 cm have been cited in guidelines as potential indications for aortic valve replacement. However, variability of such measurements is large and limits their utility in patient follow-up. The high reproducibility of 3D volumetric assessment of LV volumes and EF with CMR and the quantitative accuracy of

CMR phase contrast velocimetry for assessment of regurgitant flow and regurgitant fraction offer great promise for improved assessment of patients with aortic regurgitation. However, large-scale studies to define optimal use of CMR measurements in clinical decision making are required to provide the evidence on which systematic use of CMR for this purpose should be based.

Case 4   Ischemic Cardiomyopathy

The patient is a 76-year-old white man with remote medical history of single-vessel coronary disease (medically managed) admitted for decompensated congestive heart failure and noted to have nonsustained ventricular tachycardia on telemetry. The patient is referred for CMR for evaluation of viability (Figs. 3-10 and 3-11). Quantitative results are: EDVi: 264 ml/m^2; ESVi: 228 ml/m^2; LVMi: 132 g/m^2; LV EF: 14%, mass/volume ratio: 0.5.

Comments

These data represent the most advanced stage of ischemic cardiomyopathy, combining marked chamber dilation with severe systolic dysfunction, because of extensive old infarction, very severe postinfarction remodeling, and, perhaps, recurrent or chronic ischemia producing myocardial hibernation in residual viable myocardium. As in Case 2, the association of more spherical ventricular shape with impaired LV systolic function is clearly seen. In addition to the contribution of reduced contractility of viable myocardium to impaired systolic function here, the low mass/volume ratio also contributes to reduced systolic function because of afterload excess, as discussed in the patient with aortic regurgitation. In fact the low overall mass/volume ratio here, combined with the fact that much of the LV "myocardial" mass in this patient is noncontractile scar, results in an even lower ratio of *viable* myocardium to chamber volume than seen in the patient with aortic regurgitation, so there is inherently more marked afterload excess than the mass/volume ratio might suggest. Not even normal myocardium in this amount, in relation to chamber volume, could deliver a normal ejection fraction in this setting. Note that in contrast with the aortic regurgitation ventricle shown previously, this ventricle is more spherical than normal, especially in the two-chamber plane. Increased sphericity is a frequent concomitant of severe systolic dysfunction of any cause.

A number of therapeutic considerations are underscored by the imaging results in this patient. First, the patient is clearly a candidate for an implantable defibrillator by MADIT II criteria, although it should be noted that EF in MADIT II was obtained with other imaging tech-

niques. Second, the patient may be a candidate for surgical ventricular remodeling, based on more detailed analysis of the extent of transmural apical scar. Finally, the patient might conceivably benefit from percutaneous intervention to improve regional function in the basal anterior wall, basal and mid-inferior wall, and septum, which appear viable but dysfunctional, provided that the locations of obstruction are sufficiently proximal to influence basal myocardial function.

Many types of risk stratification and pivotal treatment decisions in the management of patients with ischemic heart disease depend on determinations of LV EF and assessment of myocardial viability in dysfunctional myocardial segments. However, there are important limitations to common clinical noninvasive methods for EF determination in this population, including 2D echocardiography (Fig. 3-12), planar radionuclide ventriculography, and even gated SPECT imaging in patients with large infarctions that produce "missing" myocardial segments.

These sobering results suggest that reassessment of the role of LV EF in risk stratification of patients with ischemic heart disease and LV dysfunction, using more reliable 3D technologies such as CMR would be highly desirable.

Transmural extent of infarct scar is a reliable predictor of reversibility of myocardial dysfunction and effectiveness of regional revascularization. CMR viability imaging, combined with SSFP cine imaging in similar planes is an optimal high-resolution method for such evaluations. Thus, CMR can set the stage for improved decision making with respect to revascularization. CMR is superior to stress echocardiography and thallium-SPECT for detection

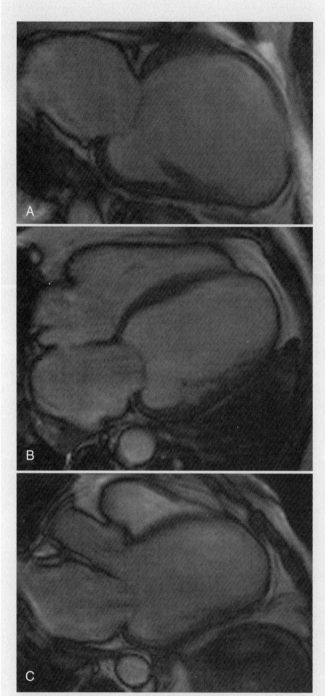

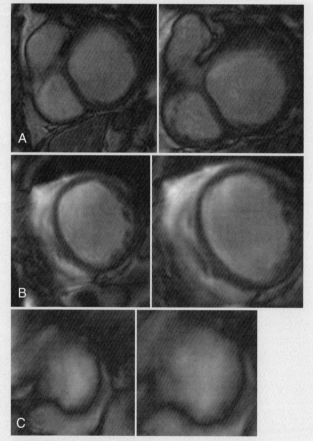

■ **Figure 3-10** Long-axis end-diastolic cine images in four chamber, LVOT plane, and two-chamber views are shown. The left ventricle is dilated in all views. Left ventricular wall thickness is normal in the basal anterior wall but abnormally low in the mid-anterior and entire apical region, which also showed transmural delayed hyperenhancement. Delayed enhancement in other planes confirms extensive apical transmural scar. There was also a jet of mitral regurgitation seen in the LVOT view. The left atrium is markedly dilated. Invasive coronary angiography is performed and showed complete occlusion of the left anterior descending with evidence of collateralization and 99% occlusion of the posterior descending artery in a left-dominant circulation.

■ **Figure 3-11** Cine SSFP left ventricular short-axis end-diastolic (*left*) and end-systolic images (*right*) for the patient with ischemic cardiomyopathy depicted in Figure 3-10. There is severe left ventricular dysfunction with severe global hypokinesis and mid-anterior and apical akinesis.

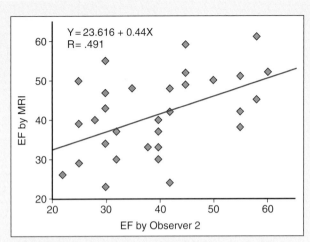

■ **Figure 3-12** Comparison of 3D CMR EF (*vertical axis*) with echo observer EF (*horizontal axis*) in 31 patients with recent acute myocardial infarction (unpublished data). There is poor agreement between the two methods. When the ability to detect patients below a cutoff value for EF of 30% or 40% by CMR is examined, echo misclassifies up to one third of patients. Substitution of echo quantitative biplane Simpson's rule EF for observer EF does not improve the results. Similar results have been found in multiple other studies of patients with recent or old MI and those meeting MADIT II criteria for implantation of a defibrillator. Planar radionuclide ventriculography is superior to echo in this study, with *r* = 0.69.

and evaluation of extent of myocardial scar. It compares favorably with PET for viability assessment, but can detect small subendocardial scars, not seen with PET, because of its superior spatial resolution.

In this patient, even before viability imaging, the association of marked wall thinning with segmental akinesis make it evident that this is ischemic heart disease with extensive infarction. However, it should be noted that subendocardial infarction of small extent on viability imaging may not result in any abnormality of LV wall thickness or systolic thickening and endocardial excursion. Thus in patients who present with a dilated, uniformly thinwalled and symmetrically hypokinetic left ventricle, the possibility of ischemic cardiomyopathy with minimal infarct scarring and extensive and severe myocardial hibernation cannot be excluded on SSFP cine imaging alone, and viability as well as stress perfusion imaging may be required to obtain an accurate etiologic diagnosis. Studies of clinic populations diagnosed as dilated nonischemic cardiomyopathy have shown a significant incidence of failure to diagnose ischemic heart disease as the correct etiology. The correct diagnosis may be made in many instances via detection of small subendocardial infarcts on viability imaging that have not produced segmental contraction abnormalities.

Case 5   **Dilated Nonischemic Cardiomyopathy**

This 66-year-old white man with a past medical history of rheumatoid arthritis presents with a protracted upper respiratory illness that has evolved into progressive dyspnea over the course of 1 month and was treated with a course of steroids and antibiotics. A 12-lead ECG shows left bundle branch block. A 2D echocardiogram shows a dilated left ventricle with severe systolic dysfunction with estimated LVEF of 30%. Invasive coronary angiography shows no evidence of coronary artery disease. The patient is referred for CMR to further assess biventricular structure and function and determine whether there is evidence of fibrosis, inflammation, or infiltrative disease (Figs. 3-13 and 3-14). Quantitative results are as follows: LVEDVi: 226 ml/m²*; LVESVi: 197 ml/m²*; LVMi: 124 g/m²*; LVEF: 13%*, mass/volume ratio: 0.5*; RVEDVi: 113 ml/m²*; RVESVi: 93 ml/m²*; RVMi: 34 g/m²; RVEF: 18%*, mass/volume ratio: 0.3.

Comments

The left ventricle is markedly dilated, with mild LVH. Left ventricular systolic function is profoundly depressed with relatively uniform wall motion. As in Cases 2 and 4, the association of more spherical shape with impaired systolic function is again evident. There is a low mass/volume ratio, again indicating that afterload excess, in addition to reduced myocardial contractility, contributes to LV systolic dysfunction here. The left atrium appears mildly enlarged. In addition, on delayed enhancement imaging two small areas of mid-wall myocardial hyperenhance-

ment are identified in the basal lateral wall and basal inferior septum, respectively. The absence of segmental wall thinning and the presence of uniform segmental systolic dysfunction point toward a diagnosis of dilated cardiomyopathy; and mid-wall hyperenhancement, combined with the absence of subendocardial hyperenhancement, support the idea that this is unlikely to be ischemic heart disease. Note that the prior echocardiographic EF of 30% correlates poorly with CMR findings. In patients with heart failure, CMR is now the imaging modality of choice for initial assessment because of its unique ability to quantitate structure and function of both ventricles while pro-

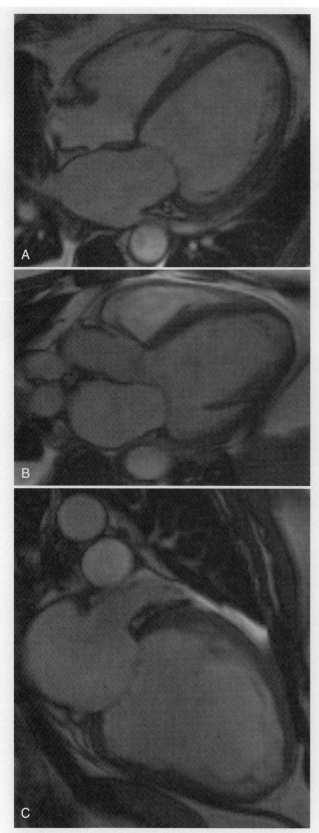

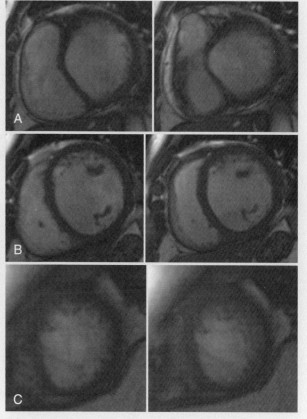

■ **Figure 3-13** Cardiac function is evaluated using TrueFISP cine imaging in long- and short-axis right and left ventricular planes. Dark blood imaging using HASTE is performed. After gadolinium contrast injection, delayed hyperenhancement imaging is performed. Left ventricular end-diastolic long-axis images in the four chamber, LVOT, and two chamber planes are shown.

■ **Figure 3-14** Left ventricular end-diastolic (*left*) and end-systolic (*right*) short-axis images at the basal, mid-ventricular, and apical levels are shown.

viding unique tissue characterization data that shed light on the etiology of myocardial disease. Patterns of delayed enhancement reliably differentiate ischemic necrosis or scar (subendocardial to transmural hyperenhancement) from nonischemic dilated cardiomyopathy (no enhance-ment, mid-wall or subepicardial enhancement consistent with fibrosis or inflammation). Emerging data suggest that, as is also true in ischemic cardiomyopathy, the extent of hyperenhancement in dilated nonischemic cardiomy-opathy has important prognostic implications.

Case 6   Hypertrophic Cardiomyopathy

An asymptomatic 50-year-old white man with a past medical history significant for morbid obesity and sleep apnea was referred for cardiac evaluation before gastric reduction surgery. Cardiovascular examination is pertinent for a 3/6 long mid-systolic murmur at the aortic area and left sternal edge. A 12-lead EKG shows left ventricular hypertrophy and T-wave inversions in the lateral leads. A 2D echocar-diogram demonstrates moderate asymmetric left ventricular hypertrophy with mild to moderate mitral regurgitation. The patient is referred for CMR (Figs. 3-15 and 3-16). Quantitative results are as follows: LVEDVi: 80 ml/m²; LVESVi: 26 ml/m²; LVMi: 136 g/m²; LVEF: 68%, mass/volume ratio: 1.75.

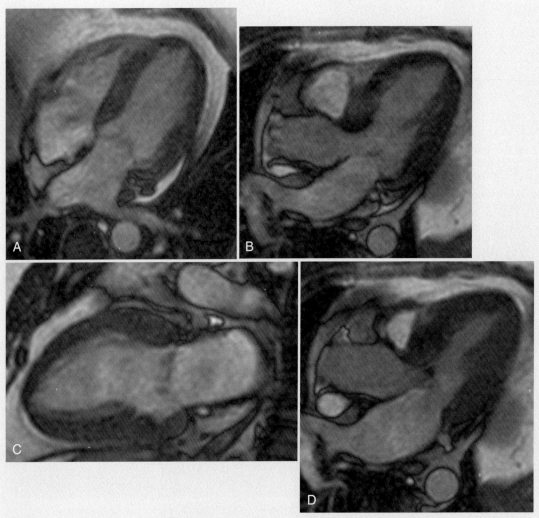

■ **Figure 3-15** TrueFISP cine imaging in the long- and contiguous short-axis planes is performed. Dark blood imaging using HASTE and flow imaging using gradient echo and phase contrast imaging are performed. Delayed hyperenhancement imaging is also obtained. Left ventricular end-diastolic long-axis images in the four-chamber and two-chamber planes (*left*) and long-axis images in the LVOT plane at end-diastole and -systole (*right*) are shown.

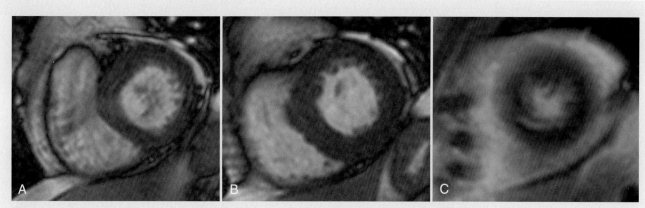

■ **Figure 3-16** Left ventricular end-diastolic short-axis images at the basal, mid-ventricular, and apical levels.

Comments

CMR shows evidence of severe asymmetric left ventricular hypertrophy. The maximal myocardial thickness was found in the anterior basal septum (2.1 cm), upper septum (1.7 to 1.9 cm), and anterior wall (1.9 to 2.0 cm). The distal anterior wall, lateral, and inferior walls are only mildly hypertrophied (1.2 to 1.3 cm). There is also evidence of systolic anterior motion of the anterior mitral leaflet striking the anterior septum in the LVOT plane at end-systole, suggesting a significant resting gradient. There is moderate mitral regurgitation. The left atrium is mildly dilated. Delayed hyperenhancement does not show any evidence of scar or fibrosis.

Hypertrophic cardiomyopathy (HCM) is the most common genetic cardiovascular disease. A subset of these patients is at significant risk of increased cardiovascular morbidity and mortality. Clinical presentation, family history, and noninvasive testing play essential roles in risk stratification, follow-up, and treatment. CMR is now the noninvasive imaging modality of choice in this disorder because it provides both accurate assessments of regional and global left ventricular hypertrophy and can also characterize the extent and location of fibrosis by delayed enhancement. Both hypertrophy and fibrosis appear to be predictors of cardiovascular risk in HCM. Emerging data suggest that increased LV mass by CMR is associated with increased risk and poor clinical outcomes, whereas the presence and possibly extent of delayed hyperenhancement are also predictors of adverse outcomes.

SUGGESTED READING

Reichek N, Gupta D: Hypertrophic cardiomyopathy: CMR imaging changes the paradigm. J Am Coll Cardiol 2008;52:567-568.

Chapter 4

Measuring Regional Function

Nael F. Osman, Alexander Jehle, and Frederick H. Epstein

KEY POINTS

- Myocardial strain is potentially a better measure of regional contractile function than motion of the endocardial border or tissue velocity, because strain directly quantifies the change in shape of regions of myocardium.

- The most common elements of the strain tensor used to quantify regional left ventricular function are circumferential shortening (E_{cc}), radial thickening (E_{rr}), and longitudinal shortening (E_{ll}).

- CMR methods to assess strain or strain rate include myocardial tagging, harmonic phase analysis (HARP), displacement encoding with stimulated echoes (DENSE), strain-encoded imaging (SENC), and velocity-encoded phase contrast. These methods can be classified as tissue tracking techniques.

- Myocardial tagging, which was developed nearly 20 years ago, is the most widely used and well-validated CMR tissue tracking technique.

- HARP is an automated image analysis method that greatly reduces the time required to quantify displacement and strain from tagged images.

- DENSE is a cardiac magnetic resonance (CMR) tissue tracking method in which displacement, rather than velocity, is encoded into the signal phase. This is achieved by acquiring the displacement-encoded stimulated echo. In practice DENSE and refined HARP methods employ similar physics and analysis algorithms.

- SENC directly images strain normal to the imaging plane.

- CMR tissue tracking methods that quantify myocardial strain have potential application to all heart diseases that alter regional contractile function. The most common example is ischemic heart disease.

- CMR tissue tracking measurements of the temporal evolution of regional strain also may be useful in the assessment of mechanical dyssynchrony.

This chapter discusses the quantification of cardiac function, specifically the "mechanical," or contractile, function. Nearly all heart diseases lead to contractile dysfunction of the left ventricle (LV). Depending on the specific disease, contractile function may be impaired throughout the LV, or the degree of dysfunction may vary significantly by region. The clinical finding of contractile dysfunction is typically made by qualitative visual assessment of cine images acquired using echocardiography, radionuclide scintigraphy, or CMR. Although qualitative assessment of cine images is the clinical standard, these methods are subjective and observer dependent. In addition to conventional cine imaging, echocardiography and CMR can perform quantitative tissue tracking to quantify regional contractile function. Reliable and easy-to-use quantitative methods could potentially reduce subjectivity and variability in the assessment of regional function. Quantitative echocardiographic techniques include tissue Doppler imaging and speckle tracking. Quantitative CMR techniques include myocardial tagging, HARP, DENSE, SENC, and velocity-encoded phase contrast.

Quantitative assessment of function requires accurate techniques to *measure* the regional function. The capacity to "measure" the regional function must be well understood. Measuring the function of some region in the heart muscle can be described by more than one quantity and in relation to its muscle's contraction and relaxation. Typical motion measurements are selected to be universal, so researchers, physicians, and technicians from different backgrounds may understand these measurements without confusion or further explanation. Obviously, because the function of the heart muscle (myocardium) is mechanical, the terms used are based on mechanics and physics.

This chapter specifies the measurements used to describe the regional function. Specifically, it discusses the quantities' velocity, displacement, and strain. A group of secondary measurements are discussed as well. The chapter then describes different CMR methods that can help one obtain some of these mechanical measurements. The focus is mainly on MR tagging, DENSE, and SENC. For each method, the chapter describes the basic concept, the measurements that can be obtained, the expected measurements in healthy population and variations in selected populations of cardiac diseases, and some of the limitations and considerations.

WHICH QUANTITIES DESCRIBE REGIONAL FUNCTION?

There are many quantities that can be used to measure regional function, but the focus here is on three quantities: velocity, displacement, and strain. Secondary measurements that can be obtained from these basic ones, such as strain rate or rotation, are also discussed.

VELOCITY: HOW FAST IS THE WALL MOVING?

Qualitative assessment of regional function is usually done by observing the speed at which the ventricular wall appears to move in cine, whether it is obtained using echocardiography, CT, or CMR. The quantity to describe the speed of the wall is the velocity, which is measured as a distance covered by a moving object per second. The velocity has a direction, or mathematically, it is not a scalar but a vector. Given that, it is useful to measure the motion in a specific direction to become meaningful. In the case of LV, it is plausible to measure the velocity of the wall as measured in the radial direction toward the center of the ventricle. This "radial" motion describes the expected inward motion of the wall during systole to reduce the cavity inside the ventricles and eject the blood through the aortic and pulmonary valves.

The *instantaneous* velocity of a piece of tissue is measured by dividing the displacement that this piece of tissue moves in a very short period of time over that period of time. In healthy people, the instantaneous velocity at any phase of the cardiac cycle is not uniform over the regions of the heart. The peak instantaneous velocities occur in mid-systole and at early and late diastole.

DISPLACEMENT: HOW FAR DOES THE WALL MOVE?

The other measure of motion is displacement, which is the total distance a piece of tissue moves over a period of time. The motion of the wall during systole is measured by the displacement that occurs from the end-diastole to end-systole. Displacement and speed are related and can be deduced from each other. A series of velocity measurements acquired at different instants of time in the cardiac cycle can be added to measure the overall displacement. Conversely, velocity can be measured from a sequence of displacement measurements at different instants of time. The velocity is the mathematical derivative of displacement.

The displacement at any instant in the cardiac cycle does not reflect the rate of deformation of the tissue. However, obtaining a sequence of displacement measurements at different instants during the cardiac cycle captures the dynamics of the heart.

STRAIN: A MEASURE OF CONTRACTILITY?

Although velocity and displacement describe the motion of tissue, they do not describe the deformations that occur to the tissue. A piece of noncontracting (dysfunctional) tissue can be moving very fast because of pulling (tethering) by another active piece of tissue. A healthy piece of myocardium is expected to contract and relax, causing deformations in its shape. A third quantity can measure these deformations and changes to the shape of the tissue. Strain, defined as the change in some length of a piece of tissue per unit length, can be that measure. The strain can take negative and positive values. The increase in length of a piece of tissue is measured in positive strain values, whereas a decrease in length (shortening) because of contraction (for example) is measured in negative strain values.

By definition, strain (E) is a tensor quantity, as it describes the change in shape of a one-, two-, or three-dimensional (1D, 2D, or 3D) solid element. The measured deformation strain differs according to which length, or direction, is considered. For analyzing cardiac function, the principal strains may be measured; however, it is more common to report the radial, circumferential, and longitudinal strains, because they are aligned with the natural coordinate system of the heart and are easy to interpret. Typical strain values for a normal heart are approximately −0.25 to −0.50 for radial thickening (E_{RR}), −0.13 to −0.25 for circumferential shortening (E_{CC}), and −0.13 to −0.20 for longitudinal shortening (E_{LL}). These values indicate that a small 3D element of myocardium, during systole, will stretch approximately 25% to 50% in the radial direction, shorten approximately 13% to 25% in the circumferential direction, and shorten approximately 13% to 20% in the longitudinal direction relative to its initial shape at the reference time of end-diastole. Other strain quantities are the principal strains that describe the maximum deformations (shortening and lengthening) of a piece of tissue. It is also possible to estimate the shear strains that are generated during myocardial contraction; however, the clinical use of this information is not well established. Figure 4-1 illustrates the directions of commonly used strains.

Strain in general can be measured from displacement. On the other hand, strain rate, which is the rate of change in strain, can be measured from the strain by simple derivative of time, or regional velocity using spatial derivatives. Overall, the rate of change of any quantity with time is measured, mathematically, as the time derivative. Techniques that measure the displacement (e.g., MR tagging and DENSE, which are described later) compute the strain by measuring spatial difference in displacement. However, strain can be directly imaged using SENC, without obtaining the intermediate measurements of displacement or velocity.

OTHER MEASUREMENTS

Other measures of motion can also be used to describe regional function, but in general they can be derived from the basic displacement or velocity measurements. For example, there is interest in measuring the rotation of the LV around the long axis. This is measured from the displacement by measuring the average displacement along the circumferential direction. The angular velocity is similarly measured from the velocity measurements. Another measurement is the twisting (torsion) of the LV,

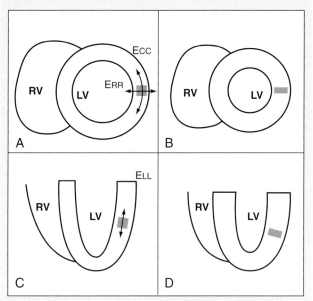

■ **Figure 4-1** Directions of commonly used strains. Assuming a square piece of tissue (gray square) in (**A**), this piece will deform during systole so that it will shorten in the circumferential direction and stretch in the radial direction (**B**). The strain in the circumferential direction is usually given the notation E_{CC}, whereas the radial strain is given E_{RR}. The longitudinal strain can be explained better in a long-axis view (**C,D**). Besides the stretching in the radial direction, the square in (**C,D**) shortens in the longitudinal direction, which is measured as the longitudinal strain E_{LL}.

which is the difference in rotation between the base and apex of the LV.

The deformation of the LV shows a twist around the long axis, seen as the rotation of the base in an opposite direction relative to the apex. This twist accompanies shortening in the longitudinal direction (from base to apex); therefore, the LV looks as if squeezed to eject the blood out of its cavity.

Obviously, the twist occurs as a result of the rotation of any point of the myocardium around the long axis. In a way, this motion (or displacement, as described earlier) is an angular motion, and could be considered a regional motion. However, it is hard to consider it to be a form of regional function, because the rotation (like displacement) could be caused by the contraction of other regions tethered to the rotating region.

MAGNETIC RESONANCE TAGGING: NONINVASIVE MARKERS

The first techniques to help detect and measure the motion inside the myocardium was by inserting small beads that were opaque to the imaging modality so it could be detected in the images and tracked to obtain the motion. Because these methods were invasive, it was solely used for research, and clinical applications were unthinkable. Moreover these physical markers interfered with the measured motion, because their existence inside the tissue would affect the regional motion. Luckily CMR provided a noninvasive alternative. CMR was shown to be capable of creating *virtual* markers inside the tissue that have exactly the same benefits for tracking the motion as the physical beads, but without the disadvantages, such as the need for surgical intervention or compromising the function.

MR tagging is the technique for doing so. Tagging has been proposed by Zerhouni et al. as a method for visualizing the motion of the myocardium, and significant improvements have been achieved by Axel. Practically, MR tagging currently is the most used CMR technique for measuring regional function of the heart. As a side note, consider one of the pitfalls of CMR, the proliferation of techniques with awkward naming. MR tagging is one of these, in which the name does not reveal the exact role of the technique. Perhaps a name such as virtual markers would have been a better description of what MR tagging actually does.

The Technique

The MR tags are generated by a special modification of the CMR scanner's pulse sequence that makes the magnetization of the tissue nonuniform so that some regions of the myocardium appear darker than others when images are acquired. These dark regions reveal that the magnetization of the corresponding tissue of the myocardium is suppressed; it stays suppressed for about 1 second before resuming its normal magnetization. Therefore, these MR tags do not last long, and the dark regions return to normal intensity across all the tissue. Hence, the MR tags gradually fade and completely disappear in about a second. During this period of time, if images are acquired in a sequence during the cardiac cycle and played as a cine movie, the MR tagging pattern appears to deform with the motion of the myocardium—similar to the motion of physical beads implanted inside the myocardium. This means that the MR tags reveal the motion inside the myocardium and, with proper design of the tagging pattern and appropriate tools, can be used to measure the motion. The exact shape of the tagged regions is called the tagging pattern, such as the line tags in Figure 4-2. Axel introduced the spatial modulation of magnetization (SPAMM) pulse sequence, which is the most efficient pulse sequence to create regular tag patterns. Moreover, SPAMM creates multiple regular tags that appear as lines (see Fig. 4-2) or rectangular grids. Because of their regular shape, it is possible to obtain the motion of the whole heart in view. Because of its simple and effective ability to produce tagged MR images, the SPAMM sequence and its variations are available on most commercial CMR scanners.

Common Tag Patterns

The use of the SPAMM pulse sequence enables the generation of a rectilinear tag patterns using a very efficient

pulse sequence. The use of 1D SPAMM generates parallel saturated surfaces orthogonal to the imaging plane. This results in parallel dark lines appearing on the acquired images. The use of two consecutive 1D SPAMM sequences generates a grid of tags composed of two sets of intersecting parallel lines. These two sets are typically designed to be orthogonal to each other. Because the motion of the heart on the plane can be described by two orthogonal sets of linear tags, a grid tag is a more efficient way to depict the in-plane motion (see Fig. 4-2). For automatic motion analysis, at least two orthogonal tag lines are needed for measuring the displacement or strain. This is double the acquisition time needed to acquire grid tag patterns. However, the line tags have better quality, described by the contrast-to-noise ratio (CNR), which is the ratio of the contrast between the bright and dark tag lines to the amount of noise in the image. Higher CNR indicates better image quality than images with lower CNR.

Analyzing Magnetic Resonance Tagged Images Using Harmonic Phase Analysis

Despite its wide availability on all CMR scanners, MR tagging is not used widely in clinical applications. This is mainly attributed to the lack of suitable methods to obtain measurements of regional function from the images. Most of the developed techniques were very time consuming, which made it very hard to apply MR tagging to studies with large number of subjects. This by itself was a great obstacle against exploring the usefulness of tagging in assessing regional function in cardiac disease.

This setback for MR tagging has been steadily changing because of two factors. First, there is a renewed interest in measuring the mechanical activities of the heart and its applications. This is more obvious in the case of determining dyssynchrony for CRT. The second and more important reason is the development of new methods that reduce the image analysis time required to measure the regional motion. The most widely used technique now is the HARP technique, which enables measuring of regional function from the tagged images produced from any of the available commercial scanners.

Examples

Figure 4-3 shows a screen shot of analyzed tagged MR images with HARP in a normal healthy heart. The technique is capable of measuring the circumferential strain. The curves have negative values, reflecting the fractional shortening in the circumferential strain. The lowest points on the curves are the maximum shortening, which is expected to occur around end-systole. Not all the regions of the myocardium reach maximum shortening at the same time—the lateral wall is slightly delayed from the septum. In the same example, a collection of points making a circular mesh can be tracked during the cardiac cycle. The overall rotation of the mesh points around the center

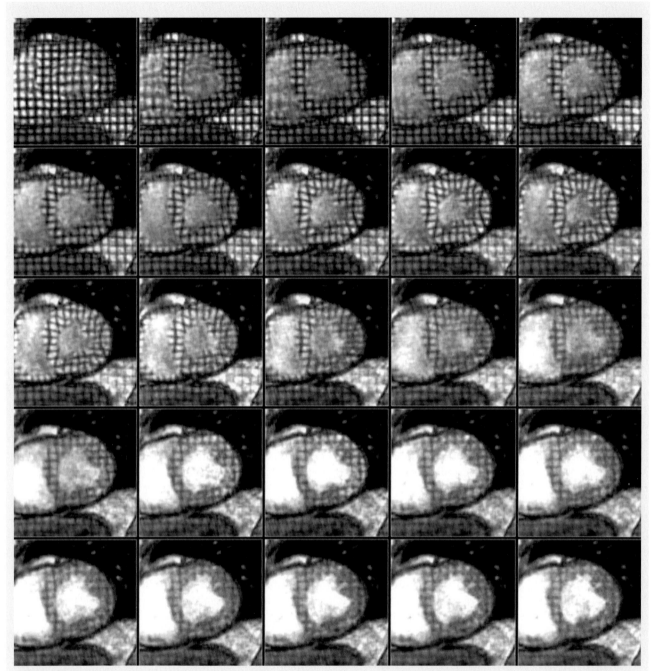

■ **Figure 4-2** Sequence of short-axis view of MR tagged heart acquired during the cardiac cycle. The grid tag pattern deforms with the tissue deformation, revealing the motion within the myocardium. Notice the fading of the tags toward the end of the cardiac cycle.

prescribes the rotation of that slice of the heart around the long axis. Figure 4-4 shows three meshes created in the basal, mid-ventricular, and apical slices of the LV.

Rotation in Acute Myocardial Infarction
Regional rotation can be measured at different locations in the myocardium, and they can show changes as a result of acute myocardial infarction. Figure 4-5 shows an example in which the anterior apical region of the heart show reduced rotation as a result of the infarction.

Dyssynchrony as Seen by Tagging
Figure 4-6 shows another example of a grid tag pattern acquired in a patient whose heart shows motion dyssynchrony.

Considerations in Pediatric Cases
The two cases presented in the following demonstrate the value of MR tagging in pediatric patients.

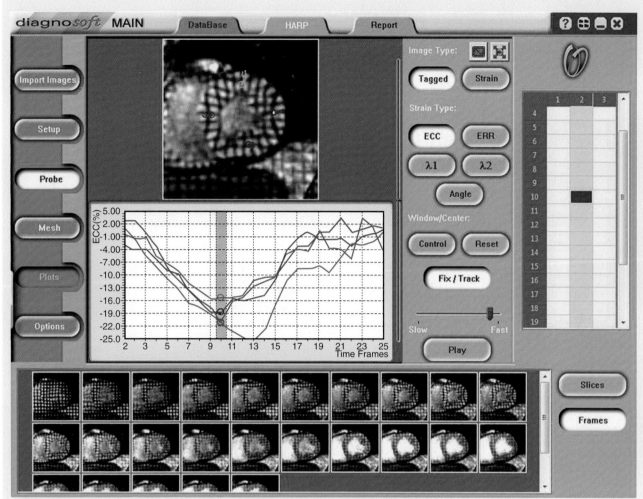

■ Figure 4-3 Screen shot of analyzed tagged MR images with HARP. The E$_{CC}$ strain was measured at four locations. The E$_{CC}$ is a negative strain in a normal heart, indicating the circumferential shortening of the wall. Note the initial systolic phase of contraction as strain gets more and more negative until it peaks. The timing for peaking is not uniform, however, and more shortening occurs in the lateral wall than the other parts. The reverse of the strain indicates the early diastolic phase, which is also different in the lateral wall.

Patient 1

Patient 1 is an 8½-year-old boy with Duchenne muscular dystrophy (DMD) but no cardiovascular symptoms. The patient has been nonambulatory for 3 years. Daily medications include Enalapril, Deflazacort, calcium, magnesium, and coenzyme Q10. The physical exam is normal. A surveillance CMR shows normal global biventricular systolic function (LVEF 67%) with normal chamber sizes. MDE imaging for fibrosis is negative. Strain analysis of tagged MR images is also performed (Fig. 4-7).

Patient 2

Patient 2 is a 24-year-old man with DMD, who has no symptoms related to the cardiovascular system, although he has had progressive respiratory difficulties requiring BiPAP ventilation and a mouthpiece ventilator. Medications include Lisinopril and Prevacid. The patient is nonambulatory. Surveillance CMR shows depressed global biventricular systolic function (LVEF 35%) with mild LV dilatation. MDE imaging for fibrosis is positive (subepicardial LV free wall). Strain analysis of tagged MR images is also performed (Fig. 4-8).

Limitations of Magnetic Resonance Tagging

Beside the general appearance of the tags, it is important to consider their quality, because it affects the accuracy of the measurements. This is dependent on the sharpness of the tags (the width of the dark tag lines) and the spacing between them.

Sharpness of the Tags

For visual reasons, it is always preferred that the tags be sharp and clearly separated from each other. This is driven by the perception that thin lines or a grid with minimal width reduces the accuracy of determining the motion orthogonal to the tag lines. However, this requirement has several drawbacks. First, the sharpness of

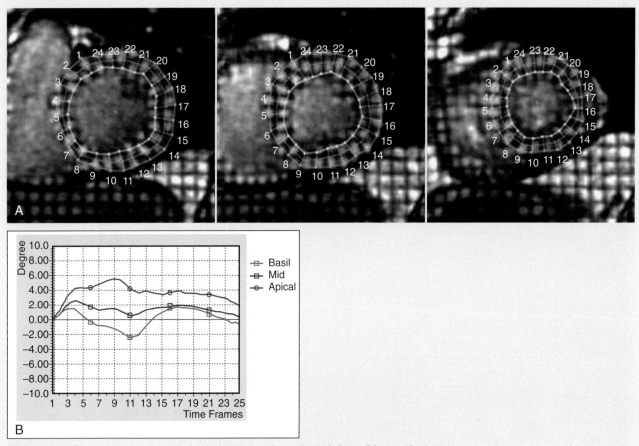

■ **Figure 4-4** Three meshes created in the basal, mid-ventricular, and apical slices of the LV. The average rotation of each mesh is shown. The rotations differ at the different levels of the LV from base to apex. Note that at early systole (until timeframe three), the three slices rotate simultaneously in the same direction, albeit at different angular speed. After that, the basal slice reverses the direction of rotation, whereas the apical slice keeps rotating in the same angular direction. This opposite angular rotations results in twisting the LV from the base to the apex, reaching maximum twisting at end-systole. Rapid untwisting occurs after end-systole so that most of it occurs in a very short period of time. This is an important feature of early diastole.

the tags is limited by the imaging resolution. A resolution that is finer than the tag's width is important, but this increases pressure on acquisition, because it requires longer imaging time. Second, the reduction in voxel size reduces the SNR and image quality. Third, to make the tag lines thinner, more complicated and longer sequences are needed to generate the tags. Finally, sharper tags are easier to identify visually but harder to detect with computers because they are very susceptible to noise and can be missed easily.

However, the minimal requirement on the sharpness of the tags is dependent on computer analysis. It is obvious that tags should be designed so that automatic analysis and quantification are more robust and reliable than being visually pleasant. The advantage of this is that in the HARP technique (discussed later), the analysis is based on the Fourier of the image and the design of tag pattern, and sharpness is irrelevant as a sinusoidal tag pattern (known as 1-1 SPAMM) becomes more favorable. As

a result, the HARP technique prefers blurred, sinusoidal tag patterns.

Spacing Between the Tags

Similar to tag sharpness, good tag separation is dependent on the analysis method. Nevertheless, it is intuitively easy to prefer smaller spacing, because it means more tag lines and better strain resolution. However, this could be at the expense of tag contrast, because the shear of the tissue within the slice causes the tags to fuse, especially in the lateral wall at end-systole. A rule of thumb used in designing tag spacing is that it should be close to the slice thickness.

Tags Fading

The rate of tags fading depends on a number of factors: T1, the imaging flip angles, and the rate of applying the RF pulses. The increase in the imaging flip angle of the RF pulses or the increase in the number of RF pulses

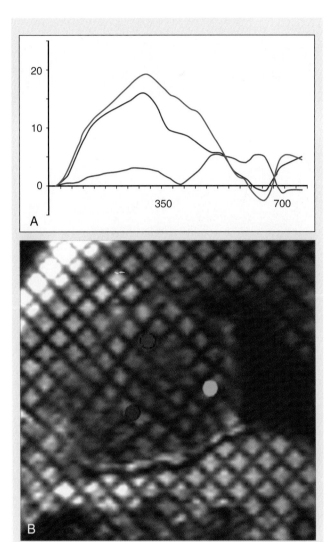

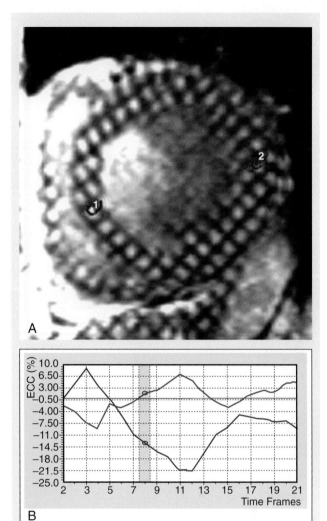

■ **Figure 4-5** Regional left ventricular apical rotation by CMR tagging in a 50-year-old man, who suffered an acute myocardial infarction. Coronary angiography showed a LAD occlusion, and the patient was revascularized by PCI. Regional LV function assessed by CMR tagging was performed 2 months after the acute infarction. The blue trace from HARP demonstrates clearly decreased regional rotation in the anterior myocardial segment compared with lateral and inferior segments. *(Courtesy of Thor Edvardsen, Rikshospitalet University Hospital, Oslo, Norway.)*

■ **Figure 4-6** Grid tag pattern acquired in a patient with motion dyssynchrony. The tagged MR images and the strain measurements can reveal the deformation of the myocardium in ways that cannot be done with conventional cines. The septum shows slight contraction early in systole (*blue curve*), which gives away and becomes dyskinetic (moving into positive values because of circumferential stretching). At the same time, the lateral wall of the LV starts contraction slightly later than the septum (around the time of the peak contraction of the septum). It proceeds to contract until it reaches maximum contraction close to end-systole. This opposite behavior of the two regions shows interventricular dyssynchrony.

applied causes the tags to fade rapidly. In most cases, the tags last long enough for systole but significantly fade in diastole, making it harder to image. In many cases, a careful adjustment of the imaging parameters can make the tag last long enough to cover the early diastole.

DISPLACEMENT ENCODING WITH STIMULATED ECHOES

The Technique

Displacement encoding with stimulated echoes (DENSE) is a fairly new technique for quantitative MR imaging of myocardial displacement and strain. The advantages of this technique include relatively high spatial resolution

compared with conventional myocardial tagging and relatively automated image analysis, similar to HARP. In DENSE, as in myocardial tagging, a precise set of RF and gradient pulses are used to tag, or encode, the tissue longitudinal magnetization. The encoding pulses are usually applied at end-diastole, on detection of the ECG R-wave, before the onset of contraction. Subsequently, a sequence of images is generated, using the encoded longitudinal magnetization, with the particular property that the phase of each image pixel is directly proportional to the tissue displacement that occurred since the time when the encoding pulses were applied. The specific MR signal generated by these RF and gradient pulses, which has the useful property that the phase of the signal is

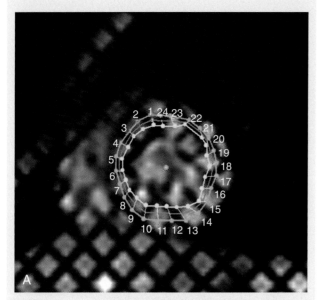

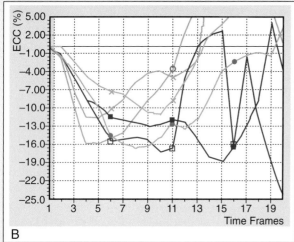

■ **Figure 4-7** This figure shows the mesh placement overlaying a tagged cine MR image on the LV. Resulting circumferential strain analysis is shown in the graph, as each of the lines represents a different region of coronary artery supply. Concentrating on the systolic portion of the graph (frames 1 to 13), regional variation in magnitude of circumferential strain is seen. The mean of all the peak circumferential strain values for this patient was −12.8% (compare with a normal child aged 5-10 years strain ≤16%). The finding of abnormal strain despite normal global EF is novel, important, and expected, given that DMD causes gradual mid-myocardial fibrosis from birth. Demonstrating abnormal strain has altered the frequency with which surveillance imaging in boys with DMD is performed, and increased aggressiveness with cardiovascular medications. (*Courtesy of William Gottliebsen and Kan Hor, Cincinnati Children's Hospital Medical Center.*)

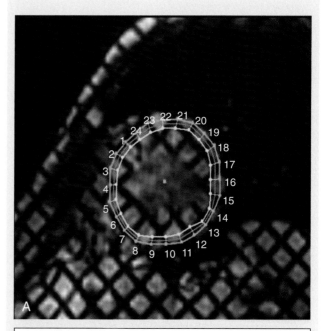

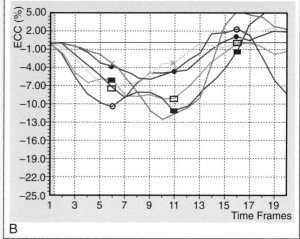

■ **Figure 4-8** This figure shows the mesh placement overlaying a tagged cine MR image on the LV. Resulting Lagrangian circumferential strain analysis are shown on the graph, in which each of the lines represents a different region of coronary artery supply. Concentrating on the systolic portion of the graph (frames 1 to 15), regional variation of circumferential strain is again seen, although magnitude of strain is reduced in all segments. In addition, peak negative strain occurs at different times for different regions, indicative of electrical systolic dyssynchrony. The mean of all the peak circumferential strain values for this patient was −6.4% (normal adult strain ≤16%). The finding of abnormal strain in the presence of severely abnormal global EF is expected, although its association with +MDE and dyssynchrony are new findings that affect further clinical therapy strategies for this patient. (*Courtesy of William Gottliebsen and Kan Hor, Cincinnati Children's Hospital Medical Center.*)

proportional to the tissue displacement, is called the stimulated echo. Thus, the technique has been coined DENSE. The stimulated echo is closely related to the signals acquired using conventional myocardial tagging, and, just as conventional tags fade with time because of T1 relaxation, the stimulated echo also undergoes exponential decay because of T1 relaxation. Because of this decay, about three fourths of the cardiac cycle can typically

be captured by DENSE before the signal-to-noise ratio becomes too low to measure tissue motion accurately.

An example demonstrating the application of DENSE CMR to imaging the heart of a normal volunteer is shown in Figure 4-9. Another example demonstrating DENSE

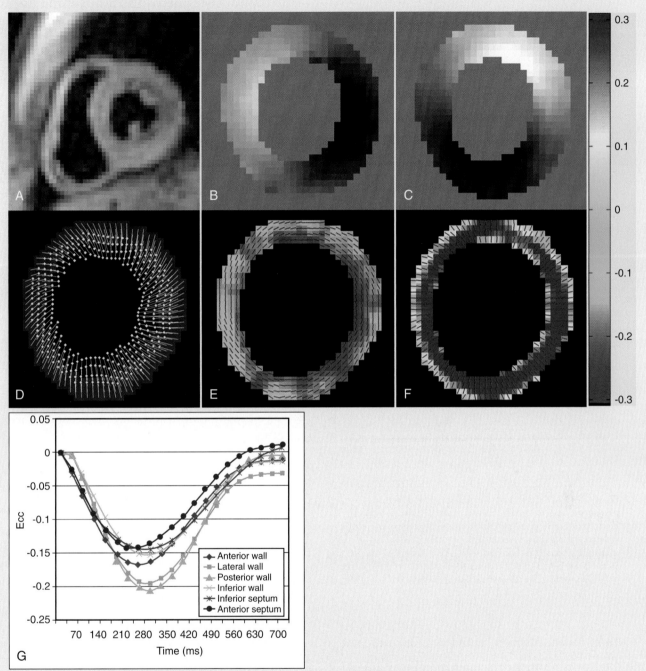

■ **Figure 4-9 A,** End-systolic magnitude-reconstructed short-axis DENSE image of the mid-ventricle, and end-systolic phase-reconstructed short-axis DENSE images encoded for 2D displacement in the septal-lateral (**B**) and anterior-posterior (**C**) directions. Non-zero values (i.e., white or black, but not gray) of the pixel phase correspond directly and quantitatively to tissue displacement. **D,** 2D displacement map created by vector combination of 1D displacement maps derived from the phase-reconstructed images, in which arrowheads represent the end-systolic position of each element of myocardium and arrow origins represent the position of each element of myocardium when tagging occurred on R-wave detection. **E-F,** Pixel-wise end-systolic first and second principal strain maps (magnitude and direction) computed from the 2D displacement map. Using the multiphase image set, example strain-time curves for circumferential shortening (E_{cc}) representing approximately three fourths of the cardiac cycle for the normal volunteer are shown in (**G**). The mid-ventricle is seen to demonstrate 14% to 21% peak circumferential shortening (normal, 13% to 25%) during systole and subsequent relaxation during diastole.

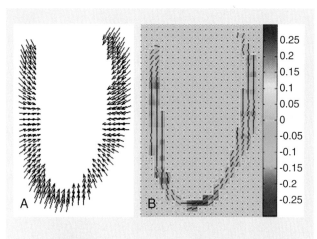

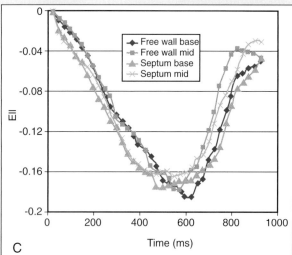

■ **Figure 4-10 A,** DENSE CMR of cardiac function applied in a long-axis view. The second principal strain (**B**) is predominantly oriented in the longitudinal direction (except at the apex), and segmental longitudinal strain (Ell) computed from this set of multi-phase images is shown in (**C**). These data demonstrate 16% to 18% peak longitudinal shortening (normal, 13% to 20%) during systole and subsequent relaxation during diastole.

CMR of cardiac function applied in a long-axis view is shown in Figure 4-10.

Examples

Ischemic Cardiomyopathy

This is a 72-year-old man with no significant past medical history who presented to an outside hospital after developing acute onset chest pain, shortness of breath, and diaphoresis. In the emergency department, he was found to have significant ECG ST elevations in leads V1 through V5. After transfer to our institution, he was emergently taken to the cardiac catheterization laboratory for treatment of a presumed anterior myocardial infarction (MI). Catheterization revealed a 100% left anterior descending (LAD) artery occlusion for which he received a bare metal stent. With the stent, TIMI grade 3 flow was

achieved, indicating complete resolution of the stenosis. Transthoracic echocardiography (TTE) performed 2 days after stent implantation demonstrated LV anterior wall and apical akinesis, with an overall LV ejection fraction of 35%. Repeat TTE 4 months after the MI showed no improvement in the anterior and apical wall motion abnormalities.

For research purposes, a cardiac MR study was performed. The cardiac MR exam included a complete stack of short-axis cine steady-state free precession (SSFP) images, three long-axis cine SSFP images (two-, three-, and four-chamber views), cine DENSE imaging in three short-axis planes (base, mid, apical views), and three long-axis planes, and late gadolinium-enhanced CMR in all short- and long-axis planes (Fig. 4-11).

Nonischemic Cardiomyopathy

This is a 52-year-old man referred to our institution for further evaluation of newly diagnosed left ventricular dysfunction. The patient described several months of progressive dyspnea on exertion, for which a TTE was performed. The initial TTE revealed global LV dysfunction, with an end-diastolic LV dimension of 6.1 cm (normal: 3.5–5.7 cm) and an overall ejection fraction of 20% to 25%. He subsequently underwent ischemic evaluation, demonstrating normal coronary artery perfusion, and was started on appropriate heart failure medications. Follow-up echocardiography several months later showed an ejection fraction of approximately 35%. For research purposes, a cardiac MR was performed (Fig. 4-12).

Pericardial Constriction

Quantitative MR tissue tracking techniques can also be used to examine the intricate wall motion abnormalities seen in patients with pericardial constriction. In this disease, chronic inflammation leads to scarring and subsequent loss of the normally elastic pericardial sac. With diminished elasticity, the pericardium loses the ability to accommodate the physiologic changes in volume associated with the normal cardiac filling cycle. Such impedance creates enhanced ventricular interdependence, an important pathophysiologic feature of constrictive pericarditis. With pericardial constriction, the hemodynamics of the ventricular chambers influences each other to a much greater degree than is normally the case. For example, in the normal heart, inspiration leads to a decrease in intrathoracic pressure, which is reflected in the cardiac chambers. However, with pericardial constriction, the rigid pericardium prevents this decrease in intrathoracic pressure to be transferred effectively to the LV. During inspiration, there is a decreased driving force from the lungs to the LV and the LV is subsequently underfilled. Furthermore, as a result of this enhanced ventricular interdependence, the right ventricle now expands into the LV in early diastole, via a shift of the interventricular septum, commonly referred to as the septal "bounce" or "shudder" (Fig. 4-13).

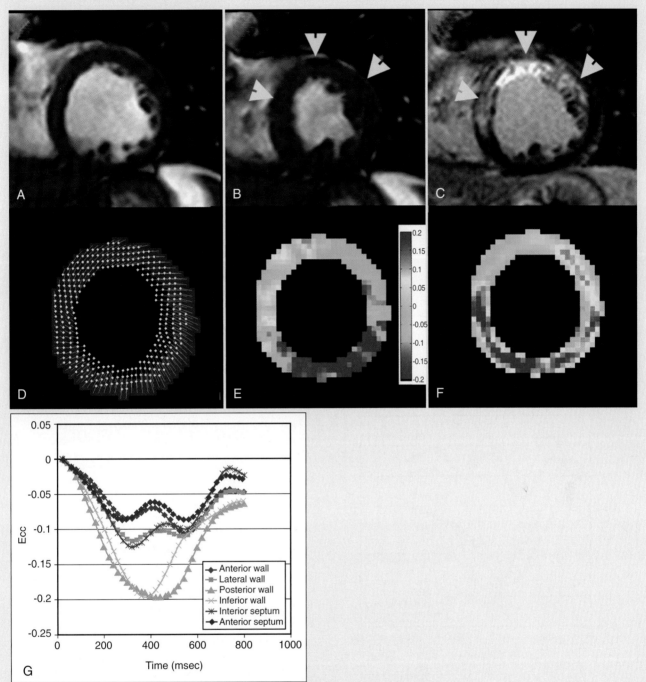

Figure 4-11 Mid-ventricular short-axis cine SSFP images at end-diastole (**A**) and end-systole (**B**) demonstrate a marked lack of wall thickening in the anterior wall that appears to extend to the anterior septum and lateral wall. Late gadolinium enhancement imaging in the same slice (**C**) shows nearly 100% transmural extent of enhancement of the anterior wall and septum, and approximately 50% transmural extent of enhancement of the lateral wall. This hyperenhancement pattern is indicative of a myocardial infarction in the distribution of the LAD. End-systolic strain maps of this same slice derived from cine DENSE CMR (**D,E**) and corresponding strain-time curves (**F**) illustrate severe dysfunction in the anterior wall and anterior septum, moderate dysfunction in the lateral wall and inferior septum, and normal contractile function in the posterior and inferior walls. This pattern of dysfunction, quantified by DENSE, correlates with the observed pattern of late gadolinium enhancement and agrees with the visual qualitative assessment of wall thickening provided in (**A**) and (**B**). As shown, a comprehensive cardiac MR evaluation helps to quantify not only the extent of tissue damage caused by the anterior myocardial infarction but also the subsequent contractile dysfunction of the LV.

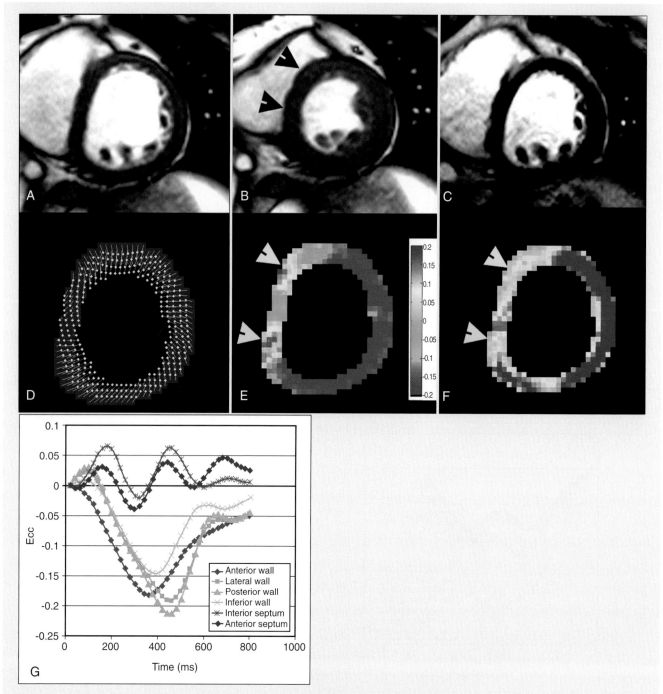

■ **Figure 4-12 A-B,** The LV myocardium is globally thinned, supporting the diagnosis of a nonischemic cardiomyopathy. As noted in Figure 4-11, ischemic cardiomyopathy usually affects the LV walls in a particular coronary distribution. This panel also demonstrates a D-shaped LV at end-diastole, representing volume overload. The diagnosis was further corroborated by the use of delayed enhancement imaging (**C**), illustrating no prior myocardial infarction or evidence of fibrosis. Cardiac MR was also instrumental in clarifying the LV ejection fraction, because patients with LV ejection fraction of 35% are candidates for implantation of a cardiac defibrillator. Using multislice cine MR, the LV ejection fraction was 38%. Quantitative imaging of strain by DENSE (**D-F**) shows severe dysfunction in the inferior and anterior septum (*arrows*), with delayed onset of shortening in the lateral, posterior, and inferior walls (**G**). The only segment with normal circumferential shortening in terms of time to onset of shortening and magnitude of shortening is the anterior wall.

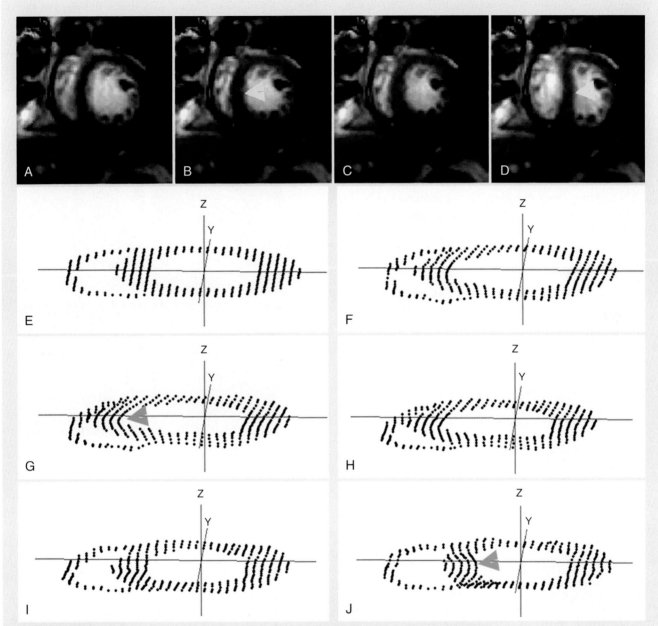

■ **Figure 4-13** This figure demonstrates the "septal bounce" of pericardial constriction using both cine
SSFP imaging and DENSE motion trajectories in a mid-ventricular short-axis view. In the systolic phase,
the septum bulges initially into the RV cavity and then "bounces" into the LV cavity during early diastole.
The diastolic septal bounce is well illustrated in both the cine (*yellow arrows*) and DENSE trajectory (*blue
arrows*) images. The septum is also shown bulging into the RV cavity in mid-systole.

Limitations of Displacement Encoding with Stimulated Echoes

Compared with conventional myocardial tagging and velocity-encoded phase contrast methods, DENSE has relatively low signal-to-noise ratio (SNR). This occurs because DENSE is based on acquiring the displacement-encoded stimulated echo, which is an MR signal that is generated from only half of the spin population that normally contributes to other commonly acquired echoes. Even though SNR is relatively low, in practice it is quite feasible to achieve fairly high spatial and temporal resolutions. For example, typical pixel size is $2.8 \times$

2.8×8 mm^3 and typical temporal resolution is 20 ms/ frame, for a total scan time of 14 heart beats per encoding direction. In our experience, such a protocol is well tolerated in heart disease patients and provides clinically useful data.

Another limitation is that DENSE is sensitive to poor ECG gating. If the ECG rhythm is very irregular or R-wave detection is poor, artifacts may occur and image quality may be poor. A third limitation is that, currently, displacement and strain analysis of DENSE images is not fully automatic. DENSE images are typically transferred to a personal computer, and semiautomated analysis methods are applied. Any given multiphase slice is typically analyzed in 3 to 5 minutes.

Strain Encoding: Imaging Contractility

Strain encoding (SENC) is another CMR technique for encoding another motion measure, the strain. Strain can be immediately encoded into the acquired images without measuring the displacement or velocity—as in the previous two techniques. The technique does not measure the strain in arbitrary direction but in a specific direction: orthogonal to the imaging plane. The encoding with SENC differs from the previous displacement encoding in DENSE as the strain measurements are not encoded in the complex phase of the image.

The Technique

Strain encoding shares the same basic ideas of MR tagging and DENSE. It encodes the tissue with patterns similar to tagging but produces images whose intensity varies according to regional contractility of the myocardium. The exact relation between the intensity and regional strain can be controlled by changing a SENC imaging parameter, called *tuning*. For example, it is possible to make the signal intensity at some region decrease as a result of contraction or vice versa, and make it brighter with contraction (Fig. 4-14). These strain-related changes in intensity and regional dysfunction can be easily viewed on the SENC images.

The raw SENC images can be further processed to produce anatomic images with coloring that indicate the

strain distribution. Figure 4-15 shows the steps of the algorithm, starting from low- to high-tuning images.

The advantages of SENC include its simplicity, as images of strain can be directly produced in real time. Also, SENC has higher in-plane resolution of strain than MR tagging, which can be very useful in assessing regional function of the right ventricle (RV) free wall.

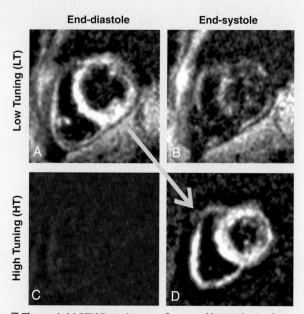

■ **Figure 4-14** SENC raw images of a normal heart obtained at end-diastole and end-systole for two different tunings. **A,** Low-tune end-diastole. **B,** Low-tune end-systole. **C,** High-tune end-diastole. **D,** High-tune end-systole. The arrow shows the shift from LT to HT at end-systole.

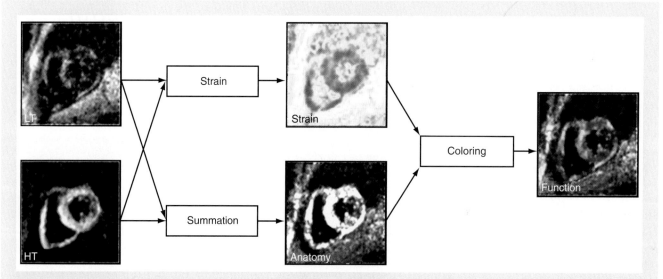

■ **Figure 4-15** Processing of raw SENC images to produce anatomic images with coloring that indicates the strain distribution. This figure shows the steps of the algorithm, starting from the low- and high-tuning images (shown in Figure 4-14, **B** and **D**). The Strain box indicates the strain computation operation from the LT and HT images, whereas the Summation box is a simple addition operation to create an anatomic image in which the heart does not fade. The anatomic image is then colored by the strain values to produce the colored functional (SENC) image. The red coloring indicates the contraction in the longitudinal direction of the heart. As can be seen, the myocardial infarct (MI) of the patient stays white, indicating dysfunction. The MI was verified by the delayed contrast enhancement image.

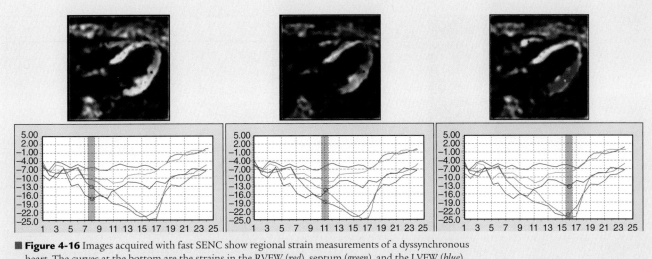

■ **Figure 4-16** Images acquired with fast SENC show regional strain measurements of a dyssynchronous heart. The curves at the bottom are the strains in the RVFW (*red*), septum (*green*), and the LVFW (*blue*). The first image is at the peak of contraction of the RVFW, the second is at the peak contraction of the septum, and the third is at the peak contraction of the LVFW.

SENC has a number of limitations versus MR tagging (HARP) and DENSE. First, it does not low the tracking of the motion of the heart. Because it only encodes the strain (contractility), the exact motion of the tissue cannot be followed. Second, SENC provides strain measurements only in the through-plane direction. Therefore, in case of short-axis images, only the longitudinal compression of the myocardium from base to apex is measured. On the other hand, circumferential shortening of the myocardium can be measured in the long-axis views of the heart (e.g., the four-chamber view).

A special pulse sequence has been developed recently to obtain SENC images in a single heartbeat. This is crucial, because it enables the acquisition of function in cases in which breath-holding is not feasible; for example, patients with pulmonary problems or pediatric cardiology. Also, it is most useful in patients with arrhythmias, in which the acquisition over multiple heartbeats as in other sequences is very difficult. Besides, the fast SENC sequence can be useful in stress tests, because it enables real-time monitoring of the patient's heart and detects changes in regional function. Figure 4-16 shows an example of images acquired with fast SENC.

Imaging Views

Because SENC just reveals the strain in the through-plane direction, it is only possible to measure the circumferential strain from the long-axis views and longitudinal strain from the short-axis views. The naming is based on the axes of the left ventricle. The long-axis is the line that goes through the LV from its base to the apex at the center, as shown in Figure 4-17.

Examples

Acute Myocardial Infarction

To study the changes in regional strain measurements post-myocardial infarction, SENC cine images were ac-

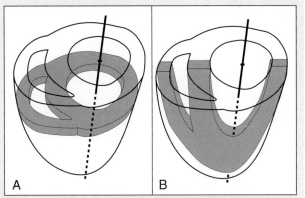

■ **Figure 4-17 A,** An imaging plane that cuts the heart orthogonally to the long axis is a short-axis plane. A short-axis plane can be at any level of the heart from the base to the apex. It is only important then to describe whether the short-axis plane is basal, mid, or apical to describe it fully. **B,** An image plane that has the long axis lying on it is a long-axis plane. There are different long-axis views, depending on their angle. (This is a four-chamber view.) If the plane cuts the left and right hearts, it is known as the four-chamber view. The two-chamber view is the long-axis plane orthogonal to the four-chamber view.

quired on long-axis planes to measure the circumferential strains. The circumferential strain was measured from the SENC images and was calculated for each segment in a modified 17-segment model. Figure 4-18 shows an example of a SENC image with large myocardial infarction. Figure 4-19 shows different circumferential strain-values in normokinetic, hypokinetic, and akinetic regions as determined with SENC-imaging.

Ischemic Heart Disease

In the case of the patient shown in Figure 4-20, wall motion analysis detected stress induced ischemia in the left ventricular apex but showed normal wall motion pattern in the lateral wall. SENC detected reduced regional

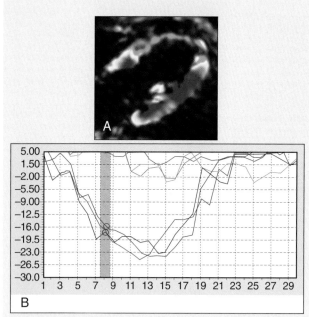

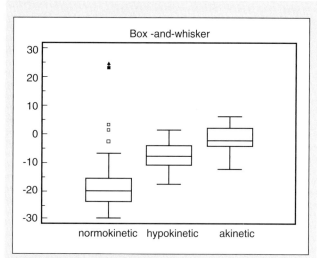

■ **Figure 4-18 A,** SENC-image of a patient with a transmural anterior myocardial infarction. The green color clearly indicates the anterior dysfunctional region, whereas in the orange-colored regions strain values are normal. **B,** Measurements from SENC can be demonstrated as strain curves. For a group of 12 patients, 252 segments were analyzed. Circumferential strain assessed with SENC was significantly reduced in regions defined as hypokinetic or akinetic by cine CMR, compared with normokinetic regions (normokinetic: $-19 \pm 8.19\%$; hypokinetic: $-8 \pm 5\%$; akinetic: $-1.3 \pm 3.9\%$, with $p < 0.001$). *(Courtesy of Mirja Neizel, Henning Steen, Evangelos Giannitsis, and Hugo A. Katus, University Hospital of Heidelberg, Germany.)*

■ **Figure 4-19** Different circumferential strain values in normokinetic, hypokinetic, and akinetic regions as determined with SENC imaging. In dyskinetic regions, peak systolic circumferential strain was reduced with a sensitivity and specificity of 90% (cutoff value -12%, ROC area 0.941, 95% CI 0.901 to 0.969). Impaired circumferential strain was also detected in regions with myocardial scar with a sensitivity of 81% and a specificity of 92% (cutoff value -10%, ROC area 0.895, 95% CI 0.849 to 0.930). The interobserver variability for SENC in these group patients was excellent ($r = 0.94$). SENC MR imaging therefore provides reliable and objective measurements of circumferential myocardial strain that could improve routine comprehensive evaluation of myocardial function and viability in patients with acute myocardial infarction. *(Courtesy of Mirja Neizel, Henning Steen, Evangelos Giannitsis, and Hugo A. Katus, University Hospital of Heidelberg, Germany.)*

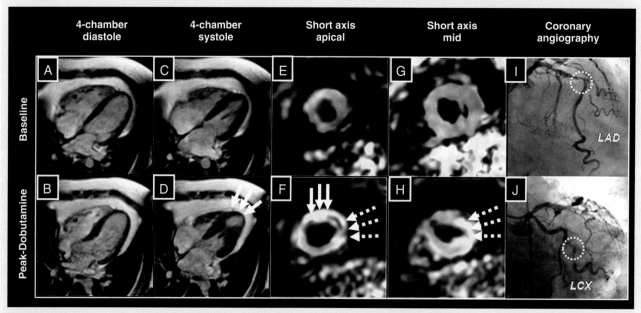

■ **Figure 4-20** Wall motion analysis detected stress-induced ischemia in the left ventricular apex but showed normal wall motion pattern in the lateral wall (**D,** *solid arrows*). SENC detected reduced regional longitudinal strain during peak dobutamine stress in both the left ventricular apex and in the mid-lateral wall (**F and H,** *solid and hatched arrows*). Coronary angiography confirmed the presence of two-vessel CAD in this patient, showing high-grade lesions (*hatched circles*) in both the left anterior descending (**I**), and in the left circumflex coronary artery (**J**). *(Courtesy of Grigorios Korosoglou, Dirk Lossnitzer, Henning Steen, Evangelos Giannitsis, and Hugo A. Katus, University Hospital of Heidelberg, Germany.)*

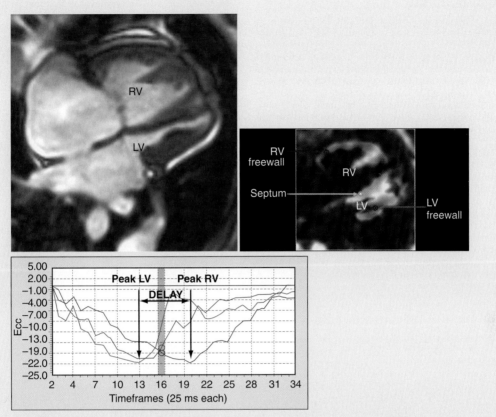

■ **Figure 4-21** SENC study showing that peak strains within normal range during development of PH do not alter, even when pulmonary artery pressure (PAP) is severely increased, RV morphology has changed, and RV function is decreased. However, a delay in time-to-peak strain of the RV free wall compared with the interventricular septum and LV free wall was detected. A time delay (125 to 225 ms) was detectable in all RV wall segments in patients with PAP > 70 mm Hg, whereas patients with moderately increased PAP (40 to 60 mm Hg) showed only regional or shorter delays (75 to 125 ms). Nevertheless, no correlation between RV peak strain and PAP could be detected. *(Courtesy of Dirk Lossnitzer, Henning Steen, Evangelos Giannitsis, and Hugo A. Katus, University Hospital of Heidelberg, Germany.)*

longitudinal strain during peak dobutamine stress in both the left ventricular apex and the mid-lateral wall. Coronary angiography confirmed the presence of two-vessel CAD in this patient.

Pulmonary Hypertension

Pulmonary hypertension (PH) is still difficult to diagnose and often remains undetected because of unspecific symptoms such as dyspnea, lethargy, and fatigue. SENC was explored as a noninvasive tool to assess RV dysfunction in patients with PH. Figure 4-21 shows an example of SENC images in PH. In a small study SENC showed that peak strains within normal range during development of PH did not alter, even when pulmonary artery pressure (PAP) was severely increased, RV morphology had changed, and RV function was decreased. However, a delay in time-to-peak strain of the RV free wall compared with the interventricular septum and LV free wall was detected. This time delay seems to be an early sign of RV dysfunction, because patients with the same PA pressure but inferior clinical state or even higher PA pres-

sure showed a decrease in RV peak strain. Given these preliminary data, SENC might be useful not only for diagnostic but also for therapeutic requirements in PAH.

Limitations of Strain-Encoded Imaging

SENC measures the region strain in the orthogonal direction of the plane. This limitation on the direction of strain measured to the image plane orientation makes it very difficult to obtain the radial strain of the LV. Measuring of the principal strains is not feasible as well. Moreover, the accuracy of the measurements depends on the right planning of the imaged views.

Because SENC images the strain only, other function quantities such as velocity and displacement are not feasible. Although the strain can be measured from MR tagging and DENSE, SENC becomes very limited, albeit more practical, for measuring regional function.

SENC shares with DENSE the problem of being a new pulse sequence not available on all CMR scanners. Experimental studies are still limited in number and further work is required to validate and verify the technique.

SUGGESTED READING

Aletras AH, Ding S, Balaban RS, Wen H: DENSE: Displacement encoding with stimulated echoes in cardiac functional MRI. J Magn Reson 1999;137:247-252.

Buonocore MH: Latest pulse sequence for displacement-encoded MR imaging incorporates essential technical improvements for multiphase measurement of intramyocardial strain. Radiology 2004;230:615-617.

Castillo E, Osman NF, Rosen BD, et al.: Quantitative assessment of regional myocardial function with MR-tagging in a multi-center study: Interobserver and intraobserver agreement of fast strain analysis with harmonic phase (HARP) MRI. J Cardiovasc Magn Reson 2005;7:783-791.

Epstein FH: MRI of left ventricular function. J Nucl Cardiol 2007;14(5):729-744.

Kerwin WS, Osman NF, Prince JL: Image processing and analysis in tagged cardiac MRI. In: Frank J, Brody W, Zerhouni E (eds): Handbook of Medical Image Processing. San Diego, Academic Press, 2000.

Kim D, Gilson WD, Kramer CM, Epstein FH: Myocardial tissue tracking with two-dimensional cine displacement-encoded MR imaging: Development and initial evaluation. Radiology 2004;230:862-871.

Masood S, Yang GZ, Pennell DJ, Firmin DN: Investigating intrinsic myocardial mechanics: The role of MR tagging, velocity phase mapping, and diffusion imaging. J Magn Reson Imag 2000;12:873-883.

McVeigh ER: MRI of myocardial function: Motion tracking techniques. J Magn Reson Imag 1996;14:137-150.

Moore CC, Lugo-Olivieri CH, McVeigh ER, Zerhouni EA: Three-dimensional systolic strain patterns in the normal human left ventricle: Characterization with tagged MR imaging. Radiology 2000;214:453-466.

Osman NF: Quantitative image analysis. In: Lardo A, Fayad ZA, Chronos NAF, Fuster V (eds): Cardiovascular Magnetic Resonance. New York, Martin Dunitz, 2003.

Osman NF, McVeigh ER, Prince JL: Imaging heart motion using harmonic phase MRI. IEEE Trans Med Imag 2000;19:186-202.

Osman NF, Prince JL: Imaging cardiac function using harmonic phase (HARP) MRI. In: Amini A, Prince JL (eds): Cardiac MRI. Philadelphia, Kluwer Academic Publishers, 2001.

Osman NF, Sampath S, Atalar E, Prince JL: Imaging longitudinal cardiac strain on short-axis images using strain-encoded MRI. Magn Reson Med 2001;46:324-334.

Pai VM, Axel L: Advances in MRI tagging techniques for determining regional myocardial strain. Curr Cardiol Rpt 2006;8:53-58.

Pan L, Stuber S, Kraitchman DL, et al.: Real-time imaging of regional myocardial function using fast-SENC. Magn Reson Med 2006;55:386-395.

Chapter 5

Size and Function of the Right Ventricle

Albert C. van Rossum and Simon C. Koestner

KEY POINTS

- Cardiac magnetic resonance (CMR) allows imaging of the entire RV without interference of ribs or lungs.

- Because of high image quality and wide field-of-view, CMR imaging is the method of choice to assess the complex geometry and function of the RV.

- RV hypertrophy that results from increased loading conditions is accurately determined by CMR.

- CMR may support the diagnosis of ARVC/D by detecting RV dilatation and focal functional abnormalities of the RV wall.

- CMR techniques may help to characterize abnormal tissue composition of hypertrophic RV myocardium.

Case 1   Anatomy of the Right Ventricle

This first section shows images of a healthy patient to demonstrate normal right
ventricular anatomy (Figure 5-1).

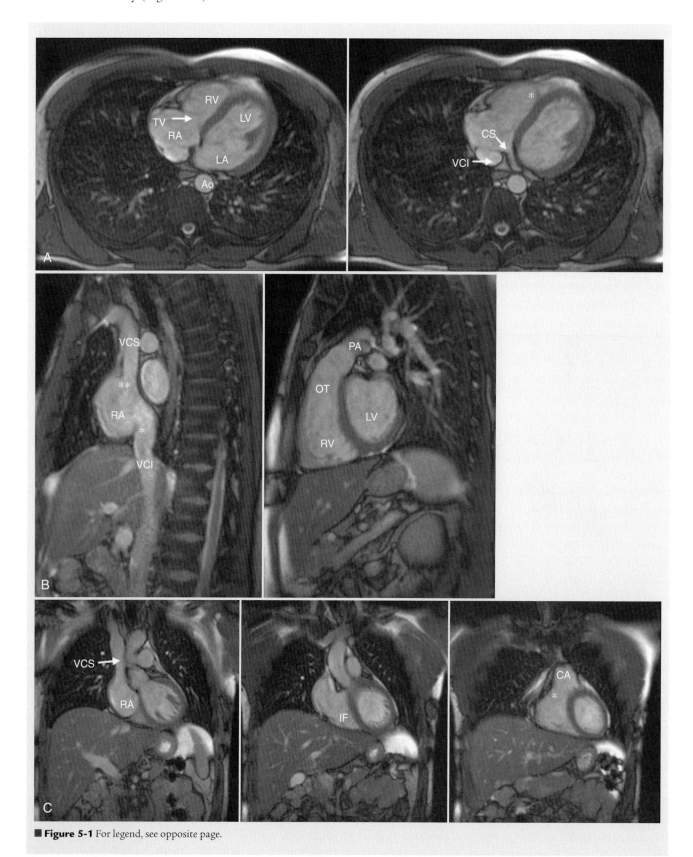

■ **Figure 5-1** For legend, see opposite page.

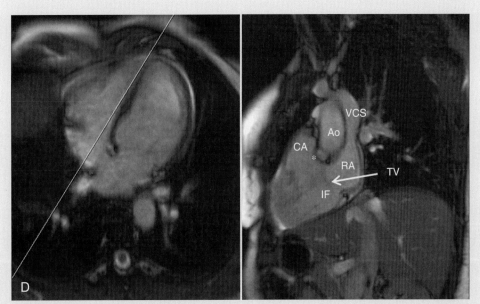

■ **Figure 5-1 A,** Transverse planes obtained with a bright-blood technique (steady-state free precession pulse sequence, SSFP). Panel A shows the right atrium (RA), right ventricle (RV), left atrium (LA), left ventricle (LV), and the descending aorta (Ao). The tricuspid valve (TV) has an insertion point displaced toward the apex compared with the mitral valve. Similar view for Panel B, with slight caudal displacement. The coronary sinus (CS) and the incoming vena cava inferior (VCI) are clearly visible. The following characteristics differentiate the RV from the LV: more pronounced trabeculae, the presence of a moderator band (*), and the more apical insertion of the tricuspid valve. **B,** Sagittal views of the right heart. Panel A, bi-caval view of the right atrium (RA) with inflow of both vena cava superior (VCS) and vena cava inferior (VCI). *: valve of inferior vena cava (Eustachii). **: crista terminalis. Panel B shows the right ventricle (RV), the right ventricular outflow tract (OT), and the pulmonary trunk (PA). The very thin structure of the pulmonary valve is barely seen at the transition of OT and PA. LV, left ventricle. **C,** Coronal views of the heart from posterior (A) to anterior (C). Panel A shows the vena cava superior (VCS) entering the right atrium (RA). On panel B, the inflow tract (IF) of the RV is depicted. The more anterior view (panel C) visualizes both the inflow and outflow tract of the RV. Compared with the LV, inflow and outflow tract of the RV are at a much wider angle. As a result, the tricuspid and pulmonary valve**s** do not share a common anatomical plane. CA, conus arteriosus; *, supraventricular crest. **D,** View of the RVOT at end-diastole, planned on the four-chamber view (see cutline). This view allows the depiction of both the inflow and outflow tract of the right ventricle. *, supraventricular crest; CA, conus arteriosus; TV, tricuspid valve; VCS, vena cava superior; Ao, Aorta; RA, right atrium; IF, inflow of the RV.

Comments

The geometry of the right ventricle (RV) is more complex than of the left ventricle (LV). The LV can be compared with an elliptic cone with two valves (mitral and aortic valves) sharing the same anatomic plane. The RV cavity is wrapped around the left ventricle and can be divided into a posteroinferior inflow portion, containing the tricuspid valve, and an anterosuperior outflow portion, from which the pulmonary trunk originates. Because of this complex geometry, CMR has become the imaging technique of choice to precisely evaluate patients with congenital or acquired disease of the right ventricle.

Case 2   **Assessment of Right Ventricular Volumes and Function**

This is a demonstration of Simpson or disk-area method for calculation of right ventricular end-systolic and end-diastolic volumes, and ejection fraction (Figure 5-2).

Comments

Today, CMR is considered the gold standard for assessment of right ventricular volumes, mass, and function, for clinical as well as research purposes. It has been shown to have a good interstudy reproducibility of functional RV parameters in healthy subjects, and in patients with heart failure or hypertrophy. However, the reproducibility of the RV measurements is lower than for the LV.

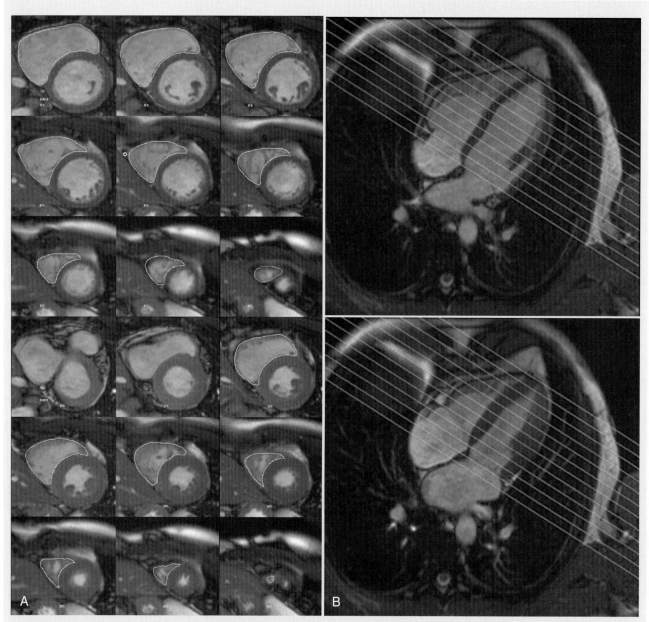

■ **Figure 5-2 A**, Nine end-diastolic and nine end-systolic short-axis images of the heart obtained with a bright-blood cine technique (SSFP), and planned perpendicular to the LV long axis of a four-chamber view (see panel B). Tracings of the endocardial contours are shown, used to calculate the RV volumes. The first and second basal end-systolic slices are not included in the calculation since these slices contain the right atrium and not the right ventricle, because of systolic long axis shortening and the anterior displacement of the tricuspid valve compared with the mitral valve. **B,** Four-chamber view at end-diastole (left) end-systole (right) with cutlines of short axis images from Figure 5-2, *A*. At end-diastole, the most basal short axis slice cuts through the mitral valve annulus and the right atrium. At end-systole, the first basal slice cuts through left and right atrium, whereas the second slice cuts through the mitral annulus and the right atrium. These differences, because of long axis shortening of the heart, must be accounted for when tracing the RV contours.

Case 3   **Right Ventricular Hypertrophy Resulting from Cardiac Amyloidosis**

A 77-year-old man presented for exertional dyspnea and atrial fibrillation for 5 months. A transthoracic echocardiogram showed a hypertrophic left ventricle with poor systolic and diastolic function. CMR was performed to retrieve the cause of the hypertrophy (Figure 5-3).

Comments

Amyloidosis results from the deposition in tissues of fibrils formed from various proteins. Involvement of the heart is frequent, leads to restrictive cardiomyopathy, and progressive heart failure, and may finally lead to death. CMR imaging has been shown to correlate well with histologic findings, with areas of late contrast enhancement demonstrating the amyloid infiltration. When compared with endomyocardial biopsy, contrast-enhanced CMR has a sensitivity of 80% and a specificity of 94% for diagnosing cardiac amyloidosis. The distribution pattern of enhanced areas is highly variable and the extent of hyperenhancement correlates with ventricular dysfunction.

Case 4   **Right Ventricular Hypertrophy Resulting from Pressure Overload**

Follow-up examination 5 years after the initial diagnosis of idiopathic pulmonary hypertension (Figure 5-4).

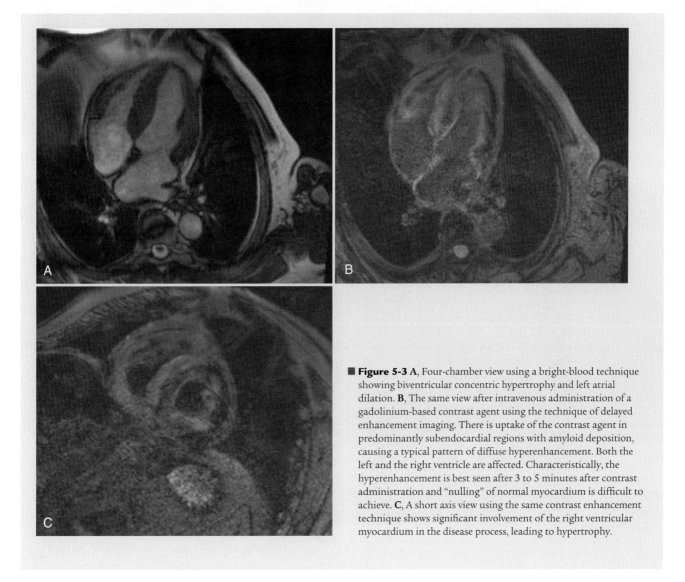

■ **Figure 5-3 A**, Four-chamber view using a bright-blood technique showing biventricular concentric hypertrophy and left atrial dilation. **B**, The same view after intravenous administration of a gadolinium-based contrast agent using the technique of delayed enhancement imaging. There is uptake of the contrast agent in predominantly subendocardial regions with amyloid deposition, causing a typical pattern of diffuse hyperenhancement. Both the left and the right ventricle are affected. Characteristically, the hyperenhancement is best seen after 3 to 5 minutes after contrast administration and "nulling" of normal myocardium is difficult to achieve. **C**, A short axis view using the same contrast enhancement technique shows significant involvement of the right ventricular myocardium in the disease process, leading to hypertrophy.

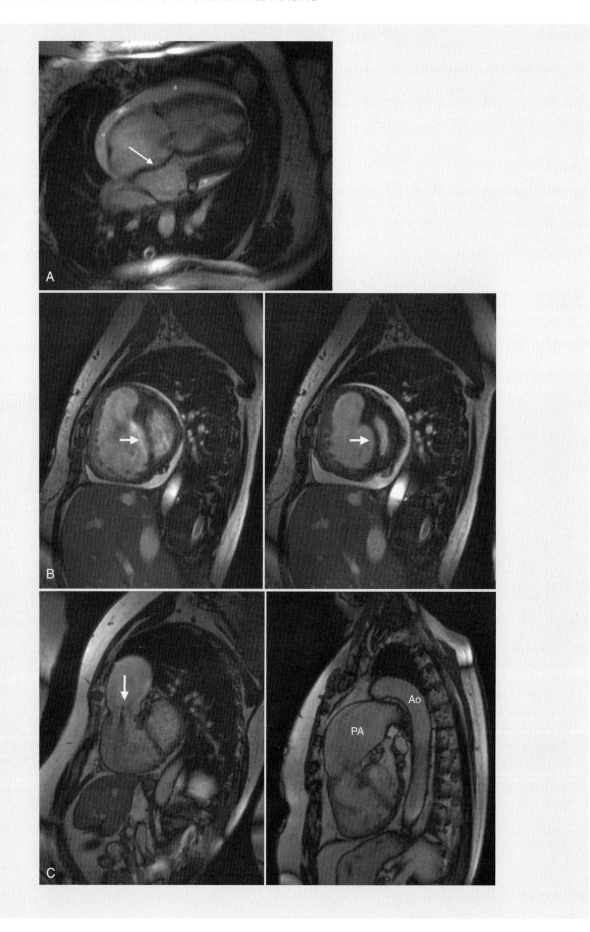

■ **Figure 5-4 A**, Bright-blood four-chamber view demonstrating pronounced hypertrophy and dilation of the right ventricle. The right to left end-diastolic diameter ratio is greater than 1, with compression of the left ventricular cavity. There is a marked dilation of the right atrium with bowing of the interatrial septum toward the left atrium because of right atrial pressure overload. Tricuspid regurgitation is apparent as a signal void into the right atrium, originating from the coaptation point of the tricuspid valve leaflets. Pericardial effusion surrounds the right atrium, right ventricle, and part of the left ventricle (*) s. **B**, End-diastolic (A) and end-systolic (B) short axis views demonstrating the flattening and bulging of the interventricular septum toward the left ventricle (*arrow*). The diastolic and systolic occurrence of septal bowing in this patient indicates both volume and pressure overload of the right ventricle. Volume overload may occur because of a left to right shunt or significant tricuspid or pulmonary regurgitation. **C**, Basal short-axis view (A) and sagittal view (B) showing the right ventricular outflow tract of another patient with pulmonary hypertension. There is a marked dilation of the right ventricle and of the pulmonary artery (PA, 60 mm diameter) leading to pulmonary valve regurgitation. The regurgitant jet is seen as a signal void originating from the coaptation point of the pulmonary valve leaflets (arrow).

Comments

Severe pulmonary hypertension caused by diseases of the lung parenchyma and/or pulmonary vasculature can lead to cor pulmonale. Right ventricular hypertrophy develops to maintain a sufficient output against high pulmonary vascular impedance. Further elevation of the pulmonary pressure leads to dilation and systolic dysfunction of the right ventricle. CMR allows the exact determination of right ventricular mass, volume, and function in patients in whom echocardiographic diagnosis may be difficult because of poor image quality in the setting of chronic obstructive pulmonary disease. Moreover, the RV shape and position in the chest can make the calculation of RV volumes and ejection fraction by echocardiography unreliable.

Case 5   **Right Ventricular Dilation and Hypertrophy Resulting from Volume and Pressure Overload in a Patient with an Atrial Septal Defect Type II**

A 64-year old patient with arterial hypertension, severe COPD, intermittent atrial fibrillation. He is referred for CMR after the echocardiographic demonstration of an atrial septal defect type II (Figure 5-5, *A*). A 39-year old patient with a known atrial septal defect (ASD) type II, referred for follow-up of RV-size and function, and calculation of the shunt size (Figure 5-5, *B-C*).

Comments

ASDs are a common cause of a left-to-right shunt, which sometimes is only diagnosed in adulthood. CMR is useful to differentiate the type of ASD and look for associated congenital defects.

CMR imaging also may be used to measure flow velocities and from these calculate volume flow in the aorta and pulmonary artery, from which in turn the Qp/Qs as well as the shunt volume in absolute terms can be extracted. These data are helpful to determine the clinical significance of a shunt. A Qp/Qs ratio of more than 1.5 is usually regarded as an indication for surgical intervention.

Case 6   **Ebstein's Anomaly**

Two cases of right heart enlargement because of Ebstein's anomaly are presented in this section (Figure 5-6).

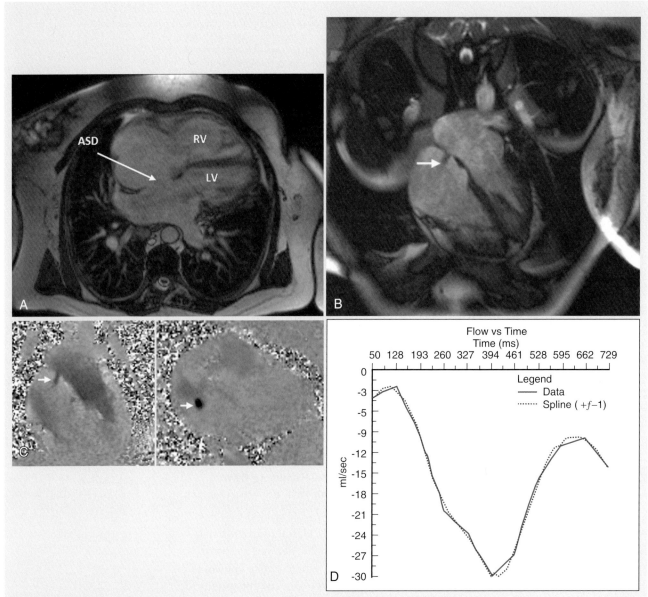

■ **Figure 5-5 A,** Four-chamber view demonstrating the enlargement of the right side of the heart and the left atrium. The ASD type II measures 32 mm (*arrow*). **B,** This patient has a smaller atrial septal defect type II (7 mm), with a left-to-right flow demonstrated by the signal void jet (arrow). Owing to this non-significant left-to-right shunt (see Figure 5-5C), there is no apparent dilation of the right heart structures. **C,** The jet (*arrow*) is also visible in this in-plane (A) and through-plane (B) phase contrast velocity images. Panel C shows the volumetric flow analysis through the ASD, made on measurements obtained from the through-plane phase contrast velocity images (as in B). In this patient, the volume of blood shunting from the left to the right atrium was calculated to be 11 ml per heart beat.

Comments

Ebstein's anomaly was first described in 1866 and occurs in about 1 to 5 per 200,000 births (less than 1% of all congenital heart diseases). Ebstein's anomaly is characterized by inferior displacement of the proximal attachments of the septal and posterior leaflets of the tricuspid valve from the atrioventricular ring, and is caused by an incomplete delamination of the ventricular myocardium during morphogenesis. Cardiac magnetic resonance is useful for determining precisely the anatomy of the right ventricle and of the great vessels, to exclude concomitant defects and assess right ventricular function. Concomitant abnormalities are frequent and include patent foramen ovale (PFO) or ASD (50% incidence in patients with Ebstein's anomaly), or less frequently ventricular septal defect (VSD), right ventricular outflow tract obstruction, aortic coarctation, patent ductus arteriosus, or mitral valve disease.

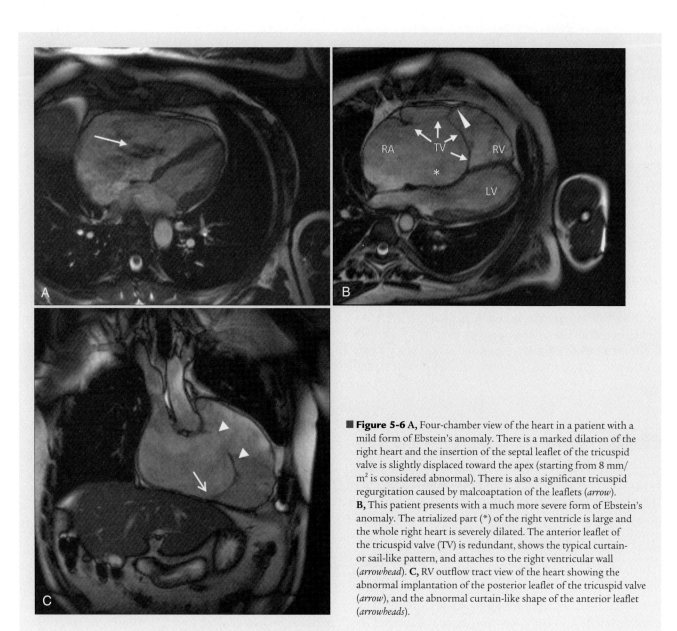

■ **Figure 5-6 A,** Four-chamber view of the heart in a patient with a mild form of Ebstein's anomaly. There is a marked dilation of the right heart and the insertion of the septal leaflet of the tricuspid valve is slightly displaced toward the apex (starting from 8 mm/m² is considered abnormal). There is also a significant tricuspid regurgitation caused by malcoaptation of the leaflets (*arrow*). **B,** This patient presents with a much more severe form of Ebstein's anomaly. The atrialized part (*) of the right ventricle is large and the whole right heart is severely dilated. The anterior leaflet of the tricuspid valve (TV) is redundant, shows the typical curtain- or sail-like pattern, and attaches to the right ventricular wall (*arrowhead*). **C,** RV outflow tract view of the heart showing the abnormal implantation of the posterior leaflet of the tricuspid valve (*arrow*), and the abnormal curtain-like shape of the anterior leaflet (*arrowheads*).

Case 7   **Right Ventricular Infarction**

A 65-year-old patient with sustained inferior myocardial infarction and signs of heart failure was referred for ventricular function and viability assessment (Figure 5-7).

Comments

CMR is a powerful tool to evaluate patients with chronic ischemic heart disease and heart failure. Whereas the cine bright-blood technique allows accurate evaluation of regional myocardial motion and global ventricular function, contrast late enhancement enables visualization of myocardial scar after infarction. A high transmural extent of scar is associated with a low likelihood of functional recovery after CABG or PCI of the infarct-related vessel.

Contrast late enhancement may reveal right ventricular infarction, which is usually associated with inferior infarction and occasionally occurs in isolation. It is more sensitive for the detection of right ventricular infarction than other diagnostic procedures (ECG, echocardiography) and has been shown to have a good interobserver reproducibility. A diagnosis of right ventricular infarction has prognostic value and is helpful in tailoring patient management.

Case 8   **Arrhythmogenic Right Ventricular Cardiomyopathy/Dysplasia**

A 37-year-old man, suspected of having arrhythmogenic right ventricular cardiomyopathy (ARVC) was admitted to the hospital with recurrent palpitations. The ECG showed a ventricular tachycardia and T-wave inversions in the precordial leads with epsilon waves after conversion to sinus rhythm. He had angiographically normal coronary arteries. The patient was referred for CMR imaging (Figure 5-8).

Comments

ARVD/C is a rare disease consisting of fibrofatty infiltration of the myocardium; it affects predominantly the right ventricle. The clinical presentation may vary with the severity of the disease. Common symptoms include ventricular arrhythmias, exercise-induced dizziness, and

sudden death. CMR allows the demonstration of regional wall-motion abnormalities, regional thinning, trabecular disarray, and fibrofatty infiltration of the myocardium. For a detailed analysis of the right ventricular free wall, the use of a small field of view with a high in-plane resolution is necessary.

Case 9   **Right Atrial Tumor**

A 67-year-old man with a history of systemic hypertension underwent a routine transthoracic echocardiogram to assess for the presence of LV hypertrophy. A right atrial mass was visualized, presumed to be an atrial myxoma by the echocardiographer. CMR examination was requested to better define the RA mass (Figure 5-9).

Comments

Primary tumors of the heart are uncommon, with an incidence of 0.02% in autopsy series. Myxomas account for 76% of all primary cardiac tumors. CMR offers several advantages for the evaluation of cardiac tumors in comparison with echocardiography. The large field of view allows one to obtain precise information on the anatomic

relations of the tumor with the surrounding extracardiac and paracardiac structures. Moreover, the use of different pulse sequences and prepulses is helpful for tissue characterization. Additional use of gadolinium-containing contrast agents allows one to assess the tumor's extent of vascularization and helps to differentiate the tumor from surrounding structures.

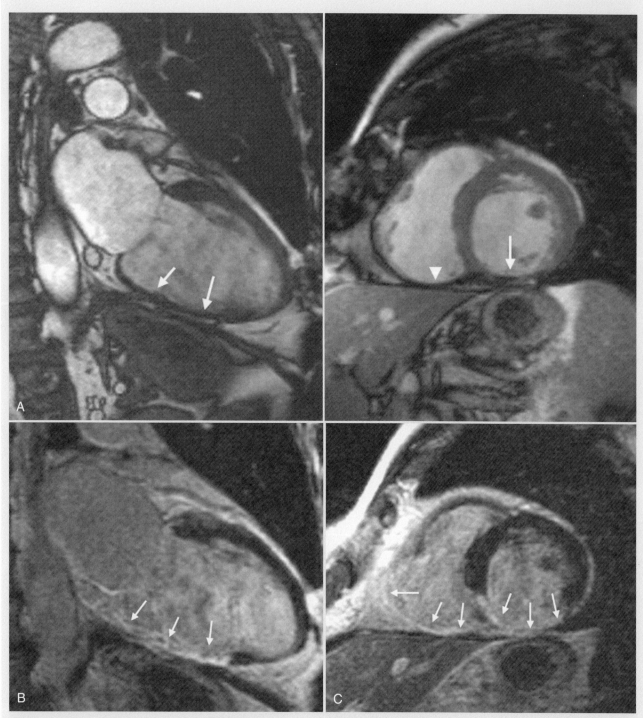

■ **Figure 5-7 A,** Bright-blood cine 2-chamber (A) and mid-ventricular short-axis (B) views of the heart. A marked thinning is visible of the basal and mid-ventricular inferior wall (*arrows*). The end-diastolic wall thickness of these segments is less than 5.5 mm and they therefore have a low probability of functional recovery after revascularization. Whereas abnormal thinning of the right ventricular wall is difficult to use as criteria, infarct involvement of the diaphragmatic segment of the right ventricle is suggested by aneurysmatic outward motion (*arrowhead*). **B,** Two-chamber view of the heart using contrast late enhancement imaging. The bright enhancement of the basal and middle segment of the inferior wall extends transmurally (*arrows*), indicating full wall thickness scar formation. This finding confirms the low likelihood of functional recovery after revascularization, as was already suggested by the wall thinning in panel A. **C,** Contrast late enhancement imaging of short axis view similar to panel B. Full wall thickness enhancement is seen of the inferior segment of the left ventricle, of the inferior segment of the interventricular septum, and of the diaphragmatic segment of the right ventricle (*arrows*), thereby confirming right ventricular infarct involvement.

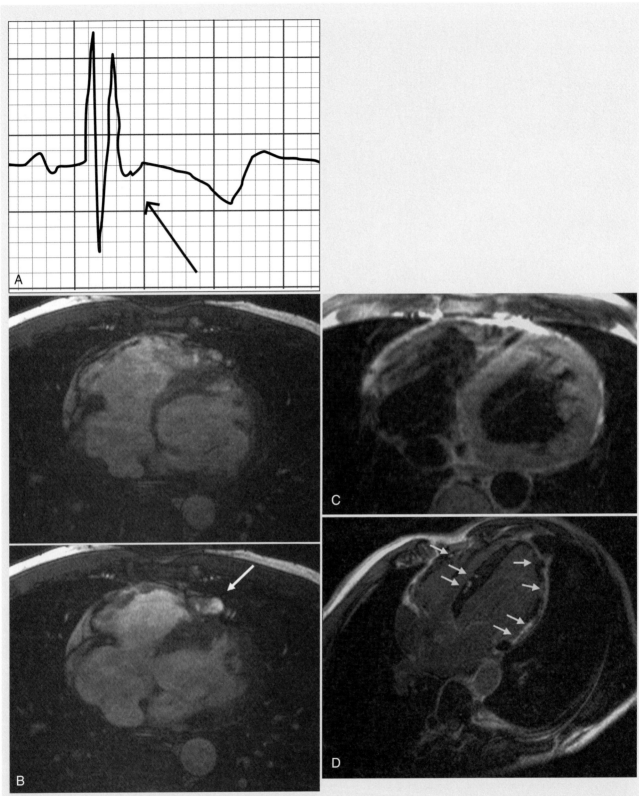

■ **Figure 5-8 A,** Lead V1 of the ECG showing a deflection after the QRS complex typical of epsilon-wave seen in ARVC (*arrow*). **B,** End-diastolic (A) and end-systolic (B) frames of transverse bright-blood cine imaging of the right ventricle. High resolution imaging (thin 4-mm slices and small field of view) allows detailed assessment of the right ventricular wall but decreases the signal-to-noise ratio (causing the grainy aspect). Apically from the moderator band focal bulging of the myocardium is seen (*arrow*), indicative of the presence of a microaneurysm, which is a typical finding in ARVC. **C,** Transverse view using a high spatial resolution T1 turbo spin-echo technique. This sequence allows the visualization of fatty tissue with high brightness. In this case, fat seems to have partly replaced the myocardium in-between the trabeculars of the moderator band. **D,** Four-chamber view using contrast late enhancement imaging for detection of regional myocardial fibrosis. Whereas transmural fibrosis is observed in the free wall of the left ventricle, spots of intramural fibrosis are seen in the interventricular septum and probably also in the right ventricular free wall (*arrows*). Thus, this patient has ARVC with biventricular involvement.

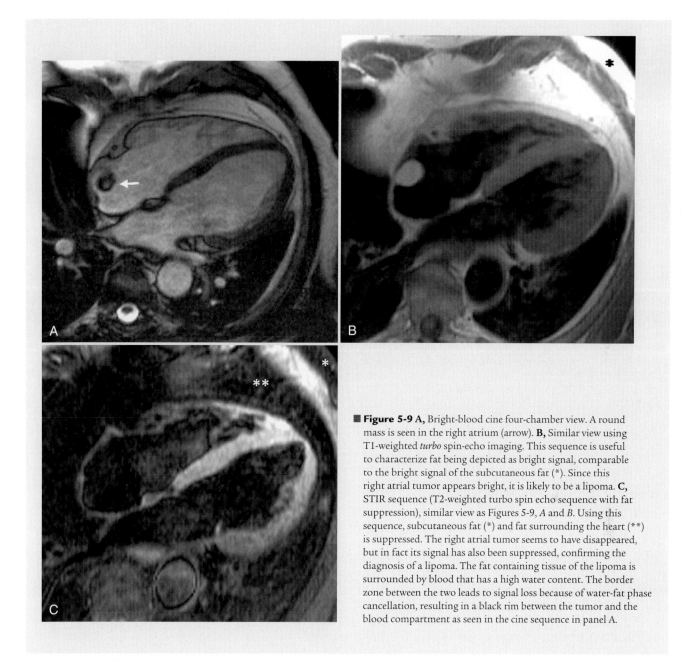

■ **Figure 5-9 A,** Bright-blood cine four-chamber view. A round mass is seen in the right atrium (arrow). **B,** Similar view using T1-weighted *turbo* spin-echo imaging. This sequence is useful to characterize fat being depicted as bright signal, comparable to the bright signal of the subcutaneous fat (*). Since this right atrial tumor appears bright, it is likely to be a lipoma. **C,** STIR sequence (T2-weighted turbo spin echo sequence with fat suppression), similar view as Figures 5-9, *A* and *B*. Using this sequence, subcutaneous fat (*) and fat surrounding the heart (**) is suppressed. The right atrial tumor seems to have disappeared, but in fact its signal has also been suppressed, confirming the diagnosis of a lipoma. The fat containing tissue of the lipoma is surrounded by blood that has a high water content. The border zone between the two leads to signal loss because of water-fat phase cancellation, resulting in a black rim between the tumor and the blood compartment as seen in the cine sequence in panel A.

SUGGESTED READING

Alfakih K, Reid S, Jones T, Sivanantham M: Assessment of ventricular function and mass by cardiac magnetic resonance imaging. Eur Radiol 2004;14:1813-1822.

Alter P, Grimm W, Rominger MB, et al.: Right ventricular myxoma. Diagnostic usefulness of cardiac magnetic resonance imaging. Herz 2005;30(7):663-667.

Babu-Narayan SV, Kilner PJ, Gatzoulis MA: When to order cardiovascular magnetic resonance in adults with congenital heart disease. Curr Cardiol Rep 2003;5(4):324-330.

Burke A, Jeudy J Jr, Virmani R: Cardiac tumors: An update. Heart 2008;94(1):117-123.

Catalano O, Antonaci S, Opasich C, et al.: Intra-observer and interobserver reproducibility of right ventricle volumes, function and mass by cardiac magnetic resonance. J Cardiovasc Med 2007;8(10):807-814.

Choi YH, Park JH, Choe YH, Yoo SJ: MR imaging of Ebstein's anomaly of the tricuspid valve. Am J Roentgenol 1994;163(3):539-543.

Conen D, Osswald S, Cron TA, et al.: Value of repeated cardiac magnetic resonance imaging in patients with suspected arrhythmogenic right ventricular cardiomyopathy. J Cardiovasc Magn Reson 2006;8(2):361-366.

Craig RJ, Selzer A: Natural history and prognosis of atrial septal defect. Circulation 1968;37(5):805-815.

Dellegrottaglie S, Sanz J, Poon M, et al.: Pulmonary hypertension: accuracy of detection with left ventricular septal-to-free wall curvature ratio measured at cardiac MR. Radiology 2007;243(1):63-69.

Grothues F, Moon JC, Bellenger NG, et al.: Interstudy reproducibility of right ventricular volumes, function, and mass with cardiovascular magnetic resonance. Am Heart J 2004;147(2):218-223.

Hundley WG, Li HF, Lange RA, et al.: Assessment of left-to-right intracardiac shunting by velocity-encoded, phase-difference magnetic resonance imaging. A comparison with oximetric and indicator dilution techniques. Circulation 1995;91(12):2955-2960.

Körperich H, Gieseke J, Barth P, et al.: Flow volume and shunt quantification in pediatric congenital heart disease by real-time magnetic resonance velocity mapping. Circulation 2004;109(16):1987-1993.

Kumar A, Abdel-Aty H, Kriedemann I, et al.: Contrast-enhanced cardiovascular magnetic resonance imaging of right ventricular infarction. J Am Coll Cardiol 2006;48(10):1969-1976.

Larose E, Ganz P, Reynolds HG, et al.: Right ventricular dysfunction assessed by cardiovascular magnetic resonance imaging predicts poor prognosis late after myocardial infarction. J Am Coll Cardiol 2007;49(8):855-862.

Maceira AM, Joshi J, Prasad SK, et al.: Cardiovascular magnetic resonance in cardiac amyloidosis. Circulation 2005;111(2):186-193.

Maceira AM, Prasad SK, Khan M, Pennell DJ: Reference right ventricular systolic and diastolic function normalized to age, gender and body surface area from steady-state free precession cardiovascular magnetic resonance. Eur Heart J 2006;27(23):2879-2888.

Marcu CB, Beek AM, Van Rossum AC: Cardiovascular magnetic resonance imaging for the assessment of right heart involvement in cardiac and pulmonary disease. Heart Lung Circ 2006;15(6):362-370.

McLure LE, Peacock AJ: Imaging of the heart in pulmonary hypertension. Int J Clin Pract 2007;61(Suppl 156):15-26.

Nijveldt R, Beek AM, Germans T, et al.: Arrhythmogenic right ventricular cardiomyopathy with evidence of biventricular involvement. CMAJ 2007;176(13):1819-1821.

O'Rourke RA, Dell'italia LJ: Diagnosis and management of right ventricular myocardial infarction. Curr Probl Cardiol 2004;29(1):6-47.

Paranon S, Acar P: Ebstein's anomaly of the tricuspid valve: From fetus to adult. Heart 2008;94:237-243.

Perugini E, Rapezzi C, Piva T, et al.: Non-invasive evaluation of the myocardial substrate of cardiac amyloidosis by gadolinium cardiac magnetic resonance. Heart 2006;92(3):343-349.

Selvanayagam JB, Hawkins PN, Paul B, et al.: Evaluation and management of the cardiac amyloidosis. J Am Coll Cardiol 2007;50(22):2101-2110.

Sen-Chowdhry S, Prasad SK, Syrris P, et al.: Cardiovascular magnetic resonance in arrhythmogenic right ventricular cardiomyopathy revisited: Comparison with task force criteria and genotype. J Am Coll Cardiol 2006;48(10):2132-2140.

Tandri H, Castillo E, Ferrari VA, et al.: Magnetic resonance imaging of arrhythmogenic right ventricular dysplasia: sensitivity, specificity, and observer variability of fat detection versus functional analysis of the right ventricle. J Am Coll Cardiol 2006;48(11):2277-2284.

Valente AM, Powell AJ: Clinical applications of cardiovascular magnetic resonance in congenital heart disease. Cardiol Clin 2007; 25(1):97-110.

Valente AM, Sena L, Powell AJ, et al.: Cardiac magnetic resonance imaging evaluation of sinus venosus defects: Comparison to surgical findings. Pediatr Cardiol 2007;28(1):51-56.

van Beek EJ, Stolpen AH, Khanna G, Thompson BH: CT and MRI of pericardial and cardiac neoplastic disease. Cancer Imaging 2007;7:19-26.

Van Wolferen SA, Marcus JT, Boonstra A, et al.: Prognostic value of right ventricular mass, volume and function in idiopathic pulmonary arterial hypertension. Eur Heart J 2007;28(10):1250-1257.

Vogelsberg H, Mahrholdt H, Deluigi CC, et al.: Cardiovascular magnetic resonance in clinically suspected cardiac amyloidosis. J Am Coll Cardiol 2008;51(10):1022-1030.

Wald RM, Powell AJ: Simple congenital lesions. J Cardiovasc Magn Reson 2006;8(4):619-631.

Chapter 6

Atria and Pulmonary Veins

Saman Nazarian, David A. Bluemke, Hugh Calkins, and Henry R. Halperin

KEY POINTS

- Magnetic resonance angiography (MRA) is an excellent imaging modality for defining pulmonary venous anatomy before pulmonary vein isolation for treatment of atrial fibrillation.

- Pulmonary vein stenosis, a possible side effect of atrial fibrillation ablation, is associated with dyspnea, cough, or hemoptysis and can be diagnosed with MRA.

- Esophageal perforation, another feared complication of catheter ablation for atrial fibrillation, typically presents with dysphagia. Early recognition and treatment is of paramount importance and can be facilitated by cardiac magnetic resonance (CMR) imaging.

- Transesophageal echocardiography (TEE) is the current standard of care for ruling out the presence of thrombus in the left atrial appendage before cardioversion or catheter ablation. The noninvasive nature of CMR compared with TEE suggests promise for its future use in thrombus evaluation.

- Because of its superior soft tissue resolution, CMR is an ideal tool for diagnosis, staging, and preprocedural planning for treatment of cardiac mass lesions.

Case 1   Right Middle Pulmonary Vein

A 65-year-old man with history of highly symptomatic persistent atrial fibrillation refractory to antiarrhythmic therapy presented for pulmonary vein isolation. Preprocedural TEE ruled out the presence of left atrial thrombus. CMR was performed prior to the procedure to plan lesion sets and obtain baseline pulmonary vein diameters (Figure 6-1). The MRA revealed a right middle pulmonary vein.

Comments

Atrial fibrillation is the most common sustained cardiac arrhythmia and is associated with increased morbidity and mortality. The identification of focal pulmonary vein triggers for atrial fibrillation has led to surgical and catheter-based ablation techniques to treat atrial fibrillation through electrical isolation of pulmonary veins from the atria. To guide the intricate lesion sets required for isolation, MRA images of the left atrium and pulmonary veins are often acquired before catheter-based pulmonary vein isolation procedures for atrial fibrillation. Three-dimensional reconstructions of such images can be merged

with an electroanatomic mapping system to provide catheter positioning information during the procedure and help guide the targeting of lesions sets. Information about variant anatomic features such as a right middle lobe pulmonary vein can change procedural plans. For example, ablation between the superior and inferior pulmonary veins is commonly performed, may cause occlusion of the right middle branch, and is best avoided in patients with such variant anatomy. Lack of information about such anatomic detail may result in pulmonary vein stenosis or occlusion, often presenting with dyspnea, cough, and/or hemoptysis.

Case 2   Pulmonary Vein Occlusion

A 39-year-old man with a 3-year history of highly symptomatic paroxysmal atrial fibrillation underwent catheter-directed pulmonary vein isolation using radiofrequency energy. Follow-up CMR images revealed mild narrowing of all pulmonary vein ostia, and occlusion of the superior branch of the left inferior pulmonary vein (Figure 6-2).

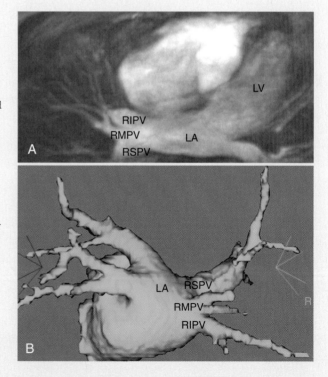

■ **Figure 6-1 A,** MRA showing pulmonary vein variant anatomy with a separate ostium for the right middle pulmonary vein. The right atrium and ventricle are visualized at the top of the image and the left atrium and ventricle at the bottom. The pulmonary veins and their tributaries are readily visualized. **B,** Three-dimensional reconstruction of MRA of left atrial anatomy in another patient with a separate ostium for the right middle pulmonary vein. Segmented three-dimensional reconstructions of the left atrium are registered with catheter positions in the left atrium and within pulmonary veins during atrial fibrillation ablation to enable accurate real-time tracking of catheter movements with respect to the preacquired image. Using the electroanatomic system's catheter positioning information, the operator can avoid delivering lesions deep in the pulmonary veins or at the ostia of small branches, thus avoiding pulmonary vein stenosis or occlusion. LA, left atrium; LV, left ventricle; RSPV, right superior pulmonary vein; RMPV, right middle pulmonary vein; RIPV, right inferior pulmonary vein.

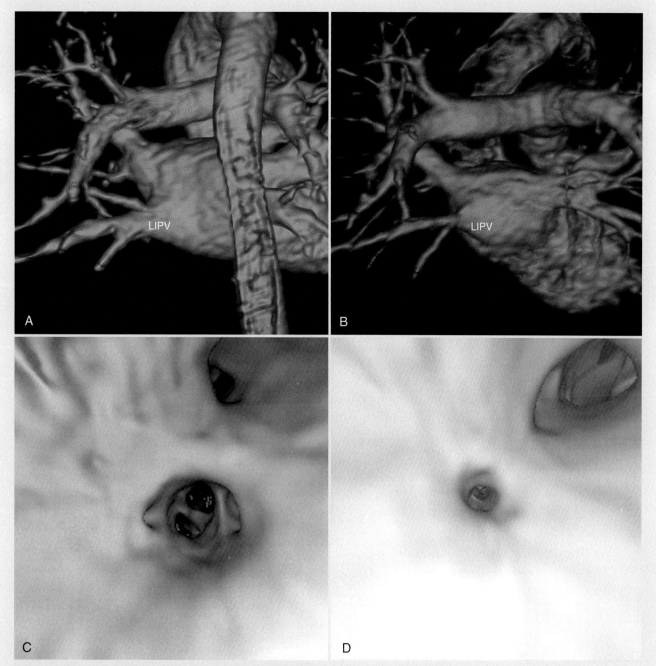

■ **Figure 6-2 A,** Preprocedural MRA of the left atrium and pulmonary veins. On this posterior view, the aortic arch and pulmonary artery are seen at the top of the image with the descending aorta's caudal course in front of the left atrium. The left inferior pulmonary vein and a small ostial branch are easily visualized. **B,** Corresponding image following radiofrequency ablation. The descending aorta is not visible allowing better visualization of the posterior left atrium and pulmonary veins. Mild narrowing of all pulmonary vein ostia and occlusion of the superior branch of the left inferior pulmonary vein is readily appreciated. **C,** Three-dimensional "catheter view" reconstruction of the preprocedural MRA of the left atrium and pulmonary veins. The view shows the ostia of the left superior and inferior pulmonary veins. Secondary branches within the left inferior pulmonary vein are appreciated from the internal view of the chamber. **D,** Corresponding image after radiofrequency ablation. Stenosis of the left inferior pulmonary vein ostium is readily appreciated and the ostial secondary branch to the right of the left inferior pulmonary vein orifice in (**C**) is no longer visible. LIPV, left inferior pulmonary vein.

Comments

Catheter ablation techniques for electrical pulmonary vein isolation have rapidly evolved over the past decade. Initial techniques relied heavily on application of radio-frequency energy onto focal triggers inside or at the ostium of the pulmonary veins. Pulmonary vein stenosis after radiofrequency catheter ablation is a relatively common complication of focal trigger ablation within the pulmonary veins, and *segmental* pulmonary vein isolation where isolation is achieved by delivery of radiofrequency energy within or at the ostium of the pulmonary veins. Patients typically present with dyspnea, cough, or hemoptysis after ablation. Newer techniques for electrical pulmonary vein isolation aim to encircle the pulmonary vein antra with lesions, thus reducing the chance of pulmonary vein stenosis. However, the complication is occasionally encountered even with antral ablation. MRAs provide a reliable means for follow-up of atrial and pulmonary vein remodeling post ablation. Three-dimensional "catheter-view" image reconstructions can also be used after registration of reconstructed images with catheter positions in the electroanatomic system. The internal view can be extremely helpful in guiding the catheter outside the ostia and at the antrum, especially in the difficult narrow anterior ridge between the left-sided pulmonary veins and the left atrial appendage.

Case 3   **Esophageal Perforation**

A 52-year-old man with symptomatic paroxysmal atrial fibrillation underwent left atrial catheter ablation for atrial fibrillation. The patient presented with dysphagia 1 week after ablation. CMR revealed evidence of esophageal perforation and a small collection of air abutting the posterior wall of the left atrium (Figure 6-3). Importantly, the left atrial wall remained intact with normal morphology and contractility. The patient was treated conservatively with fasting, total peripheral nutrition, and proton pump inhibitors, and achieved full recovery.

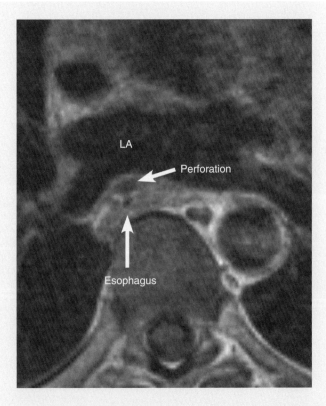

■ **Figure 6-3** Axial T1 CMR image showing the position of the esophagus immediately posterior to the left atrium. The vertebral body is visualized at the bottom of the image. The descending aorta is seen adjacent to the vertebral body. The esophagus is positioned anterior to the vertebral body and is sandwiched by the posterior left atrium and the anterior vertebral body. The ostium of the right inferior pulmonary vein is directly anterior to the anterior wall of the esophagus. Ostial ablation of the right inferior pulmonary vein was most likely responsible for thermal damage to the esophagus in this case. The esophageal perforation and a small collection of air are noted in this region.

Comments

Esophageal perforation is a recognized complication of intraoperative and percutaneous atrial fibrillation ablation. The posterior mediastinum bounded by the pericardial sac and vertebral bodies, contains the esophagus, descending thoracic aorta, azygos system, thoracic duct, and lymph nodes. Although damage to any of the structures in the posterior mediastinum is theoretically possible with application of radiofrequency energy to the posterior left atrium, esophageal damage is the only significant reported collateral damage in this region. The esophagus is not anchored in its position within the posterior mediastinum and can have variable positioning as it courses between the left atrium and vertebral body. Patients typically present with fever and chest and/or epigastric pain 1 week to 1 month after ablation. Although our patient recovered with conservative management, most cases require immediate surgery. Rapid recognition via history and confirmation with CMR or CT are warranted to prevent devastating results such as stroke and death. To avoid this complication during pulmonary vein isolation, we currently place a thermistor in the esophagus, and position it directly behind the left atrium via fluoroscopic guidance. This technique allows continuous monitoring of esophageal temperature and ablation is halted and the catheter repositioned if any temperature rise is noted. Preprocedural imaging may also aid in planning left atrial ablation lesion sets that avoid close proximity to the esophagus. However, reliance on pre-acquired images even with use of electroanatomic system registration is compromised by possible movement of the esophagus within the posterior mediastinum.

Case 4   **Left Atrial Appendage**

A 45-year-old woman with persistent atrial fibrillation was referred for evaluation of left atrium, pulmonary vein, and esophageal anatomy prior to pulmonary vein isolation. The patient also reported difficulty with swallowing, thus TEE was deferred and CMR was utilized to assess the presence of thrombus in the left atrium (Figure 6-4).

Comments

Imaging of the left atrial appendage prior to cardioversion or pulmonary vein isolation is an important step in reducing the procedural stroke risk. TEE is an invasive procedure that provides excellent resolution of the left atrium and left atrial appendage, thus allowing thrombus detection in regions that are prone to low flow and thrombus formation during atrial fibrillation. The presence of left atrial thrombus has been reported in up to 13% of patients referred for TEE in the setting of persistent atrial fibrillation. Currently, TEE is the standard of care for ruling out the presence of thrombus in the left atrial appendage. However, the noninvasive nature of CMR compared to TEE suggest promise for its future use in thrombus evaluation.

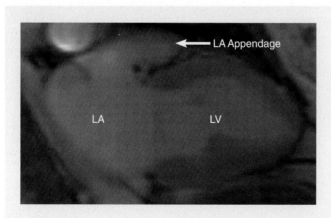

■ **Figure 6-4** A two-chamber steady-state free precession CMR image. The left atrium and ventricle are positioned at the bottom of the image. The left atrial appendage is readily visualized at the top of the image. The image shows no evidence of thrombus within the left atrial appendage.

■ **Figure 6-5** An axial steady-state free precession image at the level of the aortic root. The descending aorta is visible at the bottom of the image. Directly anterior is the left atrium. The aortic root is anterior to the left atrium. The mass is visualized adjacent to the left atrium and the aortic root. LA, left atrium; RSPV, right superior pulmonary vein.

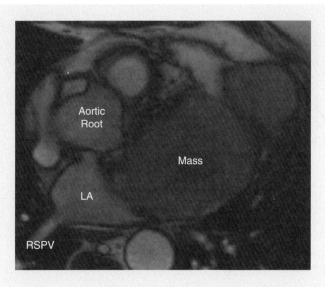

Case 5   Left Atrial Mass

A 58-year-old man presented with shortness of breath. He underwent an extensive work-up including chest x-ray and transthoracic echocardiography. Echocardiography revealed pericardial effusion and an intrapericardial mass. CMR was performed to better delineate the mass. The study revealed a mass associated with the left atrium (Figure 6-5). Biopsy revealed the mass to be a myocardial sarcoma.

Comments

Primary cardiac tumors are rare compared with metastatic disease and other lesions with cardiac mass effect such as bronchogenic cysts. The CMR image in Figure 6-5 demonstrates ready visualization of the myocardial mass associated with the left atrium. The differential diagnosis for masses abutting the left atrium includes atrial myxoma, rhabdomyoma, pericardial teratoma, lipoma, fibroma, mesothelioma, paraganglioma, and sarcomas. This mass was found to be a myocardial sarcoma. Patients with left atrial mass lesions typically present with symptoms because of obstruction of blood flow including dyspnea, orthopnea, paroxysmal nocturnal dyspnea, cough, hemoptysis, peripheral edema, fatigue, and syncope. The superior soft tissue resolution of CMR makes it an ideal tool for diagnosis, staging, and preprocedural planning for treatment of cardiac mass lesions.

SUGGESTED READING

Bertaglia E, Zoppo F, Tondo C, et al.: Early complications of pulmonary vein catheter ablation for atrial fibrillation: A multicenter prospective registry on procedural safety. Heart Rhythm 2007;4:1265-1271.

Dagres N, Kottkamp H, Piorkowski C, et al.: Rapid detection and successful treatment of esophageal perforation after radiofrequency ablation of atrial fibrillation: Lessons from five cases. J Cardiovasc Electrophysiol 2006;17:1213-1215.

Dong J, Vasamreddy CR, Jayam V, et al.: Incidence and predictors of pulmonary vein stenosis following catheter ablation of atrial fibrillation using the anatomic pulmonary vein ablation approach: results from paired magnetic resonance imaging. J Cardiovasc Electrophysiol 2005;16:845-852.

Grizzard JD, Ang GB: Magnetic resonance imaging of pericardial disease and cardiac masses. Magn Reson Imaging Clin North Am 2007;15:579-607.

Kato R, Lickfett L, Meininger G, et al.: Pulmonary vein anatomy in patients undergoing catheter ablation of atrial fibrillation: Lessons learned by use of magnetic resonance imaging. Circulation 2003;107:2004-2010.

Kottkamp H, Piorkowski C, Tanner H, et al.: Topographic variability of the esophageal left atrial relation influencing ablation lines in patients with atrial fibrillation. J Cardiovasc Electrophysiol 2005;16:146-150.

Mansour M, Refaat M, Heist EK, et al.: Three-dimensional anatomy of the left atrium by magnetic resonance angiography: Implications for catheter ablation for atrial fibrillation. J Cardiovasc Electrophysiol 2006;17:719-723.

Mohrs OK, Nowak B, Petersen SE, et al.: Thrombus detection in the left atrial appendage using contrast-enhanced MRI: A pilot study. AJR Am J Roentgenol 2006;186:198-205.

Neragi-Miandoab S, Kim J, Vlahakes GJ: Malignant tumours of the heart: a review of tumour type, diagnosis and therapy. Clin Oncol 2007;19:748-756.

Rustemli A, Bhatti TK, Wolff SD: Evaluating cardiac sources of embolic stroke with MRI. Echocardiography 2007;24:301-308.

Vasamreddy CR, Jayam V, Bluemke DA, Calkins H: Pulmonary vein occlusion: An unanticipated complication of catheter ablation of atrial fibrillation using the anatomic circumferential approach. Heart Rhythm 2004;1:78-81.

Chapter 7

Valvular Heart Disease

Marcus Y. Chen and Andrew E. Arai

KEY POINTS

- Cardiovascular magnetic resonance (CMR) can identify valvular lesions, assess their severities, and determine the consequences of the valve lesion on left ventricular function.

- CMR makes highly accurate and reproducible measurements of ventricular size, mass, and systolic function.

- CMR can provide additional clinical information in patients who have poor echocardiographic windows.

- CMR can evaluate for associated vascular abnormalities, such as the thoracic aorta, during the same evaluation.

- Accurate measurements of regurgitant volumes is performed with phase contrast CMR.

- One strength of CMR is evaluation of myocardial viability or infarction, which may contribute to the severity of valvular disease.

- Velocity-encoded phase contrast CMR can accurately estimate intracardiac shunts (Qp : Qs).

- A comprehensive CMR evaluation is not limited by ionizing radiation or nephrotoxic iodinated contrast agents and is well suited for serial assessments to determine optimal time for intervention.

Case 1 — Bicuspid Aortic Valve

This is a case of a 40-year-old woman with Turner's syndrome, hypertension, and poor echocardiographic windows (Figure 7-1).

Comments

Bicuspid aortic valve is the most common congenital cardiac abnormality, occurring in approximately 1% to 2% of the population. Bicuspid aortic valves are frequently associated with diseases of the aorta, including coarctation, dilation, or dissection. Turner's syndrome is associated with a higher incidence of both congenital bicuspid aortic valves and vascular abnormalities. In functionally bicuspid aortic valves, three commissures are present but one is fused. The fused commissure or raphe can be visualized at end-diastole and the valve appears tricuspid; however, during systole, the orifice is elliptical shaped. Additional clues for a functionally bicuspid aortic valve are an unequal size of the leaflets or eccentric position. In this case example, the truly bicuspid aortic valve has two cusps symmetrically bisecting the aortic root and no raphe at end-diastole. Quadricuspid aortic valves are an uncommon congenital cardiac anomaly found incidentally in approximately 0.013% of echocardiograms. Although quadricuspid aortic valves are a rare finding, they are associated with aortic valve dysfunction.

Most valvular abnormalities visualized by echocardiography can be assessed by CMR. CMR is useful in patients with poor echocardiographic windows. CMR can also provide additional clinical information such as left ventricular volumes, regurgitant fraction, and myocardial fibrosis or viability. High-quality angiographic assessment of the thoracic aorta can also be done without intravenous contrast during the same examination.

Case 2 — Aortic Regurgitation

This is a case involving a 50-year-old male with asymptomatic severe aortic regurgitation (Figure 7-2).

Comments

Surgical replacement for severe aortic insufficiency is indicated in asymptomatic patients based on the presence of left ventricular dysfunction (LVEF less than 55%) or abnormal chamber enlargement (end-diastolic LV internal diameter systolic diameter greater than 75 mm or end-systolic LV dimension greater than 55 mm). CMR is considered the gold standard for assessment of ventricular size, mass, and ejection fraction with little intraobserver or interobserver variability. Additionally, CMR can accurately quantify the amount of valvular regurgitation with phase-contrast techniques.

■ **Figure 7-1 A,** Systolic three-chamber steady-state free procession cine CMR (*left image*). The bright signal intensity within the ascending aorta during systole is caused by the acceleration of blood through a mildly narrowed aortic valve. Coronal aortic valve localizer image at end-diastole (*right image*). The white line depicts the imaging plane used to prescribe the aortic valve images in a short-axis orientation for panel B. **B,** Spectrum of aortic valve morphologies with short-axis cine CMR at end-diastole (*top row*) and end-systole (*bottom row*). This patient's bicuspid aortic valve (*first column*) is compared with functionally bicuspid (*second column*), normal tri-leaflet (*third column*), and quadricuspid (*fourth column*) aortic valves. Note that no raphe is evident at end-diastole in this patient's true bicuspid valve, whereas the functionally bicuspid valve has a raphe from the fused right and noncoronary cusps. During systole, the shape of the bicuspid aortic valve orifice is elliptical, as opposed to triangularly shaped in a normal trileaflet valve. The quadricuspid aortic valve has a unique X configuration at end-diastole with a square-shaped orifice during systole. **C,** Thin maximum intensity projection image of the thoracic aorta from a diaphragm-navigated ECG-gated noncontrast MRA demonstrating coarctation of the aorta. The left subclavian artery arises at the level of the coarctation.

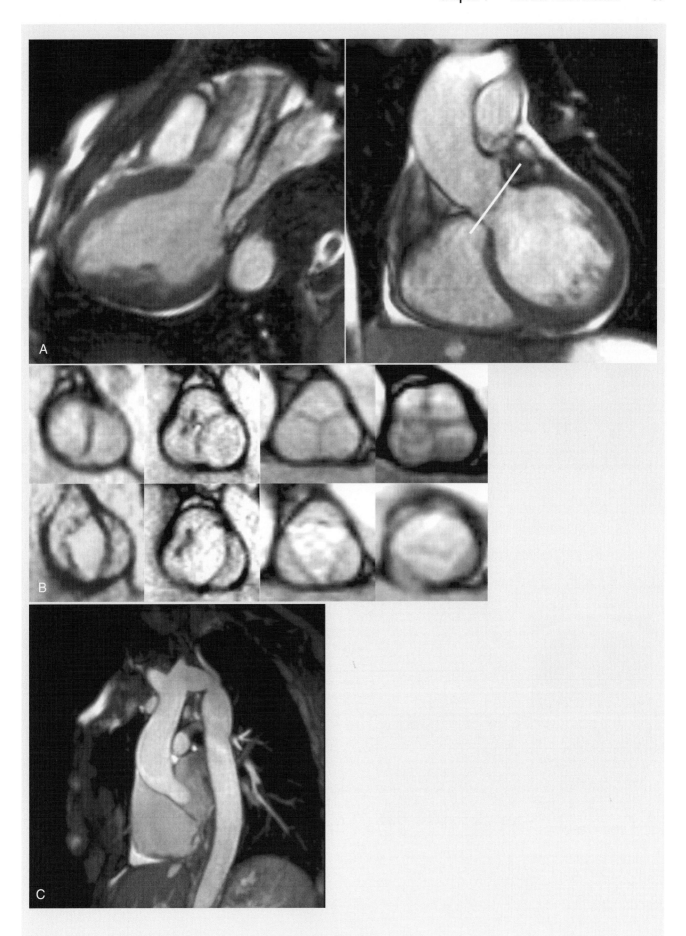

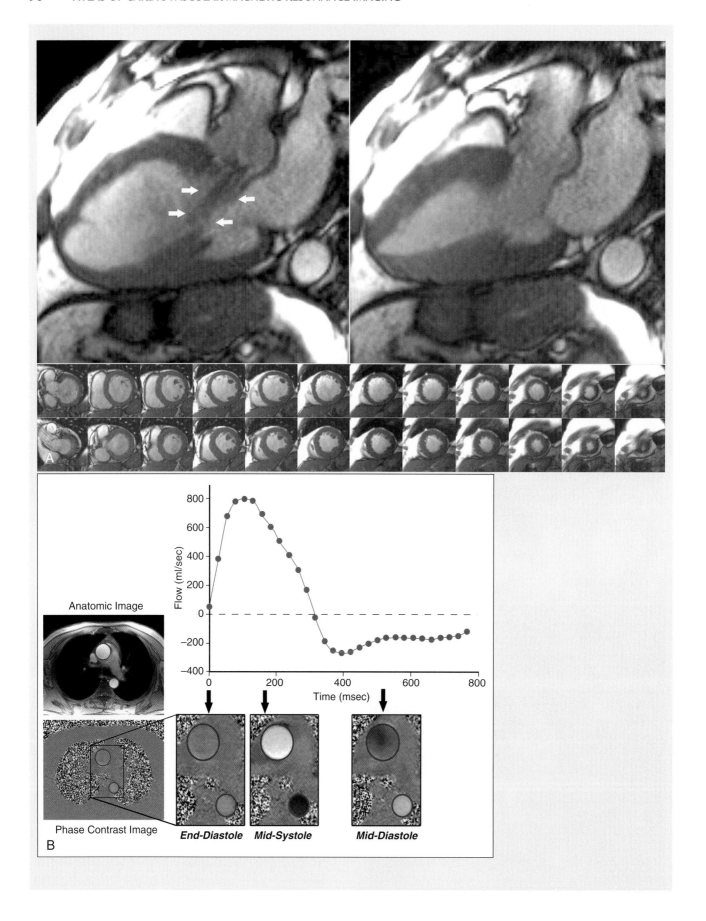

■ **Figure 7-2 A,** Cine CMR in a patient with aortic insufficiency. The three-chamber view during mid-diastole show a relatively dark signal intensity in the left ventricular outflow tract (*arrows*) that represents aortic regurgitation. The signal intensity changes are caused by dephasing and loss of signal from rapidly moving blood, but the appearance of regurgitant jets varies widely with different pulse sequences. On SSFP cine CMR, the jet size of aortic regurgitation is frequently less prominent than on color Doppler echocardiography or in-plane velocity encoded MR images. The stack of short axis images can be planimetered to measure left ventricular dimensions, volumes, and ejection fraction. In this case, the left ventricle is severely dilated (end-diastolic dimension 77 mm, end-systolic dimension 57 mm, end-diastolic volume 389 ml) with moderate eccentric hypertrophy (LV mass 283 g or 132 g/m^2, upper limits of normal less than 91 g/m^2). There is mildly reduced global systolic function (LVEF 50%). **B,** Quantification of ascending aortic blood flow (*red circle*) and descending aorta (*blue circle*) using axial ECG-gated velocity-encoded phase contrast cine CMR. Anatomic and velocity-encoded phase contrast images through the ascending aorta are obtained simultaneously at the level of the main pulmonary artery bifurcation throughout the cardiac cycle. On phase contrast images, a white signal corresponds to cranial flow and a black signal corresponds to caudal flow. The gray signal intensity of the chest wall denotes stationary tissue, and the speckled appearance of the lungs and air outside the chest wall represents noise (regions with too weak a signal for velocity measurements). At end-diastole, there is little flow in either the ascending or descending aorta. At mid-systole, there is the expected cranial flow within the ascending aorta and caudal flow within the descending aorta. However, during mid-diastole, there is aortic flow reversal caused by severe aortic valve regurgitation with caudal flow within the ascending aorta and cranial flow within the descending aorta. By integrating the velocity of all pixels within a region of interest at each time frame, blood flow can be quantified as a function of time with no geometric assumptions. This is possible because CMR can quantify velocity through the imaging plane. The graph displays ascending aortic flow versus time from all 30 velocity-encoded phase contrast images acquired across the cardiac cycle. Positive values (*above the dotted line*) represent forward flow and negative values represent reverse aortic flow. In this patient with severe aortic insufficiency, the net forward aortic volume was 165 ml per cardiac cycle with a reverse volume of 84 ml per cardiac cycle, yielding a regurgitant volume of 81 ml or a regurgitant fraction of 51%.

Case 3   Mitral Regurgitation

This is a case of a 54-year-old woman with severe aortic stenosis (Figure 7-3).

Comments

Assessment of stenotic valvular abnormalities is similar for both CMR and echocardiography. Transvalvular pressure gradients can be determined by the modified Bernoulli equation and valve area can be planimetered or derived from velocity time integrals using the continuity equation and measurement of the left ventricular outflow tract.

Case 4   Aortic Stenosis

This is a case of a 58-year-old man with shortness of breath and ischemic mitral regurgitation (Figure 7-4).

Comments

Although CMR can identify valvular abnormalities, the detection of regurgitant jets with steady-state free precession cine CMR is frequently underestimated. In-plane phase contrast CMR techniques have increased sensitivity for detecting blood flow and are comparable to color Doppler images. The regurgitant volume can be measured by directly measuring transvalvular flow or by subtracting the left ventricular stroke volume determined from a multislice Simpson's rule of ventricular function from the forward flow measurement of the ascending aorta.

Cardiac MR is able to detect and characterize small areas of fibrosis or myocardial infarction with delayed contrast enhancement. In this particular case, the delayed enhancement is useful for characterizing the etiology of mitral regurgitation as associated with an infarcted papillary muscle.

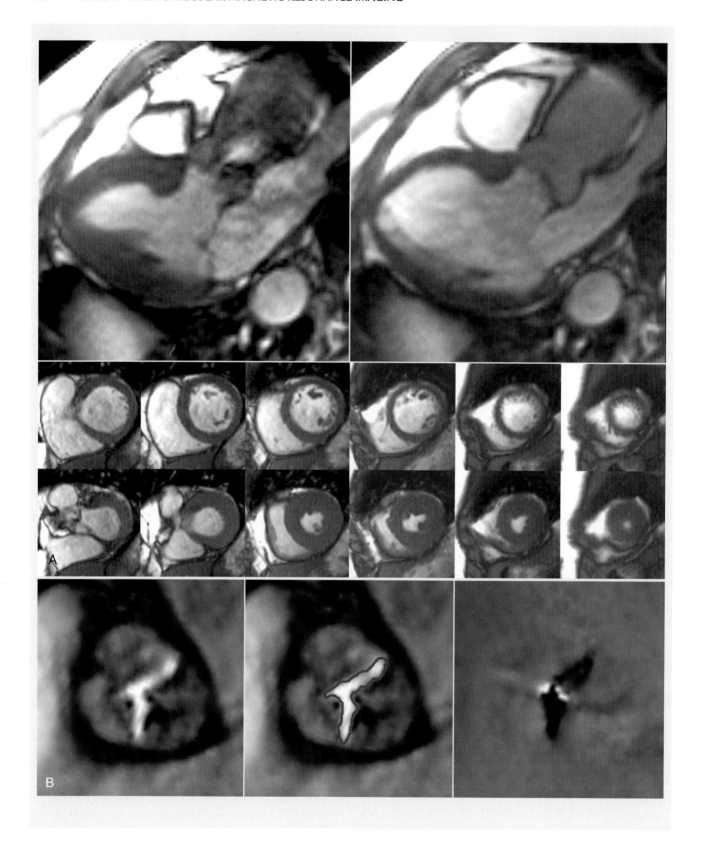

■ **Figure 7-3 A,** Aortic stenosis. Three-chamber steady-state free procession cine CMR during systole (*left image*) and diastole (*right image*). The bright and dark signal intensity within the aortic root during systole is caused by the blood acceleration and dephasing of signal intensity through a narrowed aortic valve. Planimetry of the left ventricle short-axis stack (*lower panel*) at end-diastole (*top row*) and end-systole (*lower row*) demonstrated a normal-sized ventricle (end-diastolic dimension 55 mm, end-systolic dimension 31 mm, end-diastolic volume 137 ml, LV mass 115 g) with normal systolic function (LVEF 70%). **B,** Short axis end-systolic image of the aortic valve. Note the trileaflet configuration (*left panel*) with fusion of the right and noncoronary cusps and a significantly reduced aortic orifice area. Planimetry (*middle panel*) of the aortic orifice was 0.5 cm². We recommend placing the region of interest at the transition between bright blood and the dark valve rather than on the last bright pixel or the first dark pixel at the edges of the orifice. Through-plane phase contrast imaging (*right panel*) demonstrates flow toward the head (*black*) with aliasing (*white speckles*) at a velocity encoding of 5 m/s signifying a peak velocity of greater than 5 m/s or peak aortic valve gradient greater than 100 mm Hg with the modified Bernoulli equation ($4 \times v_{max}^2$).

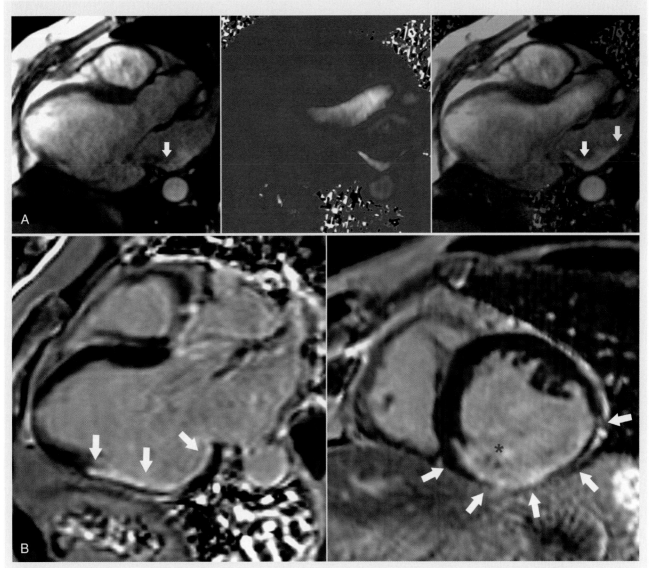

■ **Figure 7-4 A,** Ischemic mitral regurgitation. Systolic three-chamber cine CMR (*left panel*), in-plane phase contrast (*middle panel*), and fusion image (*right panel*) of both cine CMR and phase contrast images. The size and severity of the mitral regurgitation (*white arrow*) is underestimated on cine CMR. In-plane phase contrast CMR techniques can identify blood flow velocities similar to color Doppler echocardiography. The length and width of the mitral regurgitation jet is better visualized with phase contrast techniques (*yellow arrow, right panel*) and reaches the posterior atrial wall. **B,** Phase sensitive delayed enhancement three chamber (*left panel*) and mid-short axis view (*right panel*) demonstrating a nearly transmural myocardial infarction involving the inferior and inferolateral walls (*arrows*). After administration of gadolinium contrast, areas of infarcted myocardium or fibrosis appear bright because of delayed washout of contrast relative to normal myocardium. A portion of the posterior-medial papillary muscle (*asterisk*) is infarcted and likely contributes to this patient's mitral regurgitation.

Case 5   Rheumatic Valvular Heart Disease

This is a case of a 27-year-old man with rheumatic valvular heart disease (Figure 7-5).

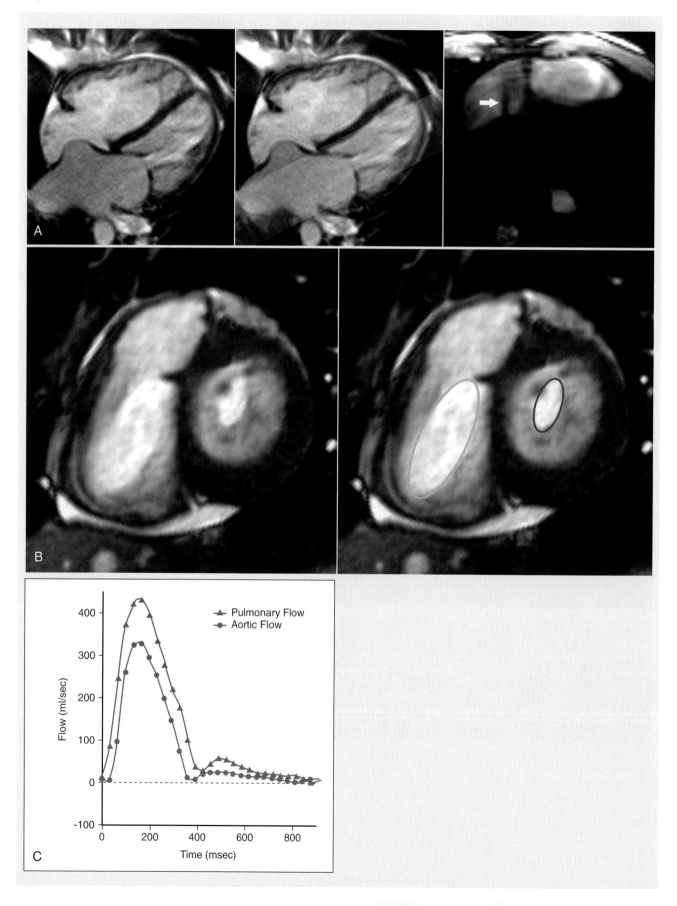

■ **Figure 7-5 A**, Images of a patient with moderate mitral stenosis and Lutembacher syndrome. The mitral valve leaflets have limited excursion and the aneurysmal interatrial septum bows toward the right side because of the elevated left atrial pressure as seen on the four chamber cine CMR during diastole (*left panel*). The right ventricle is enlarged raising the possibility of a left-to-right shunt. The middle panel and right panel illustrate how a blood saturation band can be used to detect a left-to-right shunt. A saturation band (*depicted in yellow*) is placed over the left-sided cardiac chambers on the cine CMR image (*middle panel*). Blood that encounters the saturation band appears dark. On a corresponding diastolic saturation band image (*right panel*), the blood within the left atrium and ventricle has very low signal intensity (*black*) and a majority of blood within the right atrium and right ventricle has higher signal intensity (*gray*). There is a jet of dark blood (*arrow*) passing through the aneurysmal interatrial septum. This jet represents a left-to-right shunt consistent with an atrial septal defect. **B**, Short axis cine CMR demonstrating the mitral and tricuspid valve orifices during diastole. Note the significantly smaller area of the mitral valve (*highlighted in red*) compared with the tricuspid valve (*highlighted in green*). The mitral valve planimetered area was 1.5 cm^2, corresponding to moderate valvular stenosis. **C**, Blood flow quantification over time for one cardiac cycle from velocity-encoded, phase-contrast cine CMR scans of the pulmonary artery (*blue*) and proximal aorta (*red*). The net forward blood flow was 114 ml from the pulmonary artery and 73 ml from the aorta (systemic circulation), yielding a significant Qp:Qs ratio of 1.6:1.

Comments

Lutembacher syndrome is the combination of mitral stenosis and an atrial septal defect with left-to-right shunting. Most cases are caused by rheumatic mitral stenosis. Similar to echocardiography, CMR can measure mitral valvular area with planimetry or through measurements of the pressure half time from the E and A waves. One additional strength of CMR is the ability to noninvasively measure the shunt fraction or Qp:Qs ratio with phase contrast techniques.

The blood saturation technique is a noncontrast agent dependent method to detect intracardiac shunts. One must use care not to misinterpret coronary sinus flow, which also appears dark and moving into the right atrium. The fact that coronary sinus flow is detectable indicates that the method is sensitive to blood flow on the order of less than 4% of cardiac output. In cases in which coronary sinus flow may be seen, the saturation bands can be moved to cover all of the pulmonary veins. One must also be careful to avoid saturating blood in the inferior and superior vena cava.

The blood saturation technique is specifically sensitive to the primary direction of blood flow through an atrial septal defect. It can also be used to detect ventricular septal defects and anomalous pulmonary veins.

SUGGESTED READING

Beerbaum P, Korperich H, Barth P, et al.: Noninvasive quantification of left-to-right shunt in pediatric patients: Phase-contrast cine magnetic resonance imaging compared with invasive oximetry. Circulation 2001;103:2476-2482.

Bellenger NG, Davies LC, Francis JM, et al.: Reduction in sample size for studies of remodeling in heart failure by the use of cardiovascular magnetic resonance. J Cardiovasc Magn Reson 2000;2:271-278.

Bonow RO, Carabello BA, Kanu C, et al.: ACC/AHA 2006 guidelines for the management of patients with valvular heart disease: A report of the American College of Cardiology/American Heart Association Task Force on Practice Guidelines (writing committee to revise the 1998 Guidelines for the Management of Patients With Valvular Heart Disease): developed in collaboration with the Society of Cardiovascular Anesthesiologists: endorsed by the Society for Cardiovascular Angiography and Interventions and the Society of Thoracic Surgeons. Circulation 2006;114:e84-e231.

Caruthers SD, Lin SJ, Brown P, et al.: Practical value of cardiac magnetic resonance imaging for clinical quantification of aortic valve stenosis: Comparison with echocardiography. Circulation 2003;108:2236-2243.

Dall'Armellina E, Hamilton CA, Hundley WG: Assessment of blood flow and valvular heart disease using phase-contrast cardiovascular magnetic resonance. Echocardiography 2007;24:207-216.

Ho VB, Bakalov VK, Cooley M, et al.: Major vascular anomalies in Turner syndrome: Prevalence and magnetic resonance angiographic features. Circulation 2004;110:1694-1700.

Holt NF, Sivarajan M, Mandapati D, et al.: Quadricuspid aortic valve with aortic insufficiency: Case report and review of the literature. J Cardiol Surg 2007;22:235-237.

Honda N, Machida K, Hashimoto M, et al.: Aortic regurgitation: Quantitation with MR imaging velocity mapping. Radiology 1993;186:189-194.

Hundley WG, Li HF, Lange RA, et al.: Assessment of left-to-right intracardiac shunting by velocity-encoded, phase-difference magnetic resonance imaging: A comparison with oximetric and indicator dilution techniques. Circulation 1995;91:2955-2960.

Hundley WG, Li HF, Willard JE, et al.: Magnetic resonance imaging assessment of the severity of mitral regurgitation: Comparison with invasive techniques. Circulation 1995;92:1151-1158.

Keenan NG, Pennell DJ: CMR of ventricular function. Echocardiography 2007;24:185-193.

Kim RJ, Wu E, Rafael A, et al.: The use of contrast-enhanced magnetic resonance imaging to identify reversible myocardial dysfunction. N Engl J Med 2000;343:1445-1453.

Kupfahl C, Honold M, Meinhardt G, et al.: Evaluation of aortic stenosis by cardiovascular magnetic resonance imaging: Comparison with established routine clinical techniques. Heart 2004;90:893-901.

Lin SJ, Brown PA, Watkins MP, et al.: Quantification of stenotic mitral valve area with magnetic resonance imaging and comparison with Doppler ultrasound. J Am Coll Cardiol 2004;44:133-137.

Maceira AM, Prasad SK, Khan M, Pennell DJ: Normalized left ventricular systolic and diastolic function by steady state free precession cardiovascular magnetic resonance. J Cardiovasc Magn Reson 2006;8:417-426.

Wald RM, Powell AJ: Simple congenital heart lesions. J Cardiovasc Magn Reson 2006;8:619-631.

Weber OM, Higgins CB: MR evaluation of cardiovascular physiology in congenital heart disease: Flow and function. J Cardiovasc Magn Reson 2006;8:607-617.

Weinsaft JW, Klem I, Judd RM: MRI for the assessment of myocardial viability. Cardiol Clin 2007;25:35-56.

Chapter 8

Myocardial Masses

Jennifer A. Dickerson and Subha V. Raman

KEY POINTS

- The diagnosis of an intracardiac mass requires definition of location, extent, hemodynamic effect, and tissue characteristics. Cardiovascular magnetic resonance (CMR) is ideally suited to provide this information.

- CMR may provide sufficient tissue diagnosis of masses such as lipoma and thrombus. Additional features in other cases may help refine the differential diagnosis but may not obviate the need for tissue procurement, particularly for treatment planning for malignant masses requiring histopathologic characterization.

- Benign tumors tend to obey tissue boundaries, whereas malignant processes are more likely to cross tissue planes.

- Malignant tumors of the heart are greater than 20 times more likely to represent metastatic disease versus primary cardiac tumors.

- Certain normal cardiac structures may be mistaken for abnormal cardiac masses; in such instances, delineating the anatomy helps define the diagnosis.

- Hemodynamic effects of masses are best assessed with cine imaging or velocity-encoded acquisitions, such as in cases of masses that may intermittently impair valve function due to obstruction.

- Contrast enhancement with first-pass T1-weighted imaging and delayed post-gadolinium imaging may provide information on the vascularity and fibrotic components of a mass.

- Delayed post-gadolinium imaging with a sufficiently long inversion time (greater than 600 ms) greatly facilitates the recognition of intracardiac thrombus.

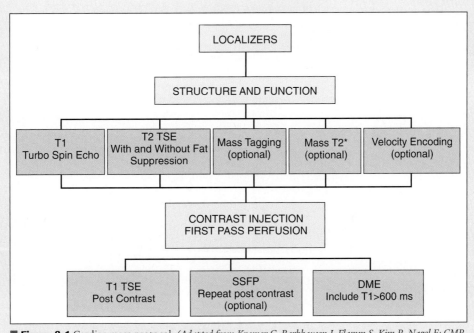

■ **Figure 8-1** Cardiac mass protocol. *(Adapted from Kramer C, Barkhausen J, Flamm S, Kim R, Nagel E: CMR Image Acquisition Protocols, Version 1.0, March 2007, with permission.)*

This chapter illustrates the utility of cardiovascular magnetic resonance (CMR) in the diagnosis and characterization of cardiac masses. Although all possible cardiac masses are not described, we have grouped the cases into (1) normal cardiac structures that may be mistaken for a cardiac mass (Case 1); (2) benign primary cardiac masses (Cases 2-4); (3) malignant primary cardiac masses (Cases 5-6); (4) cardiac masses due to systemic malignant processes (Cases 7-9); and (5) nontumor cardiac masses (Case 10). Some pericardial processes may also be considered masses, such as pericardial cysts (see Chapter 10).

Multiple imaging modalities may be used to detect cardiac masses. CMR provides the most powerful noninvasive in vivo means of characterizing a mass based on its intrinsic tissue properties manifest as distinct signal intensities using different weightings. CMR's multiplane acquisition affords evaluation of secondary hemodynamic effects of a mass, such as impaired mitral filling caused by a large left atrial mass. Figure 8-1 illustrates typical elements of a CMR cardiac mass protocol. The basic tasks in an imaging examination of cardiac masses are localization and characterization. Localization images help direct the examiner to relevant juxtacardiac abnormalities that may be related to the mass. Here one may find pleural and pericardial effusions, mediastinal extension of masses, or evidence of hepatic involvement. Morphologic questions include extent and infiltration of the mass, size, and involvement of cardiac structures. Utilizing T1- and T2-weighted turbo spin echo (TSE) sequences, with and without fat suppression, is central to tissue characterization. T2*-weighted sequences can be used in circumstances where hematoma or thrombus may be suspected. Evaluation of the hemodynamic effect of the mass requires dynamic imaging to define valvular involvement, compression or obstruction of vascular structures, and effect on cardiac function. Myocardial tagging can be employed to assist in defining motion of the mass versus normal myocardial deformation as well as to distinguish cardiac from juxtacardiac structures. After noncontrast acquisitions are completed, visualization of the transit of gadolinium-based contrast through the heart and mass with techniques such as perfusion imaging helps to define vascularity. Postcontrast imaging with various inversion times (TIs) allows for delineation of fibrotic components as well as ready delineation of thrombus when long (greater than 600 ms) TIs are used.

NORMAL CARDIAC STRUCTURES THAT MAY BE MISTAKEN FOR A CARDIAC MASS

Case 1   **Prominent Eustachian Valve**

A 38-year-old woman with a history of hypertension, and tobacco and cocaine abuse presented to the emergency room with complaints of right foot pain. Clinical examination of the lower extremities demonstrated findings consistent with arterial embolization. Transesophageal echocardiography (TEE) was performed to evaluate

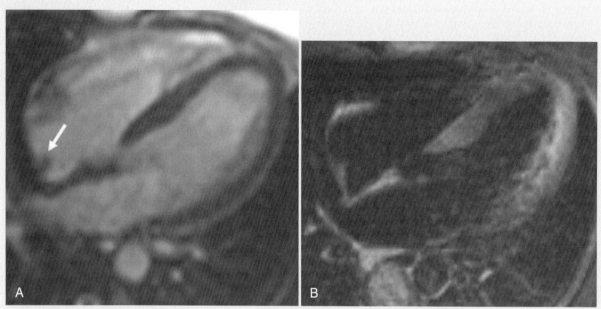

■ **Figure 8-2 A,** A still frame of a horizontal long axis steady-state free-precession (SSFP) cine acquisition sequence shows a small mass protruding in to the cavity of the right atrium (*arrow*). **B,** The dark blood short tau inversion recovery (STIR) sequence demonstrates that this mass does not suppress with fat saturation. Based on its location, CMR characteristics, and motion, this structure most likely represents a prominent Eustachian valve.

for cardiac source of emboli. TEE suggested a mass in the right atrium. CMR was performed (Figure 8-2).

Comments

CMR affords imaging of cardiac structures in limitless planes. Lack of true volumetric imaging capabilities and tissue characterization with other imaging modalities may cause certain cardiac structures to be described as abnormal cardiac masses. The term *pseudomass* denotes a normal cardiac structure that is mistaken for cardiac pathology. The Eustachian valve is present in the right atrium at the insertion of the inferior vena cava and is an embryologic remnant of the valve from the inferior vena cava that may be mistaken for a right atrial mass if prominent. Other cardiac structures that may be denoted *pseudomasses* include the crista terminalis, right ventricular trabeculation, and atrial septal aneurysm.

BENIGN PRIMARY CARDIAC MASSES

Case 2   Cardiac Myxoma

A 58-year-old man presented for cataract surgery and was found to have an abnormal electrocardiogram. Evaluation included a surface echocardiogram that was suggestive of a right atrial mass. CMR findings are shown in Figure 8-3.

Comments

Cardiac myxomas comprise 30% to 50% of all benign cardiac tumors. They typically originate from the fossa ovalis; however, they may originate from the posterior atrial wall, anterior atrial wall, or atrial appendage. Seventy-five to eighty percent are seen on the left atrial side; rarely, a cardiac myxoma arises from ventricular myocardium. They are typically solitary tumors and often pedunculated with a smooth, rounded surface. Owing to their vascularity, myxomas typically perfuse with first-pass gadolinium contrast and enhance to variable extent on delayed enhancement imaging. Myxomas can be distinguished from benign tumors such as lipomas and fibromas using T2-weighted imaging; both lipoma and fibromas are typically dark on T2 weighted images compared with the T2 enhancement characteristic of myxoma.

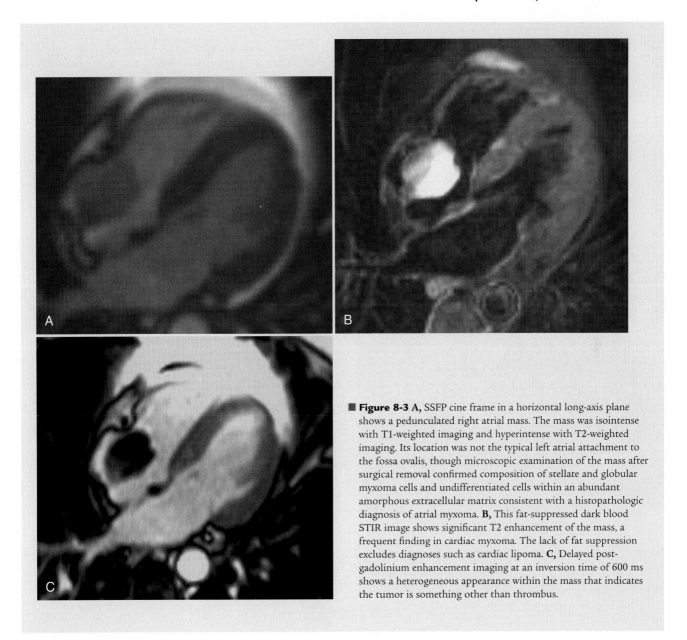

■ **Figure 8-3 A,** SSFP cine frame in a horizontal long-axis plane shows a pedunculated right atrial mass. The mass was isointense with T1-weighted imaging and hyperintense with T2-weighted imaging. Its location was not the typical left atrial attachment to the fossa ovalis, though microscopic examination of the mass after surgical removal confirmed composition of stellate and globular myxoma cells and undifferentiated cells within an abundant amorphous extracellular matrix consistent with a histopathologic diagnosis of atrial myxoma. **B,** This fat-suppressed dark blood STIR image shows significant T2 enhancement of the mass, a frequent finding in cardiac myxoma. The lack of fat suppression excludes diagnoses such as cardiac lipoma. **C,** Delayed post-gadolinium enhancement imaging at an inversion time of 600 ms shows a heterogeneous appearance within the mass that indicates the tumor is something other than thrombus.

Case 3   Cardiac Lipoma

A 63-year-old woman had a history of breast cancer as well as poorly differentiated B cell malignancy. She presented with new-onset atrial flutter underwent transesophageal echocardiography prior to cardioversion. TEE demonstrated a right atrial mass obstructing the SVC. Given her medical history, the concern for malignant extension was significant prompting CMR examination to further characterize the mass (Figure 8-4).

Comments

Lipomas are the second most common benign tumor of the heart, though less frequently encountered than lipomatous septal hypertrophy. Lipomas are typically encapsulated and have signal characteristics like that of fat, bright on T1- and T2-weighted sequences. CMR is uniquely able to make an unequivocal tissue diagnosis in the setting of cardiac lipoma by applying fat suppression that takes advantage of the known chemical shift between the resonant frequency of protons in fat compared with protons in most other tissues. Surgical pathology in this case confirmed the diagnosis of cardiac lipoma.

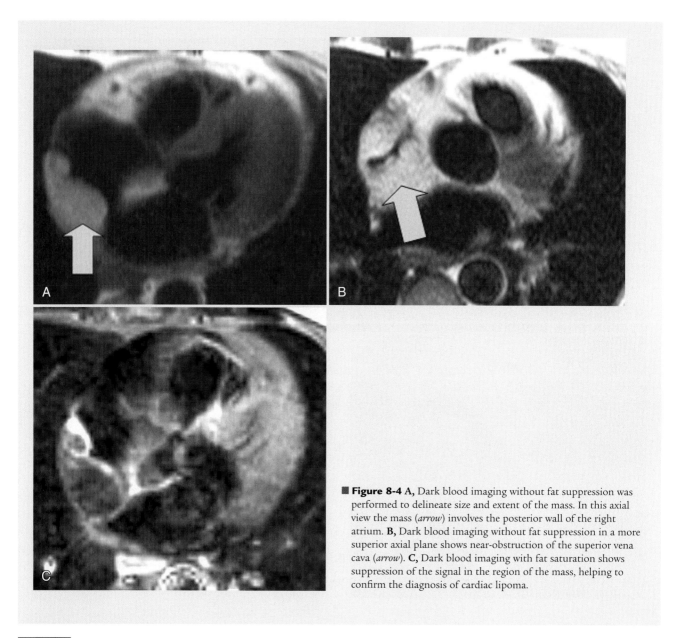

■ **Figure 8-4 A,** Dark blood imaging without fat suppression was performed to delineate size and extent of the mass. In this axial view the mass (*arrow*) involves the posterior wall of the right atrium. **B,** Dark blood imaging without fat suppression in a more superior axial plane shows near-obstruction of the superior vena cava (*arrow*). **C,** Dark blood imaging with fat saturation shows suppression of the signal in the region of the mass, helping to confirm the diagnosis of cardiac lipoma.

Case 4   Teratoma

A 24-year-old woman presented for evaluation of palpitations. Travel history to the Middle East and Central America was extensive. The patient was referred for CMR after a large mass felt to be pericardial was visualized on surface echocardiography (Figure 8-5).

■ **Figure 8-5 A-B,** Single-shot SSFP images obtained from stacks in the axial and sagittal planes, respectively, allow assessment of the size and extent of this large juxtacardiac mass. Additional coronal images (not shown) allowed comprehensive measurement that yielded 8.1 × 6.5 cm in the anterior/posterior direction and 8.0 × 8.0 cm in the cranial/caudal direction. **C,** STIR acquisition show prominent T2 enhancement, suggesting significant fluid content. The differential diagnosis at this point would include cystic masses. **D,** Delayed post-gadolinium imaging using a phase-sensitive inversion recovery sequence confirms the significant fluid content as well as intramass densities. Echinococcus was in the differential diagnosis, given the travel history, but made much less likely by negative serologies as well as absence of hepatic involvement. Also notable on this acquisition is peripheral enhancement of the mass, suggesting fibrous encapsulation versus inflammation. **E,** Chest computed tomography reconstructed in the coronal plane shows features typical for mature cystic teratoma, including intracyst fat globule (indicated by Hounsfield Units) and location. **F,** Gross appearance of the explanted mass in the operating room. Histopathologic examination confirmed the diagnosis of cystic teratoma.

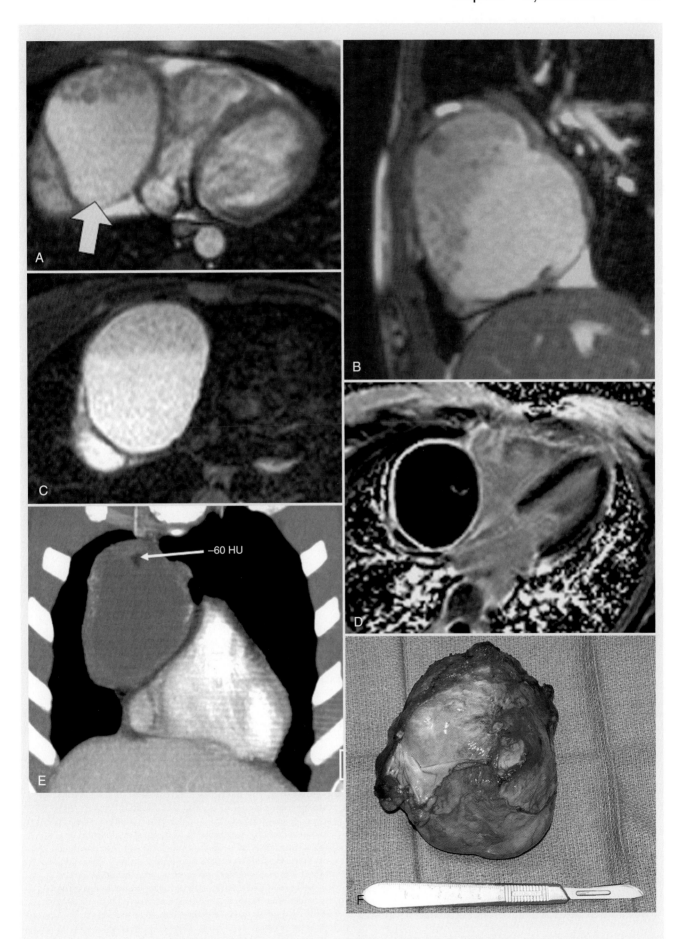

Comments

Teratomas are classically right-sided pericardial masses. They are an exceedingly rare cause of cardiac masses and most typically found in infants and children. In one case series reporting cardiac tumors in a pediatric population in a children's hospital in Canada, teratoma was present in one case in 15 years. Although a benign tumor by classification, teratomas may effect significant changes in cardiac hemodynamics via mass effect.

MALIGNANT PRIMARY CARDIAC MASSES

Case 5   Cardiac Angiosarcoma

A 44-year-old man presented with recurrent pericardial effusion and supraventricular tachycardia. Echocardiography showed the effusion as well as a right atrial mass. CMR examination was performed after the patient underwent pericardiocentesis to define the nature and extent of disease (Figure 8-6).

Comments

Cardiac tumors are 20 to 40 times more likely to represent metastatic disease (see next section) versus a primary cardiac tumor. The most common primary tumor of the heart is cardiac sarcoma, with the highest frequency being angiosarcoma. Primary cardiac lymphoma follows in frequency. CMR can be used to define the extent of disease, hemodynamic significance, and in many cases benign versus malignant classification. Definitive diagnosis needed for therapeutic planning may still require

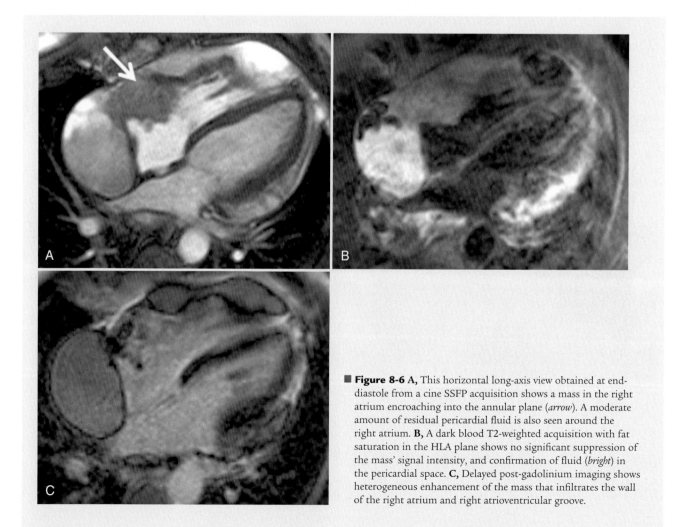

■ **Figure 8-6 A,** This horizontal long-axis view obtained at end-diastole from a cine SSFP acquisition shows a mass in the right atrium encroaching into the annular plane (*arrow*). A moderate amount of residual pericardial fluid is also seen around the right atrium. **B,** A dark blood T2-weighted acquisition with fat saturation in the HLA plane shows no significant suppression of the mass' signal intensity, and confirmation of fluid (*bright*) in the pericardial space. **C,** Delayed post-gadolinium imaging shows heterogeneous enhancement of the mass that infiltrates the wall of the right atrium and right atrioventricular groove.

tissue for histopathologic examination. Signal characteristics in this case indicated a perfused mass with irregular borders and enhancement on delayed post-gadolinium imaging. Precontrast and postcontrast signal characteristics and morphology showing crossing of normal tissue boundaries were consistent with a malignant tumor. The patient underwent median sternotomy after transvenous biopsy was nondiagnostic; tissue obtained in the operating room yielded the diagnosis of poorly differentiated angiosarcoma.

Case 6   Spindle Cell Sarcoma

A 44-year-old woman presented for outpatient evaluation of intermittent chest pain. Exercise nuclear perfusion imaging was within normal limits. Transthoracic echocardiography showed a mass in the region of the right atrium, but could not adequately define if the mass was intracardiac or extracardiac. CMR was performed for better delineation and characterization (Figure 8-7).

Comments

As with the previous case, CMR was able to demonstrate size, extent, and signal characteristics of this isolated mass that were suspicious for a malignant tumor. The presence of a localized pericardial effusion adjacent to the mass suggests contiguity of the mass with the heart. Intraoperative examination in this case confirmed dense adherence to the right ventricular free wall, and histopathologic diagnosis of the explanted mass showed spindle cell sarcoma.

CARDIAC MASSES CAUSED BY SYSTEMIC MALIGNANT PROCESSES

Case 7   Metastatic Melanoma

A 44-year-old man presented with a remote history of skin melanoma. Two years before this presentation he had undergone surgical excision of a single left ventricular metastasis, receiving chemotherapy in the interim. CMR was performed to assess for recurrence of cardiac involvement (Figure 8-8).

Comments

Secondary cardiac involvement of metastatic disease can occur from direct extension, systemic spread, or as transvenous extension. Direct extension is characteristic of lung and breast cancer, as well as mediastinal lymphoma. Systemic spread occurs with melanomas, lymphoma, and sarcomas. Transvenous extension typifies cardiac involvement due to renal and hepatic cancers.

Secondary cardiac neoplasms are 22 times more common than primary cardiac tumors. In general, metastatic tumors are hypointense relative to normal myocardium on T1-weighted images and hyperintense with T2 weighting. Cardiac melanoma is typically bright on T1- as well as T2-weighted imaging. These unique signal characteristics are thought to be due to the melanin content of this tumor type.

Case 8   Metastatic Breast Cancer

A 29-year-old woman presented for evaluation of persistent tachycardia. The past medical history was notable for invasive ductal breast carcinoma treated with surgical resection, chemotherapy, and radiation. Transthoracic echocardiography demonstrated a left atrial mass, prompting CMR examination for further characterization of thrombus versus tumor metastasis (Figure 8-9).

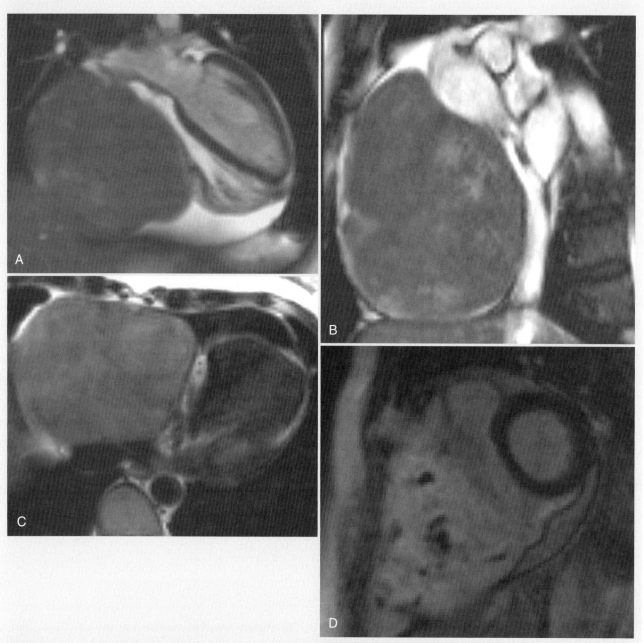

■ **Figure 8-7 A,** A still frame of an SSFP cine acquired in the horizontal long axis plane shows a large mass that measured 13 cm × 12 cm. Pericardial fluid is also noted suggesting cardiac involvement. **B,** SSFP image obtained in the sagittal plane shows that the mass obliterates the right atrium and compresses the proximal portion of the inferior vena cava. **C,** T2-weighted dark blood imaging shows heterogeneity of the mass with areas of T2 enhancement. First-pass perfusion imaging (not pictured) showed enhancement with intravenous gadolinium contrast. **D,** Delayed post-gadolinium imaging shows areas of hyperenhancement within the mass that could represent fibrotic regions.

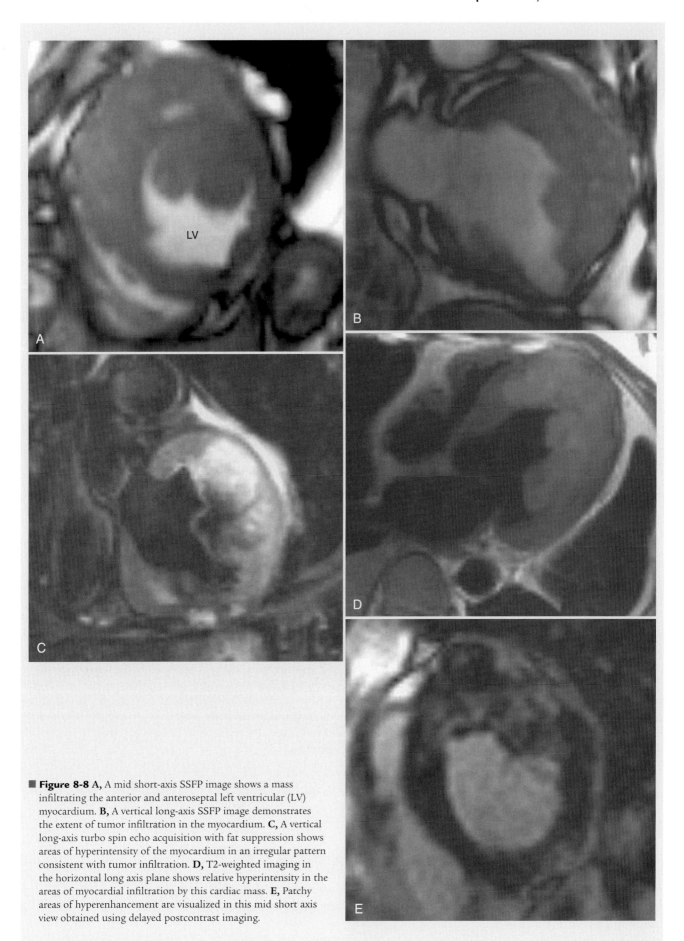

■ **Figure 8-8 A,** A mid short-axis SSFP image shows a mass
infiltrating the anterior and anteroseptal left ventricular (LV)
myocardium. **B,** A vertical long-axis SSFP image demonstrates
the extent of tumor infiltration in the myocardium. **C,** A vertical
long-axis turbo spin echo acquisition with fat suppression shows
areas of hyperintensity of the myocardium in an irregular pattern
consistent with tumor infiltration. **D,** T2-weighted imaging in
the horizontal long axis plane shows relative hyperintensity in the
areas of myocardial infiltration by this cardiac mass. **E,** Patchy
areas of hyperenhancement are visualized in this mid short axis
view obtained using delayed postcontrast imaging.

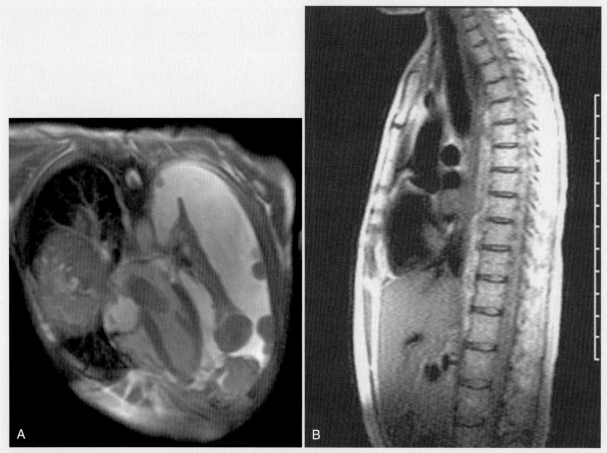

■ **Figure 8-9 A,** A horizontal long axis frame from a real-time cine acquisition shows a large mass in the left atrium measuring 5.4 × 2.5 cm. Also note the large, irregular mass in the right lung consistent with metastatic disease by prior chest computed tomography examination as well as the large left pleural effusion. Cine imaging showed significant mobility of the mass with intermittent obstruction to mitral inflow. **B,** Sagittal dark blood single heartbeat HASTE image shows the mass directly extends from the right lung mass via the right inferior pulmonary vein. Additional acquisitions were not performed due to significant dyspnea precluding detailed postcontrast characterization.

Comments

This case illustrates not only intracardiac tumor mass but also important extracardiac findings that help make the diagnosis of metastatic disease. This patient had a complex pleural effusion with nodular lung densities suggestive of metastatic disease. Rapid single heartbeat multislice acquisitions allowed demonstration of contiguity of the LA mass with the lung metastasis; direct extension is the most common cause of cardiac involvement caused by breast malignancy. In addition, central tumor necrosis with a heterogenous appearance on delayed enhancement imaging favors a malignant process.

Case 9   Erdheim-Chester Disease

A 55-year-old man with a history of Erdheim-Chester disease and atrial fibrillation experienced increasing shortness of breath. As part of his diagnostic evaluation he underwent transthoracic echocardiography that showed a large right atrial mass. CMR was ordered because of suspicion of cardiac involvement of this systemic fibrosing process (Figure 8-10).

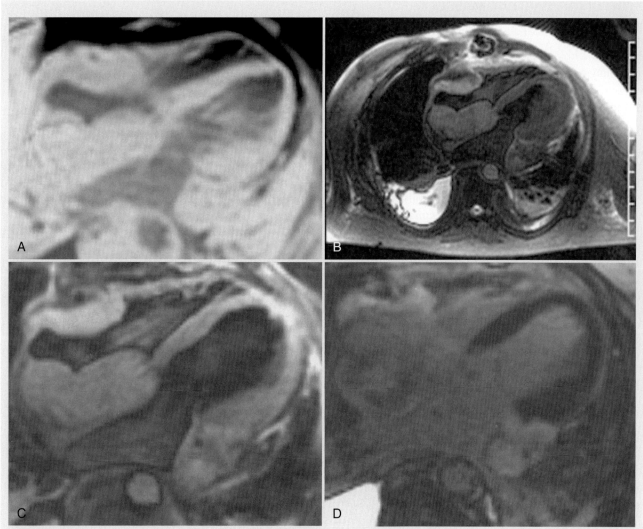

■ **Figure 8-10 A,** This frame from a real-time gradient echo cine sequence demonstrates an extensive mass infiltrating the right atrium that is relatively dark, especially compared with the bright signal from the epicardial fat. **B,** Dark blood STIR acquisition shows relatively higher signal intensity in the mass compared with the LV myocardium, but not nearly as bright as the fluid in the right pleural effusion. **C,** Delayed post-gadolinium imaging shows significant enhancement of the mass consistent with its known fibrotic pathology.

Comments

Benign masses typically do not cross tissue plane, unlike this mass that is both bulky and shows extensive myocardial infiltration. Dark blood images help to define the morphology, and fat suppression clearly excludes lipoma or lipomatous septal hypertrophy. This is an important distinction, given that lipomatous masses as well as this tumor appear bright on non–fat-suppressed T2-weighted imaging. Hyperenhancement on late post-gadolinium imaging is consistent with fibrous proliferation that is characteristic of this malignant fibrosing condition.

Together, the CMR findings of an infiltrative mass along with its precontrast and postcontrast signal characteristics are most consistent with cardiac involvement of systemic Erdheim-Chester disease. In this case surgical resection could not be considered due to the significant extent of the disease and medical comorbidities. Medical treatment with interferon α was initiated. Erdheim-Chester disease falls under the general heading of a multisystem non-X/ non-Langerhans cell histiocytic proliferative disorder with the fibrosis comprising a fine fibrillar pattern of collagen deposition with the zones of fibrosis accompanied by the aberrant histiocytic population.

NONTUMOR CARDIAC MASSES

Case 10   Intracardiac Thrombus

A 64-year-old man presented with increasing shortness of breath, 10 years after sustaining anterior wall myocardial infarction. Transthoracic echocardiography was suggestive of a thrombus in the left ventricle (LV). CMR was ordered to confirm thrombus and to assess for myocardial viability (Figure 8-11).

Comments

The clinical scenario presented carries a high pretest likelihood for the apical mass being thrombus. CMR provides a definitive diagnosis based on signal intensity on late postcontrast imaging as well as the associated extent of myocardial scar. T1 and T2 properties of thrombi are dependent on the age of the thrombus and its stage of organization. Fresh thrombi typically are hyperintense to myocardium on both T1 and T2 imaging. However, as the thrombus organizes, there is decreasing signal intensity on T2-weighted imaging. Thrombi do not hyperenhance

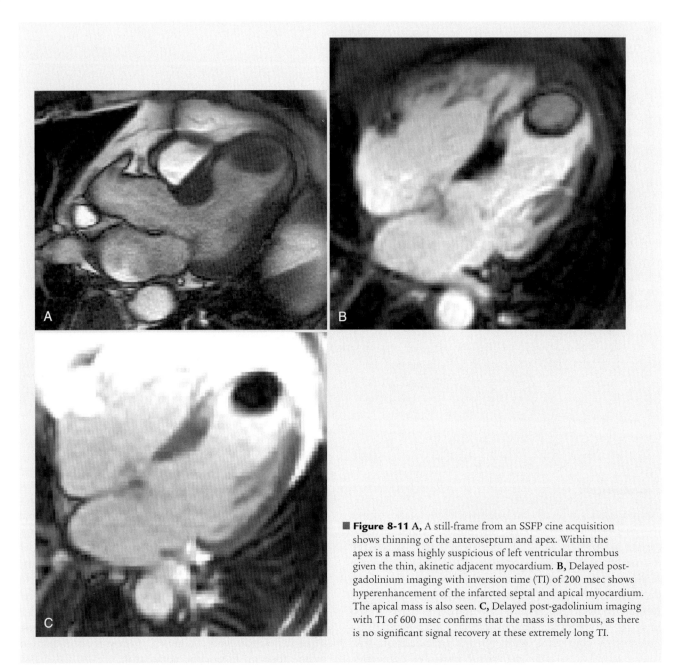

■ **Figure 8-11 A,** A still-frame from an SSFP cine acquisition shows thinning of the anteroseptum and apex. Within the apex is a mass highly suspicious of left ventricular thrombus given the thin, akinetic adjacent myocardium. **B,** Delayed post-gadolinium imaging with inversion time (TI) of 200 msec shows hyperenhancement of the infarcted septal and apical myocardium. The apical mass is also seen. **C,** Delayed post-gadolinium imaging with TI of 600 msec confirms that the mass is thrombus, as there is no significant signal recovery at these extremely long TI.

with gadolinium. The longer inversion time is use to help increase the sensitivity and specificity for the diagnosis of thrombus as illustrated in this case. CMR is the most sensitive (greater than 95%) modality to detect LV thrombus, which is important in minimizing risk of peripheral embolism after large myocardial infarction or in the setting of significant LV dysfunction. CMR is ideally suited to detect small thrombi, especially in the left ventricle, where trabeculations may hinder echocardiography.

SUGGESTED READING

Araoz PA, Eklund HE, Welch TJ, Breen JF: CT and MR imaging of primary cardiac malignancies. Radiographics 1999;19:1421-1434.

Araoz PA, Mulvagh SL, Taxelaar HD, et al: CT and MR imaging of benign primary cardiac neoplasms with echocardiographic correlation. Radiographics 2000;20:1303-1319.

Attili AK, Gebker R, Cascade PN: Radiological reasoning: Right atrial mass. AJR Am J Roentgenol 2007;188:S26-S30.

Beghetti M, Gow RM, Haney I, et al: Pediatric primary benign cardiac tumors: A 15-year review. Am Heart J 1997;134:1107-1114.

Beghetti M, Prieditis M, Rebeyka IM, Mawson J: Images in cardiovascular medicine: Intrapericardial teratoma. Circulation 1998;97:1523-1524.

Bruna J, Lockwood M: Primary heart angiosarcoma detected by computed tomography and magnetic resonance imaging. Eur Radiol 1998;8:66-68.

Dion E, Graef C, Haroche J, et al: Imaging of thoracoabdominal involvement in Erdheim-Chester disease. AJR Am J Roentgenol 2004;183:1253-1260.

Dodd JD, Aquino SL, Holmvang G, et al: Cardiac septal aneurysm mimicking pseudomass: Appearance on ECG-gated cardiac MRI and MDCT. AJR Am J Roentgenol 2007;188:W550-W553.

Fieno DS, Saouaf R, Thomson LE, et al: Cardiovascular magnetic resonance of primary tumors of the heart: A review. J Cardiovasc Magn Reson 2006;8:839-853.

Grizzard JD, Ang GB: Magnetic resonance imaging of pericardial disease and cardiac masses. Magn Reson Imaging Clin N Am 2007;15:579-607.

Gulati G, Sharma S, Kothari SS, et al: Comparison of echo and MRI in the imaging evaluation of intracardiac masses. Cardiovasc Intervent Radiol 2004;27:459-469.

Houmsse M, Raman SV, Leier CV, Orsinelli DA: Metastatic melanoma of the left ventricle: Cardiac imaging in the diagnosis and surgical approach. Int J Cardiovasc Imaging 2004;20:523-526.

Kaminaga T, Takeshita T, Kimura I: Role of magnetic resonance imaging for evaluation of tumors in the cardiac region. Eur Radiol 2003;13:L1-L10.

Kramer C, Barkhausen J, Flamm S, et al: CMR Image Acquisition Protocols, Version 1.0, March 2007. Available at: http://www.scmr.org/documents/SCMR_protocols_2007.pdf

Lam KY, Dickens P, Chan AC: Tumors of the heart: A 20-year experience with a review of 12,485 consecutive autopsies. Arch Pathol Lab Med 1993;117:1027-1031.

Meier RA, Hartnell GG: MRI of right atrial pseudomass: Is it really a diagnostic problem? J Comput Assist Tomogr 1994;18:398-401.

Raman SV, Ahmed A, Simonetti OP, Crestanello J: Tissue diagnosis with magnetic resonance imaging. Circulation 2007;116:e338.

Restrepo CS, Largoza A, Lemos DF, et al: CT and MR imaging findings of malignant cardiac tumors. Curr Probl Diagn Radiol 2005;34:1-11.

Restrepo, CS, Largoza A, Lemos DF, et al: CT and MR imaging findings of benign cardiac tumors. Curr Probl Diagn Radiol 2005;34:12-21.

Salanitri JC, Pereles FS: Cardiac lipoma and lipomatous hypertrophy of the interatrial septum: Cardiac magnetic resonance imaging findings. J Comput Assist Tomogr 2004;28:852-856.

Srichai MB, Junor C, Rodriguez LL, et al: Clinical, imaging, and pathological characteristics of left ventricular thrombus: A comparison of contrast-enhanced magnetic resonance imaging, transthoracic echocardiography, and transesophageal echocardiography with surgical or pathological validation. Am Heart J 2006;152:75-84.

Uzun O, Wilson DG, Vujanic GM, et al: Cardiac tumours in children. Orphanet J Rare Dis 2007;2:11.

Chapter 9

Pericardial Disease

Rajan A.G. Patel and Christopher M. Kramer

KEY POINTS

- Cardiac magnetic resonance (CMR) is ideally suited for imaging the pericardium because of its large field of view and ability to differentiate soft tissue based on fat and water composition.

- By CMR normal pericardium is considered less than 3 mm thick and a pericardium greater than this thickness is indicative of pathology.

- Normal pericardium appears as a rim of low signal intensity on T1- and T2-W imaging.

- In acute pericarditis T1- and T2-W spin echo (SE) sequences may generate images in which the pericardium has a moderate to high intensity signal.

- Calcified pericardium will appear dark on images generated using T1-W SE, T2-W SE, fat saturated T2-W gradient echo (GRE), and steady-state free precession (SSFP) imaging.

- On T2-W SE imaging typical pericardial cysts have a homogenous high intensity signal.

- Metastatic melanoma to the pericardium will have a high intensity signal on T1-W SE imaging owing to paramagnetic metals bound by melanin.

- In patients with isolated congenital absence of the pericardium CMR imaging with SSFP, T1-W SE and T2-W SE all will demonstrate a lack of pericardium and axial imaging will show that the heart is markedly rotated to the left.

The pericardium is a fibrous sac that surrounds the majority of the heart as it only partially covers the left atrium. The pericardium is anchored in the midline anteriorly to the sternum by superior and inferior ligaments and is also anchored to the diaphragm. The pericardial sac is composed of two layers, the visceral and parietal layers. The visceral pericardium lies on the surface of the myocardium whereas the parietal pericardium is a continuation of the visceral pericardium that is folded on top of the visceral pericardium. The space between these two layers of pericardium is referred to as the pericardial space. The surfaces of the visceral and parietal pericardium that define the pericardial space are lined with a single layer of mesothelial cells. The cells of the parietal pericardium secrete a transudative fluid into the pericardial space. Normally the pericardial space contains 15 to 50 ml of fluid. Because of its relatively low compliance the rapid accumulation of even a couple hundred milliliters of fluid can have significant physiologic consequences. On the other hand, if fluid accumulates gradually the compliance of the pericardium will increase slowly, allowing the build-up of a significant volume of fluid.

The normal function of the pericardium is to prevent the spread of infection or inflammation by direct extension from adjacent structures in the mediastinum. It my also help reduce friction between the beating heart and neighboring structures in the chest, although patients with isolated congenital absence of the pericardium do not usually develop pathology secondary to the heart abutting adjacent structures. Pathologic processes that affect the pericardium can be considered in the following categories: pericardial effusion, acute pericarditis, constrictive pericarditis, pericardial masses, and other rare conditions.

Cardiac magnetic resonance (CMR) imaging is a noninvasive imaging modality that is ideally suited for imaging the pericardium because of its large field of view and ability to differentiate soft tissue based on fat and water composition. Transthoracic echocardiography (TTE) is the workhorse of noninvasive cardiac imaging because of its portability allowing bedside exams, relatively low cost allowing widespread use, and excellent temporal resolution allowing independence from ECG gating for image acquisition. However, TTE is dependent on having an acceptable acoustic imaging window. Furthermore, the field of view is limited with TTE. It can be challenging to image posterior structures in large patients. Finally TTE cannot readily differentiate soft tissue planes unless a layer of fluid or air separates the planes. Discerning tissue type is almost impossible with TTE unless the anatomy is normal or a known variant. The pericardium itself is not well visualized with TTE.

With CMR normal pericardium appears as a rim of low signal intensity on T1- and T2-W imaging as the pericardium is largely a fibrous structure with low water content. Normal pericardium is less than 3 mm thick. Autopsy studies describe the normal pericardium to be between 0.4 and 1.0 mm thick. Sechtem et al. have reported that the average normal pericardium thickness by CMR was 1.9 ± 0.6 mm. This discrepancy may be caused by fibrous tissue that was not measured at autopsy and nonlaminar motion of the pericardial fluid resulting in an artificially thick line. By CMR normal pericardium is considered less than or equal to 3 mm thick. A pericardium seen on CMR greater than 3 mm thick is indicative of pathology.

Case 1   Pericardial Effusion

A 68-year-old woman with a history of breast cancer presented to the emergency department with a 1-week history of progressive dyspnea and lightheadedness. Her physical exam was remarkable for tachypnea, tachycardia with a blood pressure of 86/50, Kussmaul's sign, and a pulsus paradoxus of 25 mm Hg. She was given IV fluids and pericardiocentesis was performed. Two days later her symptoms began to recur and a CMR was ordered (Figure 9-1).

Comments

The differential for the etiology of pericardial effusion is broad. Common cases include neoplasm, infection (bacterial, including tuberculosis, and viral), uremia, and cardiac injury from myocardial infarction or trauma. If a pericardial effusion is sufficiently large to impair cardiac filling causing a reduction in cardiac output, then tamponade physiology is present. This is a clinical diagnosis and CMR should not be used to make this diagnosis but to corroborate it. However, if the presence of a pericardial effusion is suspected in a hemodynamically stable patient, then CMR may have diagnostic utility.

TTE is the most frequently utilized imaging modality for the visualization of pericardial effusion. This is largely because of the convenience of a bedside exam and the relatively high sensitivity and specificity of diagnosing pericardial effusion with TTE. However, loculated pericardial effusions may be difficult to appreciate on TTE. Furthermore in the immediate period after cardiac

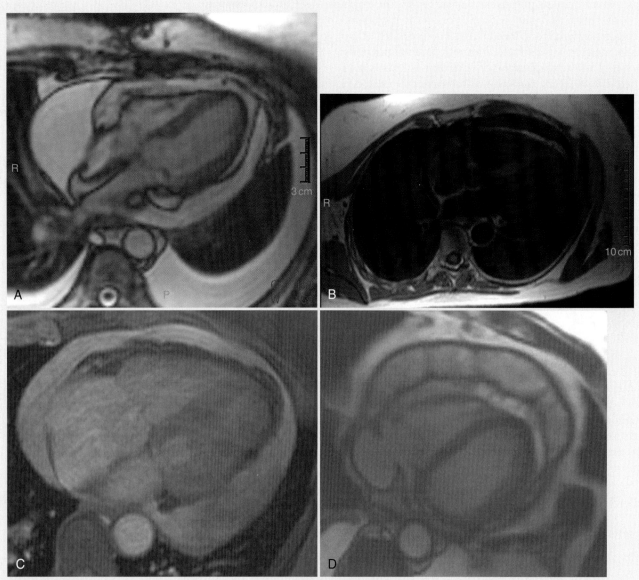

■ **Figure 9-1 A,** Four-chamber SSFP image. The patient imaged in this figure has tamponade physiology. Note the large pericardial effusion as well as bilateral pleural effusions. The right ventricle appears elongated and collapsed. **B,** Four-chamber T1-W SE image. Note that the large nonhemorrhagic pericardial effusion has a low intensity signal in contrast to the image in panel C. **C,** Four-chamber T2-W fat saturated GRE image. Note that the large pericardial effusion has a characteristic high intensity signal on GRE imaging caused by motion of the free-flowing fluid. **D,** Axial SSFP still image from a patient with metastatic cancer. Note the large pericardial effusion localized to the anterior aspect of the heart. The pericardial fluid has clearly visible septations. Bilateral pleural effusions are also visible.

surgery, air in the pleural space may reduce or eliminate acoustic windows. CMR provides a large field of view allowing localization of loculated effusions (Figure 9-1 D). Furthermore CMR is not limited by air within structures of interest.

Spin echo (SE) and gradient echo (GRE) sequences can be utilized to differentiate pericardial effusions. Hemor-

rhagic effusions are characterized by high intensity signal on T1-weighted SE images and by low intensity signal on GRE images. Nonhemorrhagic effusions are characterized by a low signal intensity of T1-weighted SE and a high signal intensity of GRE images. Malignant effusions may be accompanied by a heterogeneously thick pericardium that may have a nodular appearance.

Case 2 | Acute Pericarditis

A 64-year-old man in the cardiac care unit (CCU) with congestive heart failure (CHF) secondary to viral myocarditis developed severe chest pain. The pain was relieved by sitting upright and leaning forward and exacerbated by lying supine. The ECG was remarkable for diffuse ST elevation and PR depression. The patient was referred for CMR imaging (Figure 9-2).

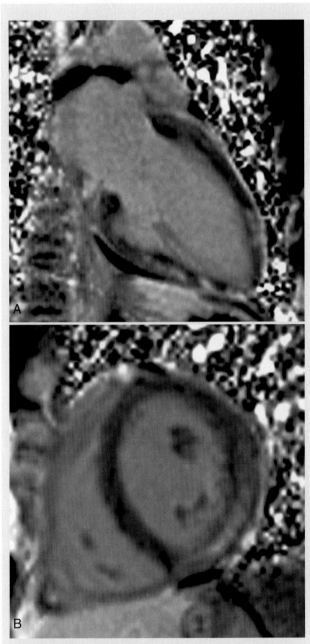

■ **Figure 9-2 A,** Two-chamber late gadolinium enhancement (LGE) phase sensitive inversion recovery GRE image. The patchy areas of mid and epi-myocardial LGE are consistent with the diagnosis of myocarditis. The anterior pericardium brightly enhances, consistent with acute pericarditis. There is a small pericardial effusion that appears dark along the inferior wall. **B,** Short axis LGE image. As in panel (**A**), a region of intramyocardial LGE is appreciated in the lateral wall as well as bright enhancement of the pericardium in the same region.

Comments

Acute pericarditis is the syndrome of the signs and symptoms caused by pericardial inflammation that lasts less than 2 weeks. The differential diagnosis for the etiology is large (Table 9-1). Many cases of acute pericarditis may actually be myopericarditis as the inflammation involves the myocardium as well as the pericardium. Dressler syndrome is the classic manifestation of this process. Twenty-four to seventy-two hours after a large transmural myocardial infarction a patient may experience local inflammation on the epicardial surface of the infarcted myocardium and the adjacent pericardium, which produces the clinical signs and symptoms of acute pericarditis. Viral myocarditis may also manifest as myopericarditis. The hallmark of this condition is elevated biomarkers such as Troponin I, in the context of the signs and symptoms of pericarditis.

As aforementioned, the fibrous composition of the normal pericardium generates a thin rim of low intensity signal on T1- and T2-W SE images. However, in acute and subacute pericarditis, not only might the pericardium appear thickened, but T1- and T2-W SE sequences may generate images in which the pericardium has a moderate to high intensity signal. Furthermore imaging using fat-saturated T1-W SE sequences after gadolinium administration may reveal enhancement of the pericardium.

TABLE 9-1 Etiology of Acute Pericarditis

Post-MI (Dressler Syndrome)
Post cardiac surgery
Post radiation therapy
Infectious etiology
    Bacterial infection
    Tuberculosis (typically presents chronically as constriction)
    Viral
    Fungal (coccidioidomycosis—Central Valley; histoplasmosis—Ohio River Valley)
    Protozoal
Connective Tissue Disease
    SLE
    Rheumatoid arthritis
    Scleroderma
    Polyarteritis nodosa
    Temporal arteritis
Drug Induced
Trauma
    Penetrating trauma to pericardium
    Post PCI with coronary perforation
    Post pacemaker lead placement with myocardial perforation
    Post CPR

Case 3   Constrictive Pericarditis

A 37-year-old man with a history of Hodgkin's lymphoma treated with mantle radiation and chemotherapy presented with a several month history of progressive shortness of breath and lower extremity swelling (Figure 9-3 A-D).

Comments

Constrictive pericarditis is the result of a chronic process resulting in a thickened pericardium with a markedly reduced compliance. Decreased pericardial compliance does not generally affect early ventricular filling. However, late diastolic filling is impaired as the rigid pericardium will not accommodate the enlarging ventricles. This results in a rapid rise in the pressure of both ventricles during diastole, the so-called square root sign on ventricular hemodynamic tracings. The reduction in preload leads to a reduction in contractility, and ultimately to a reduction in stroke volume. The pericardium functions as a rigid box with a fixed volume that isolates the heart from the thorax. Thus with respiration, right ventricular volume increases. In order to accommodate the increased right ventricular volume, left ventricular filling and volume are compromised. The opposite occurs with expiration. This phenomenon is known as ventricular interdependence and is the hemodynamic definition of constrictive pericarditis.

In the United States the leading cause of constriction is cardiac surgery, followed by mediastinal irradiation and cancer. However, worldwide the most important cause of constriction is tuberculosis (Figure 9-3 E). This is especially true in areas where tuberculosis is endemic.

CMR imaging of the pericardium demonstrating a thickness of greater than 3 mm is considered diagnostic for constriction. As many as 50% of patients will have

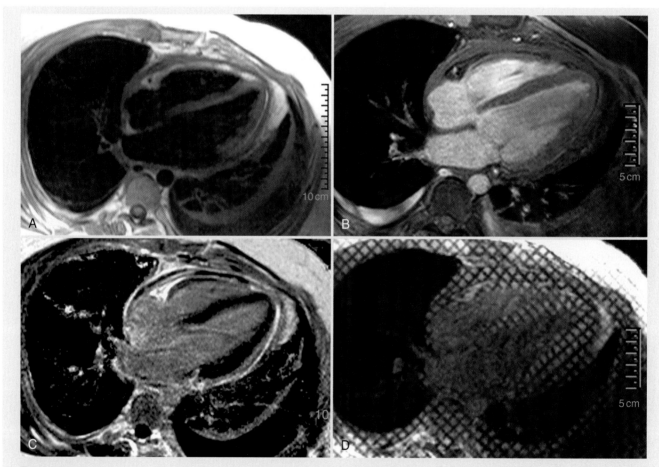

■ **Figure 9-3 A,** Four-chamber long-axis T1-W SE image from the patient in Case 3. Note the thickened gray pericardial layer that surrounds the entire heart including both the left and right ventricles. The pericardium measures 6 to 8 mm thick at its widest. **B,** T1-W fat-suppressed GRE image from the same patient in the same orientation. The thin layer of epicardial fat now appears black, leaving the gray pericardial layer to stand out. Bilateral pleural effusions are noted. **C,** Late gadolinium enhanced T1-W inversion recovery GRE image from the same patient in the same orientation. Note that there is no myocardial late enhancement, but the outer layer of the pericardium lateral to the left ventricle and right atrium demonstrates late enhancement. **D,** T1-W tagged GRE cine image from the same patient in the same orientation at end-systole. Fairly normal deformation of the tag stripes in the myocardium is noted. However, there is persistence of tag stripes in the pericardium, suggesting the presence solid fibrotic material. There is also evidence of adherence of the pericardium to the epicardium along the anterior RV surface and lateral to the LV. This is seen as lack of slippage of the epicardium along the pericardium when viewed in cine mode.

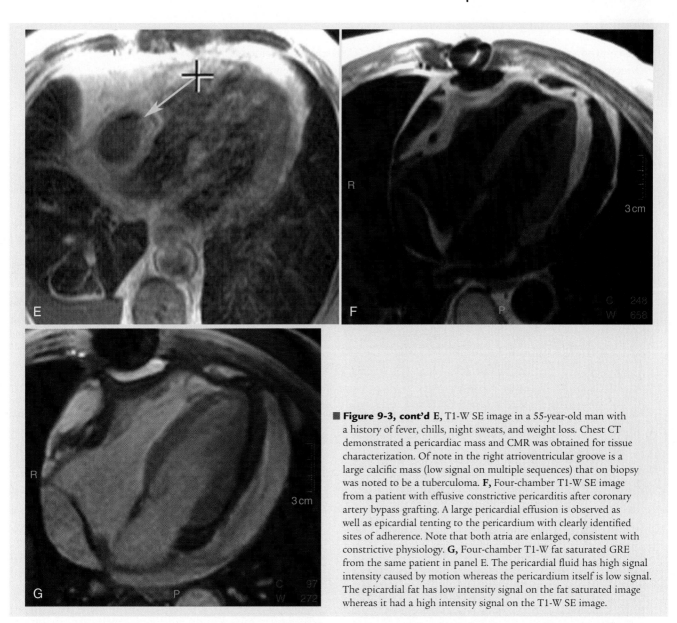

Figure 9-3, cont'd E, T1-W SE image in a 55-year-old man with a history of fever, chills, night sweats, and weight loss. Chest CT demonstrated a pericardiac mass and CMR was obtained for tissue characterization. Of note in the right atrioventricular groove is a large calcific mass (low signal on multiple sequences) that on biopsy was noted to be a tuberculoma. **F,** Four-chamber T1-W SE image from a patient with effusive constrictive pericarditis after coronary artery bypass grafting. A large pericardial effusion is observed as well as epicardial tenting to the pericardium with clearly identified sites of adherence. Note that both atria are enlarged, consistent with constrictive physiology. **G,** Four-chamber T1-W fat saturated GRE from the same patient in panel E. The pericardial fluid has high signal intensity caused by motion whereas the pericardium itself is low signal. The epicardial fat has low intensity signal on the fat saturated image whereas it had a high intensity signal on the T1-W SE image.

calcification of the pericardium that is discernible on chest x-ray. On CMR the calcified pericardium will appear dark on images generated using T1-W SE, T2-W SE, fat saturated T2-W SE, and SSFP imaging. This is most often found in the atrioventricular groove but may be localized to or distributed anywhere over the heart. The constrained ventricular filling will result in an enlarged inferior vena cava as well as a dilated right atrium and hepatic veins. With inspiration the ventricular septum will bow to the left and with expiration the ventricular septum will bow to the right because of the previously described hemodynamic changes. The latter findings can be observed with real-time imaging with the diaphragm in the plane of the imaging to view respiration. In addition, the interventricular septum must be visualized in the imaging plane, ideally in the short axis.

The treatment for severely symptomatic constriction is pericardectomy. Tagged images may be useful to the surgeon planning such an operation as they allow iden-

tification of regions at which pericardium is adherent to the myocardium. Often the differential diagnosis of constriction includes restriction. CMR can readily differentiate the two. Restriction is characterized by a thickened myocardium that may or may not have late gadolinium enhancement depending on the etiology. However, the pericardium will often be normal in thickness and composition. Masui et al. found that CMR had a sensitivity of 85%, a specificity of 100%, and a diagnostic accuracy of 93% for the diagnosis of constrictive pericarditis.

A variant of constrictive pericarditis is effusive constrictive pericarditis. Patients with this condition may present with a syndrome similar to tamponade. However, once the pericardial fluid is drained, constrictive physiology ensues. CMR imaging can be useful in determining the presence of effusive constrictive physiology as a thickened pericardium with areas of adherence to the epicardium will be observed in addition to a significant pericardial effusion (Figure 9-3 F-G).

Case 4 **Pericardial Cyst**

An asymptomatic 26-year-old woman is referred for CMR after a chest x-ray before an elective surgical procedure revealed an abnormal lobulation extending from the cardiac silhouette (Figure 9-4).

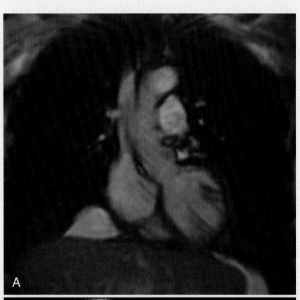

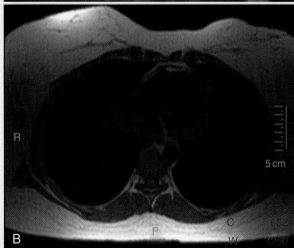

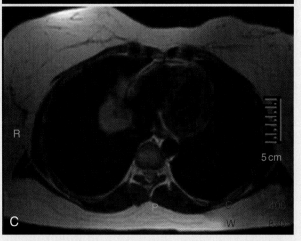

Comments

Nonmalignant masses involving the pericardium are often detected incidentally on chest x-ray or TTE. These include pericardial cysts and hematomas.

Pericardial cysts are a consequence of abnormal formation of the coelomic cavity during embryogenesis. By definition cysts are lined with a single layer of epithelial cells. Pericardial cysts are often filled with clear fluid that is often highly proteinaceous. They are most commonly observed in the costophrenic angles, especially the right. As many as 90% of pericardial cysts are in direct contact with the diaphragm. The remainder may be found at more cephalad locations. They are often discovered incidentally on chest x-ray as lobulated expansions of the cardiac silhouette. The differential diagnosis for such findings includes tumors, cardiomegaly, and ventricular aneurysms. CMR can readily make the diagnosis.

On SSFP and GRE sequences, pericardial cysts may not be easily appreciated. They also have a low intensity signal on T1-W SE. However, on T2-W SE imaging typical pericardial cysts have a homogenous high intensity signal. They do not enhance after gadolinium infusion and typically remain stable in size over time.

Pericardial hematomas can occur secondary to trauma or iatrogenesis. Medical procedures that may result in a pericardial hematoma include cardiac surgery, angioplasty with coronary artery perforation, and electrophysiology procedures such as pacemaker lead placement or atrial fibrillation ablation. Acute hematomas have high signal intensity on T1-W and T2-W SE imaging with a homogenous appearance. Subacute hematomas (1 to 4 weeks old) have a mixed high and low intensity signal appearance on T1-W and T2-W SE images. With time chronic hematomas become calcified. This results in the appearance of a dark rim and, if internal islands of calcification are present, internal areas of lower intensity signal. Pericardial hematomas do not enhance after gadolinium administration. The differential diagnosis for pericardial hematomas includes coronary fistulae and aneurysm, ventricular pseudoaneurysms, and malignant masses.

■ **Figure 9-4 A,** Coronal SSFP image from the patient in case 4. The pericardial cyst is appreciated in the right cardiophrenic space, typical location of such cysts. **B,** Axial T1-W SE image from the patient in Case 4. Note that the pericardial cyst has a low intensity signal on T1-W SE imaging. **C,** Axial T2-W SE image from the patient in case 4. The pericardial cyst in the right hemithorax has a high intensity signal in contrast to the T1-W SE image in panel B.

Case 5   **Pericardial Neoplasm**

A 70-year-old man who is a former shipyard worker presented with chest pain and weight loss. A pleural mass was noted on CXR and an enlarged cardiac silhouette was noted; a CMR was ordered for further evaluation (Figure 9-5).

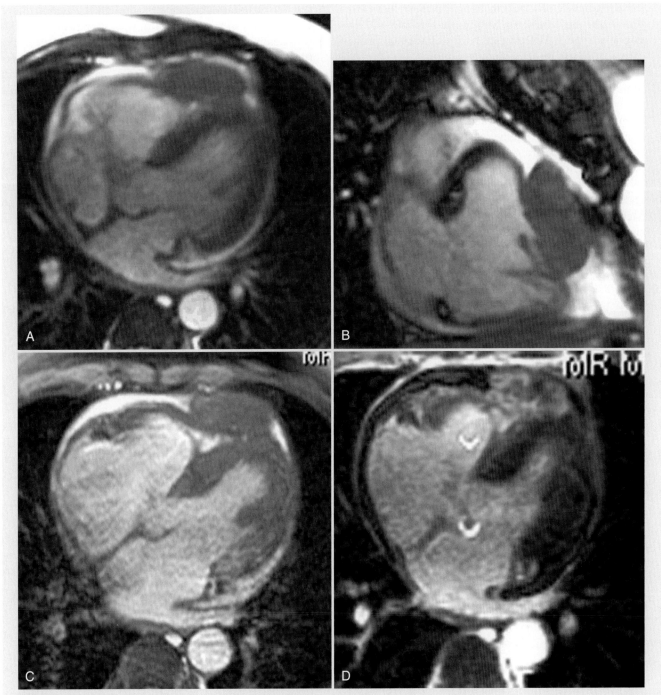

■ **Figure 9-5 A,** Axial steady-state free precession (SSFP) cine image at end-diastole in a patient with a pericardial mesothelioma. A large mass is seen in the pericardial space anterior to the RV apex. Because SSFP is T2/T1-weighted, it is not particularly useful for characterizing tissue components within a mass. **B,** Parasagittal SSFP cine image in the same patient. The mass is seen compressing the anterior free wall of the right ventricle and it measures 7 cm in the craniocaudal dimension and 2 cm in the anteroposterior dimension. **C,** Axial fat suppressed T1-W GRE image in the same orientation as panel A. Note that the mass is isointense to the myocardium. If the mass was a melanoma, it might have high signal intensity on T1-W SE imaging caused by the melanin. **D,** Axial late gadolinium enhanced T1-W inversion recovery GRE image in the same orientation. Note late enhancement of the mass consistent with fibrous scarring within the tumor.

Comments

Primary tumors of the pericardium are extremely rare. The most frequently encountered benign pericardial tumors are lipoma, hemangioma, and teratoma. The most frequently observed malignant primary pericardial tumors are mesothelioma, lymphoma, sarcoma, and liposarcoma. The CMR characteristics of various primary cardiac tumors are described elsewhere.

Metastatic disease to the pericardium is encountered more commonly than primary tumors are. As many as 10% to 12% of patients with metastatic disease have been found to have myocardial or pericardial involvement at autopsy. Nonetheless pericardial involvement is rarely the presenting syndrome of metastatic disease unless constrictive or tamponade physiology is present. In one series 42% of patients with pericardial disease and cancer had no evidence of pericardial metastases. Metastases to the pericardium may occur by direct extension, hematogenous dissemination, or lymphatic spread. Primary lung cancer is the most common metastatic lesion encountered in the pericardium, followed by breast cancer, hematologic malignancies, and melanoma. The first three neoplasms account for up to 75% of all pericardial malignant tumors.

CMR imaging is useful in diagnosing tumor type as well as ascertaining whether a thoracic tumor abuts the pericardium or penetrates through the pericardium. CMR may also prove useful in operative planning. The line delineated by the pericardium will be intact if the tumor extends up to the pericardium. If tumor has invaded the pericardium, then the pericardial line will be lost at the focal areas of tumor penetration. Additionally, a pericardial effusion may be appreciated. Most pericardial tumors have a low intensity signal with T1-W SE and a high intensity signal on T2-W SE images. The notable exception is metastatic melanoma. Melanin binds iron and other paramagnetic metals. This results in a high intensity signal on T1-W SE imaging. Furthermore, hemorrhagic pleural effusions secondary to malignancy appear bright on T1- and T2-W SE images. Finally malignant tumor tissue often contains areas of late gadolinium enhancement (LGE) caused by fibrosis within the tumor.

Case 6   Congenital Absence of the Pericardium

A 24-year-old man is referred for CMR after a chest x-ray performed before elective surgery suggests cardiomegaly (Figure 9-6).

Comments

The embryonic pleuropericardial membrane develops into the left pericardium. A commonly quoted theory explaining the development of congenital absence of the pericardium suggests that the left common cardinal vein atrophies prematurely during development. This results in poor perfusion of the left pleuropericardial membrane and failure of the left pericardium to develop. Absence of the right pericardium and complete (right and left) absence of the pericardium are very rarely observed.

Patients with an isolated absence of the pericardium are generally asymptomatic. However, absence of the pericardium can also be associated with other congenital abnormalities of thoracic structures including the heart, lungs, diaphragm, and chest wall. Cardiac abnormalities that have been described in association with congenital absence of the pericardium include atrial septal defect (ASD), patent ductus arteriosus (PDA), mitral stenosis, and tetralogy of Fallot.

Patients may be referred for CMR after a chest x-ray incidentally leads to the discovery of a leftward displaced heart. CMR imaging with SSFP, T1-W SE, and T2-W SE all will demonstrate a lack of pericardium. Furthermore, lung tissue may be observed interposed between the aorta and main pulmonary artery. Axial images will demonstrate a heart that is markedly rotated to the left.

Case 7   Ruptured Pericardium

A 40-year-old man is involved in a high speed head-on motor vehicle accident. He is experiencing severe chest pain and is having difficulty breathing. Chest x-ray and the trauma protocol CT demonstrate leftward displacement of the heart. He is hemodynamically stable 24 hours after admission and is referred for CMR (Figure 9-7).

Partial absence of the pericardium or pericardial rupture secondary to trauma can lead to myocardial herniation. This may present clinically as arrhythmias, chest pain, syncope, or occasionally sudden death. Myocardial herniation through the pericardium may be readily observed with CMR on multiple imaging sequences. Cine SSFP imaging can provide dramatic images of the myocardium prolapsing in and out of the ruptured pericardium.

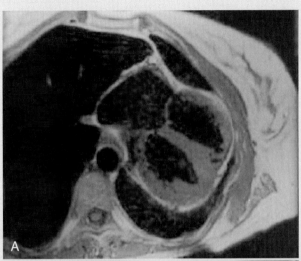

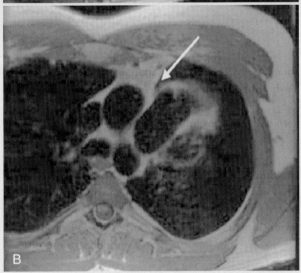

■ **Figure 9-6 A,** Axial T1-W SE image from a patient with congenital absence of the pericardium. The myocardium is significantly displaced into the left chest compromised the left lung. **B,** Axial T1-W SE image from a patient with congenital absence of the pericardium. The left atrial appendage and main pulmonary artery are rotated into the left chest. A "tongue" of lung tissue is wedged between the main pulmonary artery and the aorta (*arrow*). This finding is most consistently seen in congenital absence of the pericardium. *(From Gatzoulis MA, Munk MD, Merchant N, et al: Isolated congenital absence of the pericardium: Clinical presentation, diagnosis, and management. Ann Thorac Surg 2000;69:1209-1215, with permission.)*

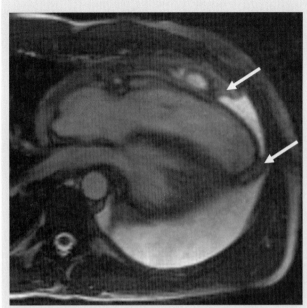

■ **Figure 9-7** Four-chamber SSFP image. The patient has a perforated pericardium with myocardial herniation. The myocardium is shifted to the left relative to its normal position within the chest. *White arrows* indicate the perforated edges of the pericardium. The right ventricle herniates out of the pericardium. A large left pleural effusion is also present.

imaging loculated pericardial effusions, acute pericarditis, constrictive and effusive-constrictive pericarditis, nonmalignant as well as neoplastic pericardial masses, and congenital as well as traumatic defects in the pericardium.

SUGGESTED READING

Chiles C, Woodard PK, Gutierrez FR, Link KM. Metastatic involvement of the heart and pericardium: CT and MR imaging. Radiographics 2001;21:439-449.

Gassner I, Judmaier W, Fink C, et al. Diagnosis of congenital pericardial defects, including a pathognomic sign for dangerous apical ventricular herniation, on magnetic resonance imaging. Br Heart J 1995;74:60-66.

Gatzoulis MA, Munk MD, Merchant N, et al. Isolated congenital absence of the pericardium: clinical presentation, diagnosis, and management. Ann Thorac Surg 2000;69:1209-1215.

Kim JS, Kim HH, Yoon Y. Imaging of pericardial diseases. Clin Radiol 2007;62:626-631.

Lewinter M, Kabbani S. Pericardial Diseases. In: Zipes D, Libby P, Bonow R, Braunwald E (eds): Braunwald's Heart Disease. Philadelphia: Elsevier Saunders, 2005:1757-1780.

Masui T, Finck S, Higgins CB. Constrictive pericarditis and restrictive cardiomyopathy: evaluation with MR imaging. Radiology 1992;182:369-373.

Oyama N, Oyama N, Komuro K, et al. Computed tomography and magnetic resonance imaging of the pericardium: anatomy and pathology. Magn Reson Med Sci 2004;3:145-152.

Pineda V, Andreu J, Caceres J, et al. Lesions of the cardiophrenic space: findings at cross-sectional imaging. Radiographics 2007;27:19-32.

Sechtem U, Tscholakoff D, Higgins CB. MRI of the normal pericardium. AJR Am J Roentgenol 1986;147:239-244.

Sparrow PJ, Kurian JB, Jones TR, Sivananthan MU. MR imaging of cardiac tumors. Radiographics 2005;25:1255-1276.

SUMMARY

TTE is the workhorse for noninvasive imaging of the heart and pericardium. However, when pericardial disease is suspected CMR may be advantageous because of the larger field of view and the capability to discern soft tissue types as well as the dependence of TTE on adequate acoustic imaging windows. CMR has utility in

Taylor AM, Dymarkowski S, Verbeken EK, Bogaert J. Detection of pericardial inflammation with late-enhancement cardiac magnetic resonance imaging: initial results. Eur Radiol 2006;16:569-574.

Vinee P, Stover B, Sigmund G, et al. MR imaging of the pericardial cyst. J Magn Reson Imaging 1992;2:593-596.

Wang ZJ, Reddy GP, Gotway MB, et al. CT and MR imaging of pericardial disease. Radiographics 2003;23 Spec No:S167-S180.

Yamano T, Sawada T, Sakamoto K, et al. Magnetic resonance imaging differentiated partial from complete absence of the left pericardium in a case of leftward displacement of the heart. Circ J 2004;68:385-388.

Chapter 10

Dilated Cardiomyopathy and Myocardial Infarction

Nikolaos Tzemos, Gabriel Vorobiof, and Raymond Y. Kwong

KEY POINTS

- Cardiac magnetic resonance (CMR) is the current golden standard for accurate assessment of ventricular volumes and global and regional function, thus providing information on prognosis.

- Extracellular accumulation of gadolinium, imaged at 10 to 30 minutes after injection, identifies areas of myocardial fibrosis commonly seen in cardiomyopathies, generally subendocardial or transmural in a coronary distribution in the case of ischemic cardiomyopathy.

- Transmural extent of LGE can predict recovery of myocardial function after revascularization in patients with coronary artery disease.

- Negative stress CMR with either adenosine or dobutamine stressors has excellent negative predictive value for subsequent coronary events.

- Noncoronary segmental distribution and midwall or epicardial involvement of LGE are atypical of myocardial infarction. This allows discrimination between ischemic and nonischemic etiologies of cardiomyopathy, which can assist in clinical decision making.

- Takotsubo cardiomyopathy is characterized by left ventricular apical dilation and regional hypocontraction, absence of first-pass perfusion abnormality, and minimal or absent concomitant subendocardial LGE.

- Because of its higher spatial and temporal resolution, CMR can offer an improved assessment for the presence and extend of ventricular noncompaction, compared with echocardiography.

- CMR can accurately quantify severity of valvular regurgitation and stenosis using phase contrast imaging. In the same study CMR can assess the physiologic impact of the valvular heart disease by providing quantitation of large vessel morphology and ventricular volumes and functions.

- CMR is the most sensitive technique for detecting clinically unrecognized small subendocardial myocardial infarctions that do not result in wall motion abnormality or ECG changes, thereby identifying patients at risk of cardiac events.

- CMR infarct imaging can provide direct information on the amount of irreversibly injured myocardium and viable myocardium, including the extent of periinfarct zone and microvascular obstruction, which are strong predictors of cardiovascular outcome in patients after myocardial infarction (MI).

Case 1   Nonischemic Cardiomyopathy

A 54-year-old woman without significant risk factors for coronary artery disease presented to our services complaining of a 4-week history of exertional dyspnea (NYHA class III) and pedal edema. The patient did not have any history of alcoholism, family history of heart disease, or sudden cardiac death. ECG showed sinus rhythm and a left bundle branch block pattern of unknown duration. Transthoracic echocardiography showed a dilated left ventricle and severe global hypokinesis with reduced ejection fraction of 25%. A coronary angiography was performed that revealed no significant coronary stenosis. CMR was performed (Figure 10-1).

Comments

Determining the etiology of heart failure is essential for directing the correct treatment and predicting survival of patients who presented with new cardiac failure. CMR can often differentiate ischemic from nonischemic etiologies by the pattern of distribution of LGE. Indeed, in patients with idiopathic nonischemic cardiomyopathy, there is often a distinct pattern of LGE presenting as patchy longitudinal midwall LGE that spares the subendocardium and subepicardium and does not conform to a coronary vascular territory, as in our current case. The transmural extent of this midwall LGE has been implicated in the pathogenesis of ventricular arrhythmias in patients with nonischemic dilated cardiomyopathy. More recently LGE has been shown to prognosticate cardiac events in patients with this condition.

Case 2   Takotsubo Cardiomyopathy

A 48-year-old woman without coronary risk factors was admitted to the emergency room following 30 minutes of severe retrosternal discomfort associated with diaphoresis. ECG showed widespread T-wave inversion in anterolateral leads. Emergency cardiac catheterization revealed unobstructed epicardial coronary arteries with LV distal akinesis resembling apical ballooning but without any intracavitary thrombus formation. CMR was performed the following day to assess the degree of ventricular dysfunction (Figure 10-2).

Comments

Left ventricular (LV) apical ballooning (Takotsubo cardiomyopathy) is a unique clinical entity characterized by transient anteroapical hypokinesis in the setting of elevated adrenergic tone, ECG abnormalities mimicking acute coronary syndrome, modest elevation of cardiac enzyme levels, and a lack of angiographically significant epicardial coronary stenoses. Although diagnosis is usually suspected by a lack of significant coronary lesion on angiography, CMR is useful in this context by providing precise evidence of LV structural changes, exclusion of concomitant significant obstructive coronary disease, assessing for any extent of myocardial necrosis, and noninvasive monitoring for recovery of ventricular function.

Case 3   Large Myocardial Infarction

A 56-year-old man with a history of anterior myocardial infarction one year ago was referred to CMR for assessment of new onset chest pain, ventricular function, and myocardial viability (Figure 10-3). During the hospitalization for his acute MI, coronary intervention of the proximal LAD was complicated with luminal dissection and as a result there was incomplete coronary revascularization of the infarct-related artery despite attempts to perform coronary stents.

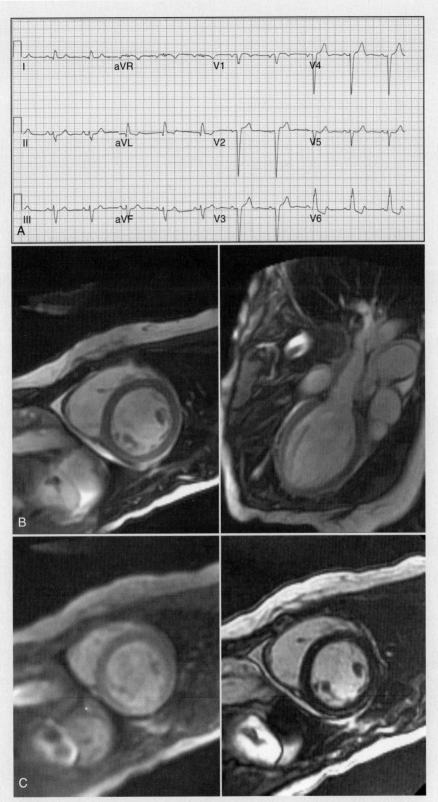

■ **Figure 10-1 A,** Electrocardiogram demonstrating sinus rhythm and left bundle branch block conduction. **B,** Cine CMR. Diastolic frames of mid short-axis and 2-chamber long axis cine steady-state free precession (SSFP) imaging which demonstrate moderately dilated left ventricular (LV) chamber and severe global hypokinesis. **C,** Contrast-enhanced CMR. Left panel shows absence of perfusion defects during first-pass gadolinium transit across the myocardium. Right panel shows a mid short-axis late enhancement (LGE) image obtained 10 minutes after gadolinium administration demonstrating midwall linear LGE, which are not confined to a coronary arterial distribution.

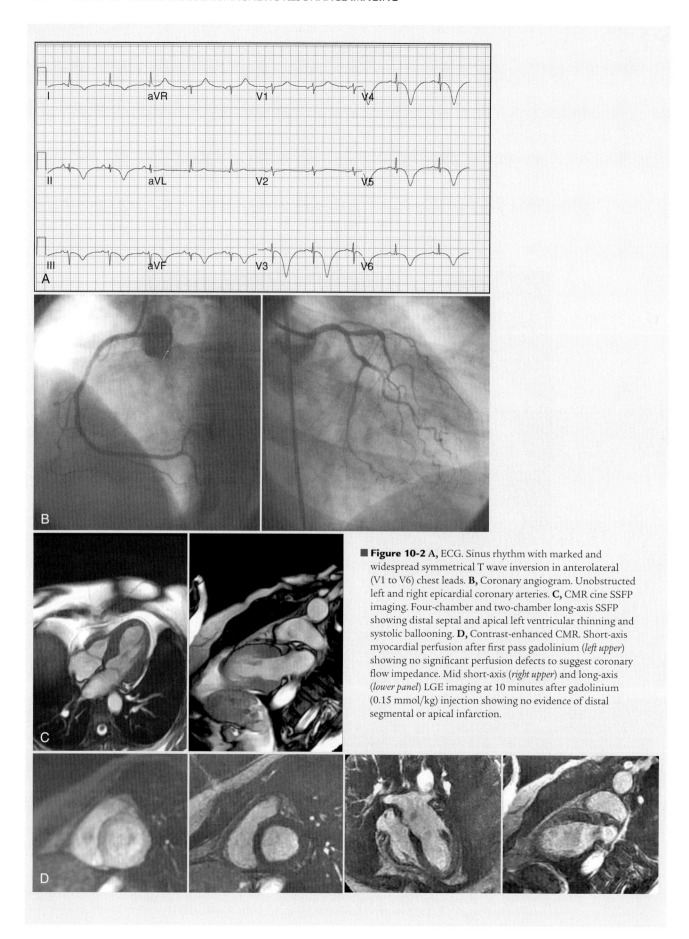

■ **Figure 10-2 A,** ECG. Sinus rhythm with marked and widespread symmetrical T wave inversion in anterolateral (V1 to V6) chest leads. **B,** Coronary angiogram. Unobstructed left and right epicardial coronary arteries. **C,** CMR cine SSFP imaging. Four-chamber and two-chamber long-axis SSFP showing distal septal and apical left ventricular thinning and systolic ballooning. **D,** Contrast-enhanced CMR. Short-axis myocardial perfusion after first pass gadolinium (*left upper*) showing no significant perfusion defects to suggest coronary flow impedance. Mid short-axis (*right upper*) and long-axis (*lower panel*) LGE imaging at 10 minutes after gadolinium (0.15 mmol/kg) injection showing no evidence of distal segmental or apical infarction.

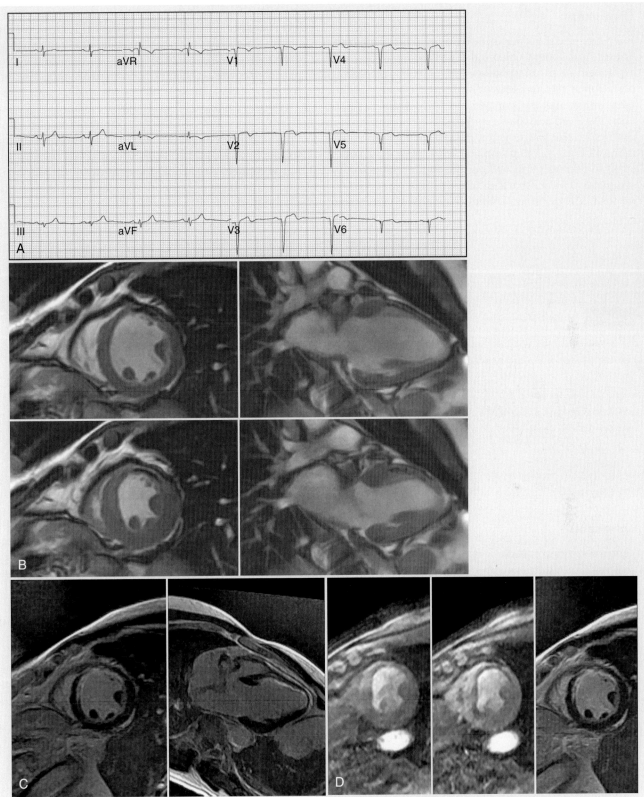

■ **Figure 10-3 A,** Resting ECG showing sinus rhythm, and evidence of old anterior MI by Q waves in leads V1 to V4 with inverted T waves. **B,** Cine SSFP imaging demonstrating a large region of anterior akinesia involving the mid to distal anterior walls (top images show the end-diastolic frames and the bottom images show the end-systolic frames of the short-axis and two-chamber long axis views, respectively). Despite the anterior MI, there is normal global LV size (81 ml/m²) and only mildly reduced LV ejection fraction of 51%. **C,** This anterior akinesia is matched by a medium-sized late enhancement consistent with a transmural MI in short-axis and long-axis views, respectively. Using a semi-automated signal intensity detection technique, the infarct size is quantified at 15% of the total LV mass. **D,** First-pass myocardial perfusion using fast gradient-echo CMR: Comparison between rest (*left image*) and during adenosine stress (*middle image*), there is marked reversibility of the perfusion defect, which involved the anterior, anteroseptal, and even the inferoseptal wall, which is not infracted (compare with the right image of late enhancement). These findings suggest evidence of periinfarct ischemia surrounding a medium-sized MI. This patient on repeat coronary angiography showed a subtotally occluded proximal left descending artery with collateral supply from the right coronary artery.

Comments

For patients with suspected or confirmed coronary artery disease, gadolinium-enhanced CMR offers a combined assessment of LV morphology and function, myocardial perfusion at rest and stress hemodynamic states, and infarct extent and transmurality for myocardial viability. Cine SSFP can provide three-dimensional imaging of the ventricular size and function at high spatial and temporal resolutions (1.5 mm in-plane and temporal resolution at 40 to 50 msec) and without the use of geometric assumption. The most widely used current stress modality for CMR perfusion studies is adenosine vasodilating stress in order to induce a visible difference in blood flow between normal and hypoperfused myocardium. In this case changes in LV morphology and function, infarct size, and transmural extent can be quantified accurately and myocardial flow reversibility reflecting ongoing coronary stenosis was depicted qualitatively. There is growing evidence of strong prognostic implication of vasodilating stress CMR in risk stratification of patients with suspected or known CAD. The excellent spatial resolution and contrast noise ratio of LGE imaging can also accurately predict regional recovery of contractile function in response to coronary revascularization after infarction.

Case 4   **Left Ventricular Noncompaction**

A 55-year-old man with no family history of cardiomyopathy or sudden cardiac death and no risk factors for ischemic heart disease presented at our emergency service because of dyspnea. He noticed progressively reduced exercise tolerance (NYHA class III) in the past 4 weeks accompanied by pedal edema. Transthoracic echocardiography was limited because of poor acoustic windows and a CMR study was requested to assess the etiology of cardiomyopathy (Figure 10-4).

Comments

Ventricular noncompaction is a rare congenital cardiomyopathy resulting from an intrauterine developmental arrest that stops compaction of the loose, myocardial fiber meshwork. The noncompacted myocardium has a "spongy" appearance with prominent trabeculations and deep intertrabecular recesses that communicate with the ventricular cavity. Two forms of ventricular noncompaction have been described: a nonisolated form associated with other congenital heart defects, such as ventricular septal defects, pulmonic stenosis or hypoplastic left ventricle and so far seen exclusively in children; and an isolated form that is often undetected. Both CMR and 2D-echocardiography identified the global and segmental dysfunction in this group of patients and these findings correlated well with the morphopathologic findings. Only CMR, however, accurately identified the characteristic features of isolated noncompacted myocardium, including the alterations in myocardial architecture and the prominent and excessive trabecular meshwork. The characteristic, discriminating feature of ventricular noncompaction is a thickened ventricular wall with two layers of hypokinetic segments: a thin (compacted) epicardial layer and a much thicker (noncompacted) endocardial layer.

Case 5   **Severe Valvular Heart Disease Leading to Cardiomyopathy**

A 23-year-old athletic woman with rheumatic heart disease and severe mitral regurgitation complained of reduced physical endurance after strenuous exercise. Transthoracic echocardiography confirmed severe mitral regurgitation into a large left atrium but LV global function and volumes could not be adequately assessed because of limited acoustic windows. CMR was performed (Figure 10-5).

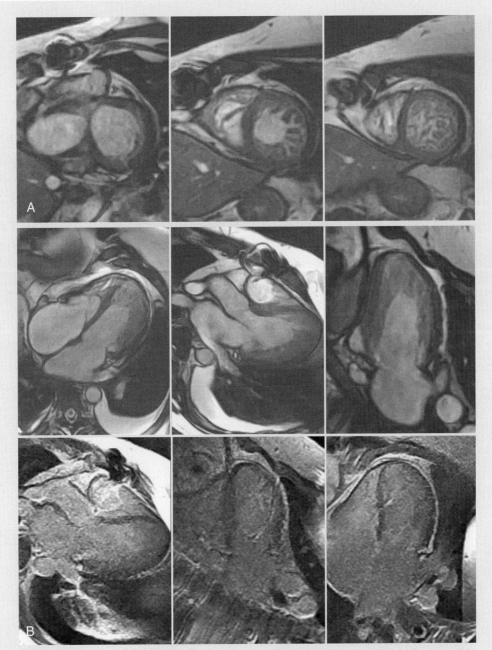

■ **Figure 10-4 A,** Short-axis cine SSFP images showing deep spongelike recesses in left ventricular walls most pronounced on the inferolateral walls and at the apex. The LV is normal in diastolic size (LV end-diastolic volume index at 87 ml/m²; normal, less than 112 ml/m²) with a moderately reduced global systolic function (LV ejection fraction calculated by volumetric calculation at 32%; normal, greater than 55%). The maximal thickness ratio of the noncompacted versus compacted region at the inferolateral wall was 3.4, which meets the diagnostic criteria of LV noncompaction in the literature. **B,** Radial long-axis views showing noncompacted mid lateral to apical walls (*top*). Ten minutes after gadolinium injection, there was no obvious LGE of the LV to indicate myocardial scar or infarction (*bottom*).

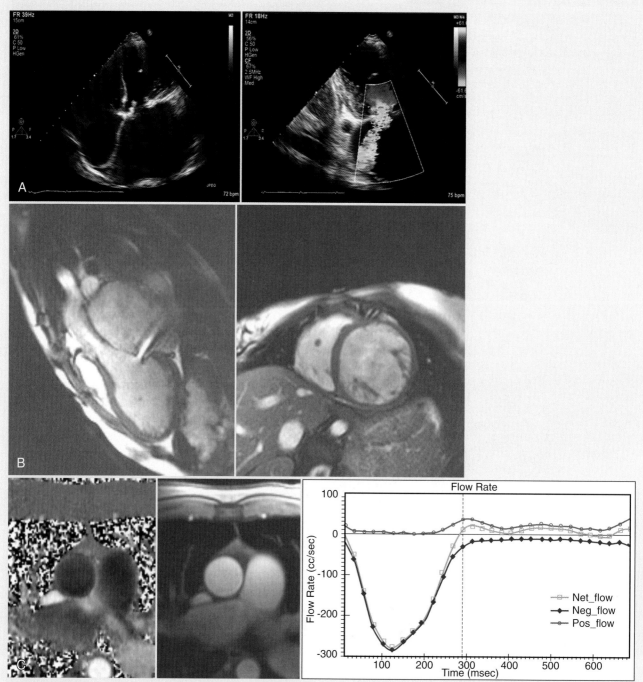

■ **Figure 10-5 A,** Echocardiogram: Left panel shows four-chamber view image, with markedly dilated left atrium, thickened mitral valve leaflets. Right panel, shows a two-chamber view image with Doppler color through the mitral valve and proximal flow acceleration. **B,** Left panel shows a horizontal long axis (four chamber) cine SSFP. The left atrium is markedly dilated with evidence of mitral regurgitation in systole, seen as signal void caused by dephasing, through the mitral valve leaflets. Right panel shows a mid short-axis cine SSFP of the dilated LV (LV end-diastolic volume index 109 ml/m²; normal, less than 99 ml/m²) with mild global hypokinesis (LV ejection fraction 54%). The LV stroke volume is determined by the difference between the LV end-diastolic volume and the LV end-systolic volume and was calculated at 125 ml in this case. **C,** Quantification of the mitral regurgitant blood flow using phase contrast imaging by CMR. Upper panel shows phase and magnitude images of the ascending aorta. Lower panel shows the measured aortic systolic flow volume of 57 ml. The blood volume of mitral regurgitation (regurgitant volume) is calculated by subtracting the aortic systolic forward flow volume from the LV stroke volume. The regurgitant fraction is then calculated as the percentage of LV stroke volume that regurgitates into the left atrium, that is, by dividing the regurgitant volume by the LV stroke volume and expressing it as a percentage.

Comments

CMR is the current noninvasive gold standard for quantification of ventricular volumes and function. In this case of a patient with severe valvular heart disease being assessed for candidacy for surgery, CMR provides reproducible quantitation of the severity of mitral regurgitation and its resultant impact on ventricular function and size. Although the severity of valvular regurgitation was qualitatively assessed by the severity of the regurgitant jet, velocity-encoded phase contrast imaging quantified regurgitant blood flow. In stenotic valvular heart disease, peak velocity across a valve obtained from phase contrast imaging can be used to estimate pressure gradient between the two connecting chambers, similar to Doppler echocardiography. Thus CMR is capable of providing a comprehensive assessment of valvular heart disease, based on reliable quantification of flow volumes and LV function; hence it can contribute to decision making regarding the need for surgical intervention or ongoing monitoring.

Case 6   Small Unrecognized Myocardial Infarction

A 52-year-old man with hyperlipidemia and positive family history of coronary artery disease (CAD) developed exercise-induced discomfort. A nuclear (SPECT) adenosine test showed no perfusion defects. He continued to complain of exertional chest pain and a dobutamine CMR was requested (Figure 10-6).

Comments

CMR currently is the most sensitive noninvasive method in detecting small myocardial scars from MI. This was made possible by the high contrast-noise ratio as a result of accumulation of gadolinium contrast in areas of infarction, when imaged at a precise time window with a novel technique that specifically suppresses the normal myocardium. This case illustrates that subtle signs of coronary syndrome including small unrecognized MI and peri-infarct ischemia, which cannot be easily appreciated by conventional wall motion or nuclear imaging, can be detected by the addition of contrast-enhanced CMR techniques.

Case 7   Large Acute Myocardial Infarction, Microvascular Obstruction, and the Peri-Infarct Zone

A 52-year-old firefighter presented to the emergency department with persistent indigestion after watching a football game. ECG showed 3 mm ST-segment depression in leads V1 to V4 and 2 mm in leads II, III and AVF. Emergency coronary arteriography was performed showing proximal left anterior descending occlusion and moderate stenosis in the mid right coronary artery. Percutaneous intervention was performed with successful revascularization of the left anterior descending artery. Four days later CMR was performed to assess LV function (Figure 10-7).

Comments

Being an extravascular class of contrast media, gadolinium-based agents penetrates interstitial space within an acute infarct zone based on relative loss of cell membrane integrity, but its entry into cells or interstitial space is prohibited by coronary vascular debris in the microcirculation. Although CMR infarct imaging can provide direct information on the amount of irreversibly injured myocardium and viable myocardium, tissue characteristics within the region of ischemic insult can be differentiated and the extent of the peri-infarct and MO quantified. Growing evidence has suggested MO and the periinfarct zone are strong predictors of cardiovascular outcome in patients after MI.

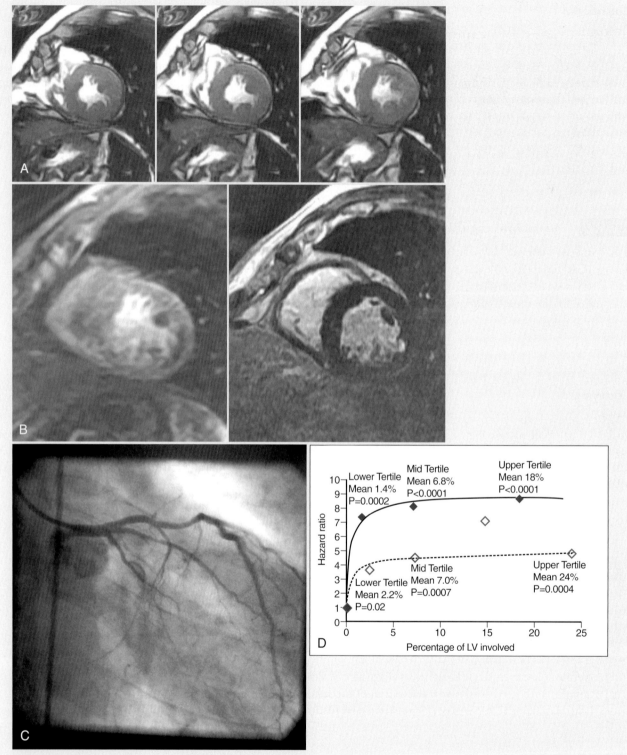

■ **Figure 10-6 A,** Basal mid short-axis cine SSFP at increasing doses of dobutamine (10-30 mcg/kg/min). At peak (right panel) there was a very subtle regional wall motion abnormality at the inferolateral wall, which was not appreciated at the time of stress cine imaging. **B,** LGE quantified to involve 1.5% of total LV mass was noted in the inferolateral wall matching the region of wall motion abnormality during stress (right panel). During first-pass myocardial perfusion at mid-dose dobutamine (20 mcg/kg/min), a perfusion defect affecting the mid inferolateral wall surrounding and involving a larger myocardial extent than the LGE region was noted. **C,** Coronary angiography after the CMR demonstrated a severe stenosis of a small nondominant left circumflex coronary artery. **D,** Our group investigated the prognostic implication of LGE in a consecutive cohort of 195 patients without a history of MI referred for CMR for assessment of ischemia. After a medium follow-up of 16 months, 16% of patients experienced cardiac events (MACE). On this graph, the hazard ratio to experiencing MACE is expressed on the y-axis, and the myocardial extent of the LV on the X-axis. Presence of LGE, which is consistent with clinically unrecognized MI, was associated with marked elevated hazards to MACE. As the LGE extent (*blue dots*) increased, the hazards to MACE progressively increased. Compared with wall motion score in tertiles calculated based on segmental extent and severity (*red diamonds*), LGE extent portended to a stronger association with MACE. In addition, we found that even a very small amount of LGE (less than 2% of the mean LV mass in the lowest tertile) was associated with a greater than sevenfold increase in MACE hazards.

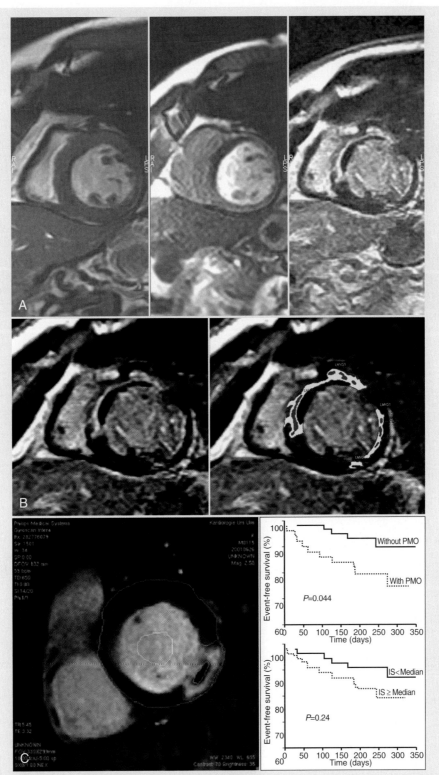

■ **Figure 10-7 A,** Left panel shows mid short-axis cine SSFP imaging a large anterior and anteroseptal akinesis but with normal wall thickness. Despite successful revascularization of the infarct related left anterior descending artery, first-pass myocardial perfusion shows a large defect in the subendocardial anteroseptal and anterior wall consistent with a large no-reflow zone (middle panel). Right panel shows LGE imaging, which shows a large enhanced region surrounding an area of hypoenhancement consistent with microvascular obstruction (MO), matching the area of hypoperfusion on first-pass perfusion. **B,** CMR can identify semiquantitatively, based on signal intensity criterion, myocardial regions of high gadolinium enhancement representing the core of the infarct (*depicted in red*) and intermediate enhancement regions representing the periinfarct zone (*depicted in yellow*). **C,** In several studies, the presence of MVO has an impact on long-term survival in patients post-AMI. In the more recent study, Hombach et al. studied 110 patients at a mean of day 6 after acute MI and defined MO as persistent MO (PMO) on LGE imaging. Forty-six percent of the patients had MO. In this paper the authors showed that PMO had stronger prognostic value than infarct size alone in predicting late LV remodeling and survival after MI. (*Adapted from Hombach V, Grebe O, Merkle N, et al: Sequelae of acute myocardial infarction regarding cardiac structure and function and their prognostic significance as assessed by magnetic resonance imaging. Eur Heart J 2005;26(6):549-557, with permission.*)

SUGGESTED READING

Fujita N, Chazouilleres AF, Hartiala JJ, et al: Quantification of mitral regurgitation by velocity-encoded cine nuclear magnetic resonance imaging. J Am Coll Cardiol 1994;23(4):951-958.

Gelfand EV, Hughes S, Hauser TH, et al: Severity of mitral and aortic regurgitation as assessed by cardiovascular magnetic resonance: optimizing correlation with Doppler echocardiography. J Cardiovasc Magn Reson 2006;8(3):503-507.

Gerber BL, Garot J, Bluemke DA, et al: Accuracy of contrast-enhanced magnetic resonance imaging in predicting improvement of regional myocardial function in patients after acute myocardial infarction. Circulation 2002;106(9):1083-1089.

Haghi D, Fluechter S, Suselbeck T, et al: Cardiovascular magnetic resonance findings in typical versus atypical forms of the acute apical ballooning syndrome (Takotsubo cardiomyopathy). Int J Cardiol 2007;120(2):205-211.

Hombach V, Grebe O, Merkle N, et al: Sequelae of acute myocardial infarction regarding cardiac structure and function and their prognostic significance as assessed by magnetic resonance imaging. Eur Heart J 2005;26:549-557.

Ichikawa Y, Sakuma H, Suzawa N, et al: Late gadolinium-enhanced magnetic resonance imaging in acute and chronic myocardial infarction. Improved prediction of regional myocardial contraction in the chronic state by measuring thickness of nonenhanced myocardium. J Am Coll Cardiol 2005;45(6):901-909.

Jahnke C, Nagel E, Gebker R, et al: Prognostic value of cardiac magnetic resonance stress tests: adenosine stress perfusion and dobutamine stress wall motion imaging. Circulation 2007;115(13):1769-1776.

Kim RJ, Wu E, Rafael A, et al: The use of contrast-enhanced magnetic resonance imaging to identify reversible myocardial dysfunction. N Engl J Med 2000;343(20):1445-1453.

Kizilbash AM, Hundley WG, Willett DL, et al: Comparison of quantitative Doppler with magnetic resonance imaging for assessment of the severity of mitral regurgitation. Am J Cardiol. Mar 15 1998;81(6):792-795.

Kwong RY, Chan AK, Brown KA, et al: Impact of unrecognized myocardial scar detected by cardiac magnetic resonance imaging on event-free survival in patients presenting with signs or symptoms of coronary artery disease. Circulation 2006;113(23):2733-2743.

Mahrholdt H, Wagner A, Judd RM, et al: Delayed enhancement cardiovascular magnetic resonance assessment of nonischaemic cardiomyopathies. Eur Heart J 2005;26(15):1461-1474.

McCrohon JA, Moon JC, Prasad SK, et al: Differentiation of heart failure related to dilated cardiomyopathy and coronary artery disease using gadolinium-enhanced cardiovascular magnetic resonance. Circulation 2003;108(1):54-59.

Mitchell JH, Hadden TB, Wilson JM, et al: Clinical features and usefulness of cardiac magnetic resonance imaging in assessing myocardial viability and prognosis in Takotsubo cardiomyopathy (transient left ventricular apical ballooning syndrome). Am J Cardiol 2007;100(2):296-301.

Nazarian S, Bluemke DA, Lardo AC, et al: "Magnetic resonance assessment of the substrate for inducible ventricular tachycardia in nonischemic cardiomyopathy. Circulation 2005;112(18): 2821-2825.

Petersen SE, Selvanayagam JB, Wiesmann F, et al: Left ventricular noncompaction: insights from cardiovascular magnetic resonance imaging. J Am Coll Cardiol 2005;46(1):101-105.

Schwitter J, Wacker CM, van Rossum AC, et al: MR-IMPACT: comparison of perfusion-cardiac magnetic resonance with single-photon emission computed tomography for the detection of coronary artery disease in a multicentre, multivendor, randomized trial. Eur Heart J 2008;29(4):480-489.

Weiford BC, Subbarao VD, Mulhern KM. Noncompaction of the ventricular myocardium. Circulation 2004;109(24):2965-2971.

Wu KC, Zerhouni EA, Judd RM, et al: Prognostic significance of microvascular obstruction by magnetic resonance imaging in patients with acute myocardial infarction. Circulation 1998;97:765-772.

Yan AT, Shayne AJ, Brown KA, et al: Characterization of the periinfarct zone by contrast-enhanced cardiac magnetic resonance imaging is a powerful predictor of postmyocardial infarction mortality. Circulation 2006;114:32-39.

Chapter 11

Hypertrophic Cardiomyopathy

Andrew S. Flett and James C. Moon

KEY POINTS

- CMR employs multiple techniques in HCM patients to assess LV/RV cardiac function, hypertrophy, morphology, flow, velocities, perfusion, and fibrosis.

- Clinical application includes detecting early phenotype expression, characterizing established disease, distinguishing phenocopies, and potentially aiding in risk stratification both for sudden death and heart failure.

- In early disease or apical HCM, CMR may detect areas of hypertrophy missed by echo. The presence of LGE may also aid diagnosis.

- The extent of LGE is correlated to clinical risk markers for sudden death, progression to heart failure and is predictive of nonsustained VT; thus, LGE may aid in risk stratification.

- CMR can be useful in patients with outflow tract obstruction when there are complicating factors such as multilevel obstruction, RV obstruction, aortic membranes, or poor echo windows.

- CMR may aid in the diagnosis of phenocopies of HCM.

- Patients with progressive disease almost invariably have extensive LGE.

- CMR, like all other imaging modalities, has certain pitfalls that are important to be aware of when interpreting scans.

Recent advances in cardiovascular magnetic resonance (CMR) have resulted in its emergence as a useful tool in the evaluation of the patient with hypertrophic cardiomyopathy (HCM) and one that is likely to play an increasing role in the future. The combination of multiple techniques in one scan builds up a sophisticated picture of LV/RV cardiac function, hypertrophy, morphology, flow, velocities, perfusion, and fibrosis.

HCM is a common genetic disease affecting 1 in 500 of the population, manifested by increased myocardial mass, in the absence of loading conditions (hypertension, aortic stenosis) sufficient to cause the abnormality. The most common etiology is an autosomal-dominant disorder caused by mutations in genes that encode cardiac sarcomeric proteins. The pathologic hallmarks of the disease are myocardial hypertrophy, myocyte disarray (usually in association with myocardial fibrosis) and small-vessel disease. Accurate and timely diagnosis relies on several factors including the family history, ECG and echo parameters, and importantly, the screening of families when a proband is identified. Clinical sequelae include systolic and diastolic dysfunction, myocardial ischemia, arrhythmia, abnormal vascular responses, and skeletal muscle dysfunction. Serious complications include thromboembolism, heart failure, infective endocarditis, ventricular arrhythmia, and sudden death. Treatment is designed to reduce symptoms and complications when possible and to prevent disease-related sudden death.

Clinical uses of CMR in HCM include detecting early phenotype expression, characterizing established disease, and distinguishing phenocopies. The potential exists to aid risk stratification both for sudden death and heart failure.

EARLY DISEASE

The first signs of phenotypic expression in HCM may be difficult to detect with imaging. In families with HCM, an individual with an affected first degree relative has a 50% pretest probability of gene carriage. The presence/absence of an abnormal ECG is helpful and may strongly suggest disease expression but does not confirm the diagnosis. The traditional gold standard test to assess LV mass—2D echocardiography—has several limitations in this regard. It is reliant on adequate acoustic windows and the fixed probe on the chest wall necessitates oblique short axis cross sectioning of the LV. In addition, although the distribution of hypertrophy in HCM is often diffuse it may frequently be segmental, confined to relatively small regions of the LV chamber that may be obscured or have inadequate border definition on echo. In familial cases, in particular where the ECG is abnormal and the echo normal, cine CMR, which does not have these limitations, may detect missed hypertrophy, occurring in up to 5% of cases in some series (Figures 11-1 and 11-2).

An intriguing suggestion is that there may be prephenotypic expressions of sarcomeric protein mutation carriage in minor cardiac morphologic abnormalities—for example crypts (also described as clefts or recesses), particularly at the inferior RV insertion points. Small changes in piloting (Figure 11-3) may reveal these. A few may be part of the normal spectrum, but multiple clefts (Figure 11-4) may be more significant.

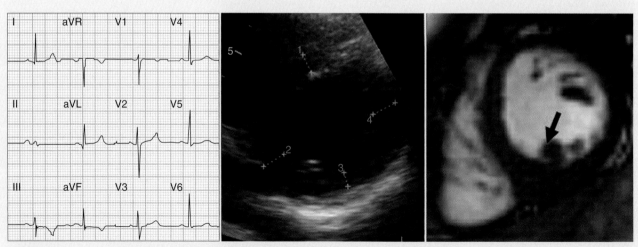

■ **Figure 11-1** Echo may overlook localized LVH. Here, basal inferoseptal hypertrophy is clearly present on CMR. Often it is difficult to differentiate RV from LV structures; false tendons and trabeculation complicate matters further. Note the location of the hypertrophy matches the T-wave inversion.

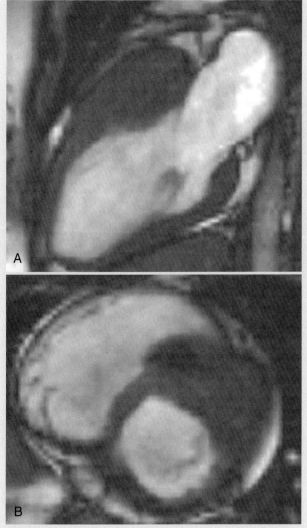

■ **Figure 11-2** Localized, basal, anteroseptal hypertrophy can be missed on echocardiography.

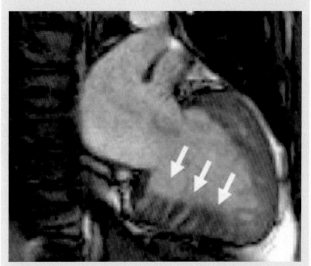

■ **Figure 11-4** Multiple clefts. The significance of these is unclear. These may represent a form of left ventricular noncompaction, sarcomeric protein disease, or may just be an extreme of normal variance.

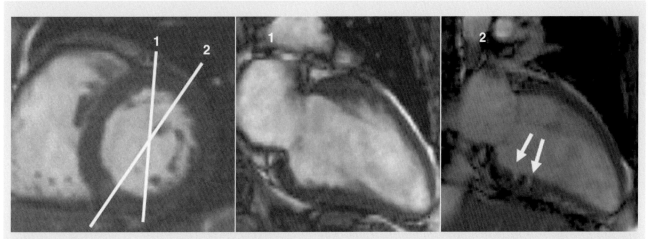

■ **Figure 11-3** Clefts in HCM—the orientation of the slice is critical. On short axis images, the presence of clefts should be suspected by a paler appearance at the RV insertion point (clefts are narrower than the slice thickness). Long-axis images with a minor rotation of the imaging plane demonstrate these (compare 1 and 2).

APICAL INVOLVEMENT

CMR may help the detection of hypertrophy missed by echo. This is particularly true for the apex where echo views are frequently technically challenging because of near field artifact. In patients suspected to have apical hypertrophy (unexplained repolarization abnormalities on ECG, particularly negative T waves anteriorly) CMR may elucidate missed hypertrophy. Additionally, apical cavity obliteration, microaneurysms, thrombus, and LV noncompaction can be identified (Figure 11-5).

PATIENTS AT RISK

Risk stratification in HCM remains challenging. Current risk factors for sudden death include family history of sudden cardiac death (SCD), syncope, nonsustained ventricular tachycardia (NSVT), abnormal blood pressure response to exercise, and severe left ventricular hypertrophy. Applying these risk factors unfortunately does not adequately stratify some patients, who may only have one or no risk factors and still die suddenly. Conversely many patients with defibrillators never require a shock.

With the use of contrast agents based on gadolinium-DTPA (Gd-DTPA), focal areas of fibrosis can be identified. Gd-DTPA is an extracellular contrast agent and accumulates in areas of scar making the area brighter on CMR—a phenomenon called late gadolinium enhancement (LGE) or delayed enhancement. This is familiar from myocardial infarction where the LGE occurs in coronary artery territories and its distribution in the LV wall reflects the sequence of myocardial ischemia, occurring from the endocardium spreading in a wavefront to the epicardium dependent on the degree of transmurality of the infarct. A similar scarring process occurs in HCM, but the mechanism is less well understood. Correlations have been made between histology and in vivo imaging,

showing that LGE, like myocardial infarction, represents increased focal fibrosis rather than disarray (Figure 11-6).

However, in HCM, the extent of LGE and its distribution is different from myocardial infarction and highly variable but does occur in recognizable patterns (Figures 11-7 and 11-8). LGE is common in HCM, occurring in up to 80% of patients, and represents focally increased fibrosis and sometimes complete replacement scarring. Post mortem studies of hearts of patients with HCM have shown greater extent of fibrosis in patients with NSVT. The extent of LGE and hence fibrosis is correlated to clinical risk markers for sudden death, progression to heart failure, and is predictive of NSVT. Therefore, it is plausible that LGE imaging could provide the direct in vivo visualization of the substrate (scar, fibrosis) for sudden death; a highly attractive scenario. The clinical significance of this is not yet fully established and outcome data are needed. Currently extensive LGE in young patients is probably the most concerning finding. It may be most clinically useful in patients possessing a single risk factor for sudden death where clinical management is unclear. The presence of extensive LGE may help those difficult decisions regarding the insertion of a defibrillator.

OBSTRUCTION

Left ventricular outflow tract obstruction occurs in up to 20% of HCM patients at rest. Significantly more than this exhibit obstruction on stress and both of these are readily assessed by rest and stress echocardiography. CMR can be useful when there are complicating factors such as multilevel obstruction, RV obstruction, aortic membranes, or poor echo windows. It is also helpful for establishing the precise anatomy of obstruction and of the mitral valve as well as demonstrating the area of systolic anterior motion (SAM) of the mitral valve

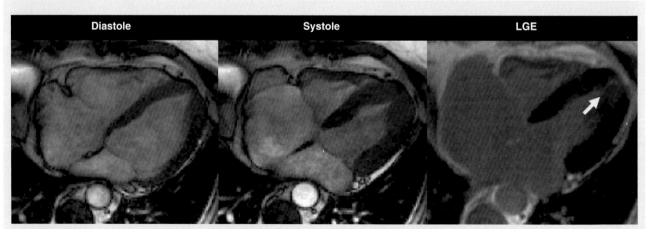

■ **Figure 11-5** Apical cardiomyopathy, not identified by echocardiography. Four-chamber view with apical cavity obliteration in systole and limited apical LGE (*arrowed*). Several apical crosscuts should be taken if apical HCM is suspected with reduced slice thickness (5 mm) to ensure the true apex is identified.

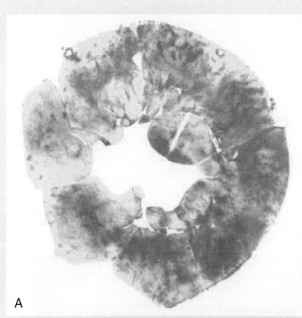

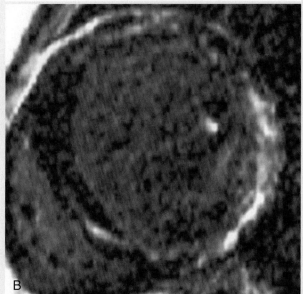

■ **Figure 11-6** LGE represents areas of increased focal fibrosis in HCM. **A,** histologic slice demonstrating extensive red, collagen staining. **B,** from the same patient, in vivo CMR LGE uptake in the same segment. Note: The ex-vivo imaging is "supra-systolic" so has a smaller cavity and thicker wall than the in vivo diastolic LGE image.

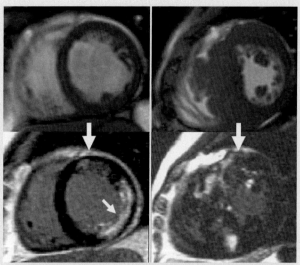

■ **Figure 11-7** LGE imaging in MI (**left**) versus HCM (**right**). Myocardial infarction produces LGE in (a) coronary artery territories and (b) in a specific distribution from endocardium to epicardium reflecting the wavefront of necrosis as it progresses. LGE in HCM may occur in several characteristic patterns. It tends to occur in areas of hypertrophy (unless there has been thinning in progressive disease) and may be based anywhere in the wall (epicardial to endocardial).

TABLE 11-1 Phenocopies of Sarcomeric HCM

Storage diseases
Anderson-Fabry disease
Glycogen storage diseases
Mucopolysaccharidoses
Mitochondrial myopathies
Syndromes (Noonan's, Friedreich's ataxia)

Physiologic hypertrophy
Increased afterload (hypertension, aortic stenosis, outflow tract obstruction)
Athlete's heart
Ethnic variants
Compensatory hypertrophy (after remote MI)

Infiltration
Amyloid
Senile Amyloid

Aging
Sigmoid septum

with septal contact before surgery or alcohol ablation (Figure 11-9).

CMR with contrast can delineate the precise extent of necrosis after alcohol ablation as areas of LGE and microvascular obstruction. It is also useful in the follow-up of these patients particularly if they fail to respond adequately to therapy. A residual septal bulge SAM: septal contact remote from the ablation/myectomy site also can be seen sometimes (Figure 11-10).

PHENOCOPIES

Other conditions may present with left ventricular hypertrophy (LVH) and cause diagnostic difficulty (Table 11-1). CMR, at least in the early stages, may help refine the differential diagnosis, pointing to specific etiologies (Table 11-2). End-stage disease processes may all culminate in the final common pathway of fibrosis, dilatation, impaired systolic function, and atrial dilatation (Figure 11-11).

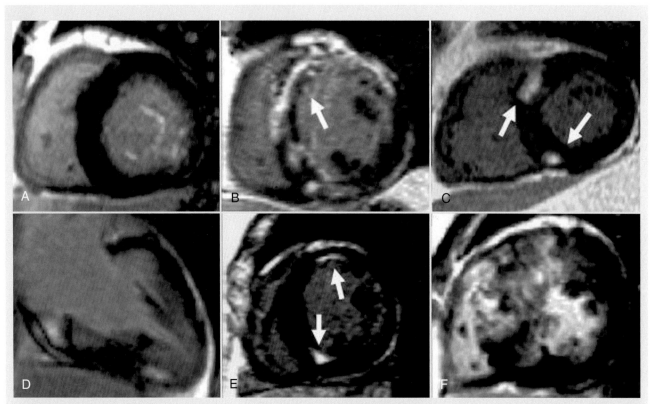

■ **Figure 11-8** Different patterns of LGE. **A,** Hypertrophy but no LGE. Myocardium appears homogenously black. **B,** Progressive disease with heart failure. Extensive LGE involving at least 20% of myocardium (here 50%), traversing multiple coronary artery territories. Additional features may include dilated LA, impaired long axis function, LV thrombus, and aneurysm formation. **C,** RV insertion point (HCM). A common finding, small amounts may be benign. **D,** Apical HCM with LGE occurring in the hypertrophied apex, sparing the base. **E,** Subendocardial (HCM). **F,** High-risk (HCM). Extensive LGE sometimes in association with impaired LV function or thinning.

TABLE 11-2 Characteristic Patterns on CMR Occurring in HCM Phenocopies

PHENOCOPY	CAVITY	FUNCTION AND HYPERTROPHY	LEFT ATRIUM	LGE
Sarcomeric HCM	Small, cavity obliteration	Reduced thickening, supranormal EF, can be systolic impairment, concentric, asymmetric hypertrophy, outflow tract obstruction	Variable, often enlarged	Highly variable, in pattern and extent; may be absent
Hypertension	Normal	Normal, long axis reduction; more concentric	May be enlarged	None unless coronary disease
Athletes heart	Large, but resolves with deconditioning	Supranormal thickening concentric (eccentric LVH less than 15 mm) in proportion to cavity	Normal	None
Amyloid	Normal	Reduced, particularly in long axis, effusions. Concentric	Often large	Global; subendocardial the most common pattern; difficult to image; dark blood pool
Fabry's disease	Normal	May be reduced. More concentric. Obstruction less common	May be large	Inferolateral in early disease progressing to extensive LGE
GSDIIIa	Unknown	Unknown. Can lead to severe systolic failure, RV involvement	Unknown	Progresses to extensive LGE

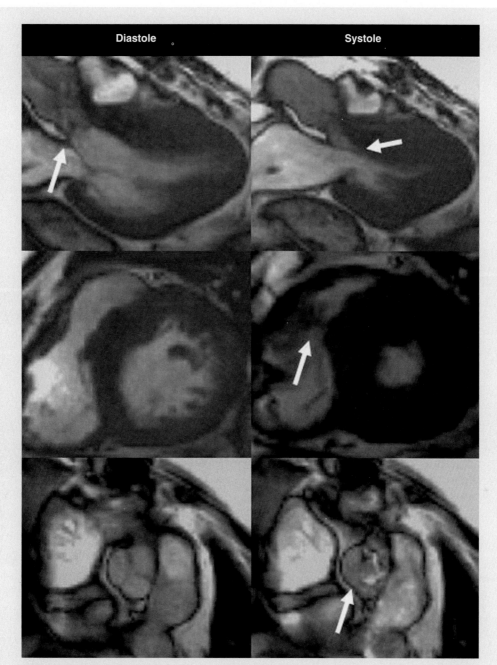

■ **Figure 11-9** Complex multilevel obstruction. **Top left,** Subaortic membrane (*arrowed*). **Top right,** Left ventricular outflow tract obstruction with SAM (*arrows*). **Middle,** Right ventricular outflow tract obstruction with turbulent flow (*arrows*). **Bottom,** Restricted noncoronary cusp motion (*arrows*).

Phenocopy examples include storage disorders such as Anderson-Fabry's disease (AFD), amyloid, and athlete's heart. In the latter, hypertrophy is concentric (eccentric), wall thickening appears supranormal, and the hypertrophy is not at the expense of cavity size—cavities are large and there is no late gadolinium enhancement. The others can be more difficult. Typically AFD patients have basal inferolateral LGE in the early stages (Figure 11-12), but this may be absent.

Cardiac amyloidosis is an uncommon disease characterized by deposition of amyloid protein in the myocardium, causing apparent hypertrophy and a restrictive cardiomyopathy. The pattern of LGE is subendocardial, affecting all four chambers diffusely in up to 70% of cases and resulting in high myocardial Gd-DTPA concentrations (particularly at the endocardium) making blood and myocardium null synchronously (both appear dark).

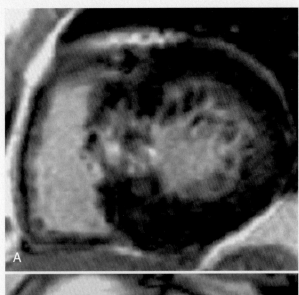

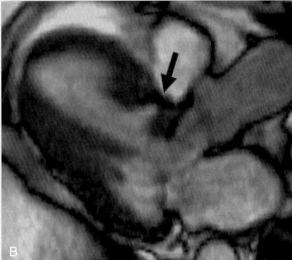

■ **Figure 11-10 A,** Acute myocardial infarction of alcohol septal ablation demonstrating transmural LGE. Note that in this case, the acute infarct has dark islands of microvascular obstruction where no gadolinium has entered the myocardium. **B,** A follow-up ablation patient several years post septal ablation showing thinning of the septum. However, in this case, there is a residual missed septal bulge causing recurrent LVOTO.

PROGRESSIVE DISEASE

The natural history of HCM over time often includes some wall thinning, cavity size increase, and a reduction in ejection fraction. In some (up to 3% prevalence) progression to severe heart failure occurs. Some patients progress to systolic impairment and a "dilated cardio-myopathy-like" burnt out stage, also known as progressive disease. This may result in marked cavity dilatation, systolic impairment, and thinning of previously hypertrophied walls. The natural history of HCM can be profiled in families where individuals of different ages are at different stages of disease expression (Figure 11-13). Patients with progressive disease almost invariably have extensive late gadolinium enhancement (Figure 11-14).

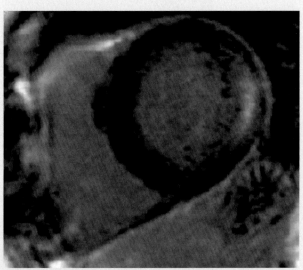

■ **Figure 11-12** Typical focal basal infero-lateral LGE in Anderson Fabry disease. LGE can occur in any pattern, however, and distinguishing from HCM is not possible.

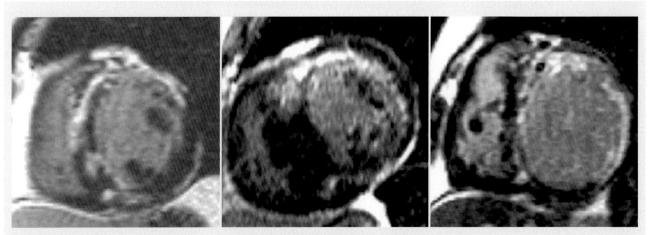

■ **Figure 11-11** Fibrosis as a final common pathway: sarcomeric HCM (**Left**), AFD (**Middle**), glycogen storage disease IIIa GSDIIIa (**Right**).

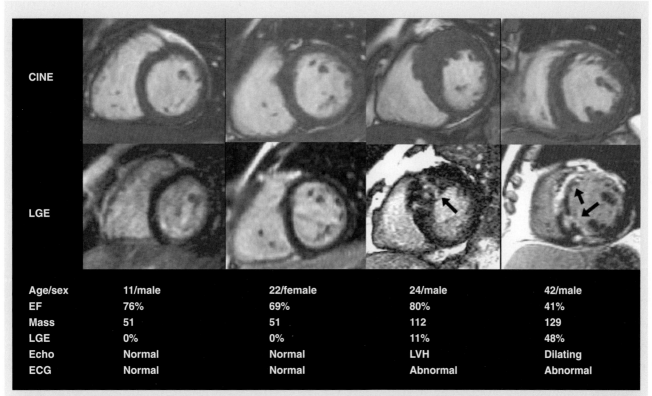

Age/sex	11/male	22/female	24/male	42/male
EF	76%	69%	80%	41%
Mass	51	51	112	129
LGE	0%	0%	11%	48%
Echo	Normal	Normal	LVH	Dilating
ECG	Normal	Normal	Abnormal	Abnormal

■ **Figure 11-13** Natural history of HCM. Single family with hypertrophic cardiomyopathy at different ages and degrees of phenotypic expression. On the left, an asymptomatic carrier with normal investigations, moving thorough mild expression with LVH and ECG changes and small amounts of LGE (*arrowed*) to the patient on the right with a dilating, failing ventricle and extensive LGE (arrows).

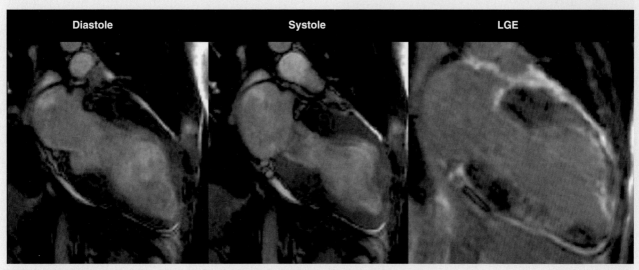

■ **Figure 11-14** Progressive disease in HCM. Poor LV systolic function, basal hypertrophy, apical thinning, and extensive diffuse LGE.

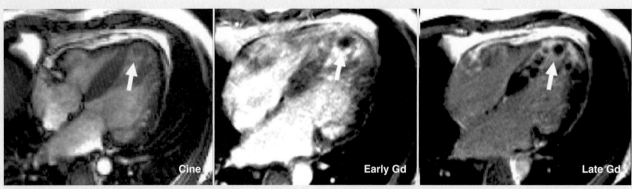

■ **Figure 11-15** Thrombus confirmed by early Gd imaging in progressive disease. Gd does not enter avascular tissue and hence, thrombus appears black, forming on thinned, aneurysmal/akinetic myocardium. Early Gd imaging should be performed in all patients with suspected recent infarction, severe LV dysfunction, and other prothrombotic conditions (e.g., malignant hypereosinophilia) to elucidate thrombus.

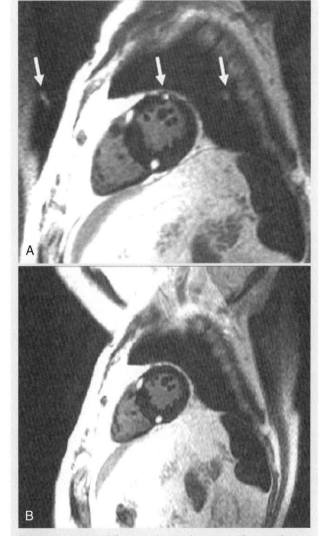

■ **Figure 11-16** Pitfalls: nonischemic ghosting artifact. **A,** Three apparent areas of LGE can be seen. **B,** After a phase encoding direction swap, only the two genuine areas remain. There appears to be a cyst in the lung ghosting across the image

Rarely in advanced disease when thinning has occurred and regional systolic function is poor, LV thrombus may form (Figure 11-15).

PITFALLS

Bad Piloting in Apical Hypertrophic Cardiomyopathy

In patients with suspected apical cardiomyopathy, it is important to ensure that adequate care is taken in the piloting of the long-axis views. Small errors in piloting can lead to erroneous impressions of wall thickness at the apex along with the potential to miss apical microaneurysms or overestimate cavity obliteration. Several long-axis cross-sections through the LV at reduced (5 mm) slice thickness should be taken to ensure the true apex is interrogated.

Late Gadolinium Enhancement Artifact

Apparent areas of LGE may sometimes be seen, with no abnormality present. This represents artifact induced by ghosting from areas of high signal elsewhere such as cerebrospinal fluid. This can be removed by placing a saturation band over the area of high signal or by inducing a phase encoding direction swap (Figure 11-16).

Diffuse Interstitial Expansion

The late gadolinium enhancement technique relies on differential areas of fibrosis. This is because the magnet operator sets the MR parameter for its detection based on the normal signal intensity of myocardium to set the nulling point (or black point) of myocardium. If fibrosis is very diffuse then the operator will set abnormal myocardium as nulled resulting in missed LGE (Figure 11-17). Patient optimization of LGE is outlined in Table 11-3.

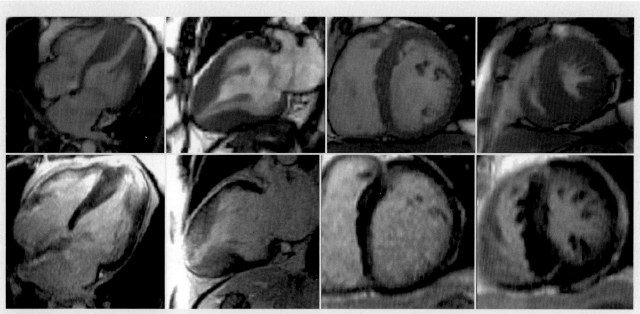

(*arrows*).

■ **Figure 11-17** Diffuse interstitial expansion in HCM. Long axis views show LGE toward the apex; this is not seen in the apical short axis image. This is because the LGE imaging relies on the operator nulling the majority of the myocardium. In the apical SA view, all the myocardium has a degree of diffuse interstitial expansion—and all is nulled (apart from some RV insertion point LGE). This highlights a

TABLE 11-3 Patient Optimization of LGE

PATIENT CHARACTERISTIC	STANDARD IR-FLASH	MODIFIED IR-FLASH	STANDARD IR-FISP	MODIFIED IR-FISP
Normal	Trigger 2 Segments 23 20-degree flip angle 115-140 lines (14 heart beats)		Trigger 2 Segments 65 50- to 60-degree flip angle 130 lines (12 heart beats)	
HR less than 800 ms		Trigger 3 Segments 19-21 Flip angle 22 degrees	Trigger 3 or 4 Segments 45	Trigger 3 or 4 Segments 45
HR variable		Trigger 3 (if possible)		Trigger 3 or 4 Consider systolic scanning
For endomyocardium				Scan in systole; acquisition window low as possible: segments 30 Wait until blood pool down
Severe fluid ghosting				Increase FOV; switch PE direction; use presaturation bands. Consider shorter scan or single shot.
Poor breath-hold				Segments 65 or single shot 1 average

Terminology here is Siemens based. For a conversion to other scanners see http://www.scmr.org/technologists/documents/crossvendorlexicon.pdf and http://radiographics.rsnajnls.org/cgi/content/full/e24/DC1

CONCLUSION

CMR combines a variety of different techniques to provide clinically useful information in HCM. It is established in the clinical management of patients with roles ranging from diagnosis to risk stratification, prognosis, planning surgical procedures, and differentiating phenocopies.

SUGGESTED READING

Choudhury L, Mahrholdt H, Wagner A, et al: Myocardial scarring in asymptomatic or mildly symptomatic patients with hypertrophic cardiomyopathy. J Am Coll Cardiol. 2002;40:2156-2164.

Moon JC, Fisher NG, McKenna WJ, Pennell DJ: Detection of apical hypertrophic cardiomyopathy by cardiovascular magnetic resonance in patients with non-diagnostic echocardiography. Heart. 2004;90:645-649.

Moon JC, McKenna WJ, McCrohon JA, et al: Toward clinical risk assessment in HCM with gadolinium CMR. J Am Coll Cardiol 2003;41:1561-1567.

Rickers C, Wilke NM, Jerosch-Herold M, et al: Utility of cardiac magnetic resonance imaging in the diagnosis of hypertrophic cardiomyopathy. Circulation 2005;112:855-861.

Valeti US, Nishimura RA, Holmes DR, et al: Comparison of surgical septal myectomy and alcohol septal ablation with cardiac magnetic resonance imaging in patients with hypertrophic obstructive cardiomyopathy. J Am Coll Cardiol 2007 Jan 23;49(3):350-357.

Chapter 12

Iron Cardiomyopathy

John C. Wood and Nilesh Ghugre

KEY POINTS

- Iron cardiomyopathy remains the leading cause of death in transfusional siderosis.

- Heart and endocrine gland iron overload occurs from chronic exposure to nontransferrin bound iron.

- Different organs have unique kinetics of iron uptake and clearance.

- Serum ferritin and liver iron are useful but insufficient markers of cardiac and endocrine risk.

- Cardiac magnetic resonance (CMR) can be use to quantitate iron deposition in many tissues, including the heart.

- CMR visualizes the safely stored iron, so patients may be presymptomatic, but relative risk of organ complications increases proportionally to the amount of stored iron.

- Annual measurements of liver iron, cardiac iron, and cardiac function are becoming the standard of care in transfusional siderosis.

- Cardiac toxicity is completely reversible in most situations with intensive chelation, although full recovery may take years.

DISEASE RESPONSIBLE FOR IRON OVERLOAD

Table 12-1 lists the most common diseases responsible for primary (nontransfusional) iron overload as well as the most common forms of secondary (transfusional) siderosis. Hemochromatosis types 1 to 4 represent hyperabsorption syndromes. Genetic defects in key iron regulatory proteins lead to loss of negative feedback of iron absorption. Primary iron ingestion, outside of acute overdosing, is generally restricted to cultures that perform fermentation in iron vessels. Some porphyrin pathway defects are associated with hepatic and extrahepatic iron accumulation. Liver disease, resulting from alcohol, hepatitis, and metabolic syndromes, often produces isolated hepatic siderosis. Cardiac iron has been well documented in hereditary hemochromatosis, particularly types 1 and 2, but is otherwise relatively uncommon in nontransfusional siderosis. Thalassemia major and sickle cell disease are among the most common genetic disorders in the world. Because genetic heterozygosity conveys a survival advantage for malaria, disease prevalence is greatest in the Middle East, Mediterranean, Africa, India, China, and the Far East. Iron overload in myelodysplastic syndromes is becoming more problematic as improved chemotherapeutic regimens lengthen life expectancy from the primary disease. Similarly, improved outcomes in a number of cancer therapies have increased the number of survivors bearing large transfusional iron stores. Cardiac iron overload is relatively common in all forms of transfusional siderosis, depending on the intensity and duration of transfusional support.

TABLE 12-1 Etiologies of Primary and Secondary Hemochromatosis

NONTRANSFUSIONAL IRON OVERLOAD	TRANSFUSIONAL IRON OVERLOAD
Hereditary Hemochromatosis	Thalassemia major
Type 1: HFE	Sickle cell disease
Type 2: Hemojuvelin, Hepcidin	Myelodysplastic syndromes
Type 3: TFR2	Blackfan-Diamond syndrome
Type 4: Ferroportin	Congenital dyserythropoietic anemia
Iron ingestion	Pure red cell aplasia
Heme metabolism disorders	Iatrogenic marrow suppression
Liver disease	

ORGANS AFFECTED BY IRON OVERLOAD

The anterior pituitary, particularly gonadotrophic cells, appear to be the most sensitive organs to iron deposition (Table 12-2). However, iron deposition occurs in all endocrine organs with variable clinical penetrance. Liver damage includes fibrosis, cirrhosis, and hepatocellular carcinoma, although clinical manifestations are generally delayed compared with the other disorders. Cardiac iron deposition occurs in approximately two thirds of adults with thalassemia major and remains the leading cause of death. Prevalence of iron-mediated complications is less well characterized in other forms of transfusional siderosis. Early diagnosis has greatly reduced organ complications in nontransfusional siderosis.

IRON ADSORPTION AND TRANSPORT

Inorganic iron (Fe^{2+}) enters the body via dimethyl transferase 1 (DMT1) in the enterocyte with assistance of the colocalized reductase duodenal cytochrome B (DCytB). A separate transporter, heme carrier protein 1 (HCP1), is responsible for transporting heme moieties resulting from breakdown of animal products. Within the enterocyte, free iron interacts with the iron storage protein ferritin as well as iron response elements that regulate iron-trafficking gene expression. Iron export through the apical membrane occurs through a transmembrane channel known as ferroportin and its colocalized reductase, haephestin. Figure 12-1 illustrates the paths of iron adsorption and transport.

The second major source of intravascular iron is through red blood cell phagocytosis in hepatic and splenic macrophages. Free iron is pumped out of intracellular lysosomes via DMT1 (assisted by a reductase, STEAP1) and exported across the plasma membrane via ferroportin. A circulating reductase, ceruloplasmin, assists in oxidizing and loading the exported iron onto transferrin.

Transferrin shuttles iron to the bone marrow for subsequent red cell synthesis and to the liver for storage. In the liver, transferrin binds to a transferrin receptor complex consisting of transferrin receptor 1 (TFR1), transferrin receptor 2 (TFR2), hemojuvelin (HJV), and hfe protein. Upon binding, transferrin-TFR1 complexes are

TABLE 12-2 Organs Affected by Iron Overload

ORGAN	CONSEQUENCE	AGE OF ONSET	POPULATION PREVALENCE
Pituitary	Hypogonadism, growth failure	Childhood	35%-55%
Pancreas	Diabetes	Adulthood	6.4%-10%
Thyroid	Hypothyroidism	Adulthood	9%-10.9%
Parathyroid	Parathyroidism	Adulthood	unknown
Adrenal	Adrenal insufficiency	Adulthood	unknown
Liver	Fibrosis, cirrhosis, malignancy	Adulthood	14%
Heart	Arrhythmia, heart failure	Adolescence	≈10%
Bone	Arthritis, osteoporosis	Adulthood	Variable

internalized into lysosomes and the TFR1 is recycled. The latter constituents of the TFR complex represent an iron-sensing element that regulates production of the hormone hepcidin. When transferrin saturation is high, hepcidin levels rise. Circulating hepcidin causes internalization of ferroportin in enterocytes and macrophages, lowering transferrin saturation and free iron levels.

In addition to transferrin saturation, hepcidin is positively regulated by the inflammatory cytokines interleukin 1 and interleukin 6, leading to low circulating iron levels during infections or other times of stress. This

represents the primary mechanism of the anemia of chronic disease. Hepcidin is negatively regulated by GDF15, an erythroblast-derived protein produced during severe anemia and during pregnancy. This facilitates iron absorption and transport to the bone marrow. The iron hyperabsorption observed in thalassemia intermedia syndromes is produced through this mechanism.

IRON STORES AND FLUXES

Normal iron uptake from the gut is around 1 mg/day and balances iron losses through sloughing of intestinal endothelia (Figure 12-2). Most of the iron (1800 mg) is consumed in the production of red blood cells in the marrow (lumped together as the "Erythron"). Muscle holds approximately 300 mg, mostly in the form of myoglobin. Liver has a dynamic repository of approximately 1000 mg. With such small iron input, there must be efficient iron recycling of senescent red blood cells by reticuloendothelial macrophages. Under normal conditions transferrin is only 30% to 40% saturated and there is no nontransferrin bound iron (NTBI). Extrahepatic organs do not take up significant amounts of transferrin bound iron. Chronic transfusion therapy adds approximately 0.3 to 0.5 mg/kg/day of iron (18 to 30 times the normal flux) into the erythron, overwhelming spontaneous elimination mechanisms. Transferrin carrying capacity saturates, producing toxic NTBI. NTBI is taken up readily by extrahepatic tissues, causing oxidative damage. NTBI also readily enters the liver and is significantly more toxic to the liver than transferrin bound iron, stimulating fibrosis and inflammation.

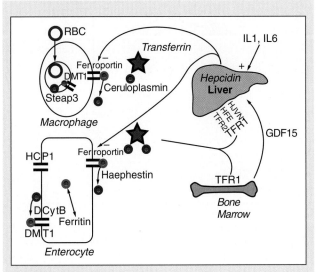

■ **Figure 12-1** A schematic illustrating the paths of iron adsorption and transport.

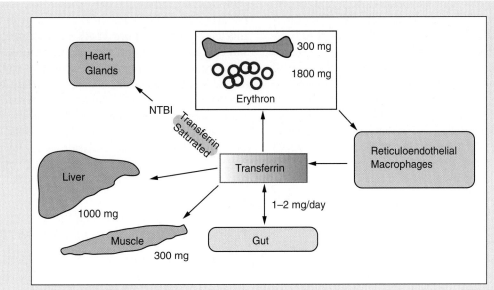

■ **Figure 12-2** Schematic illustrating iron stores and fluxes in normal subjects.

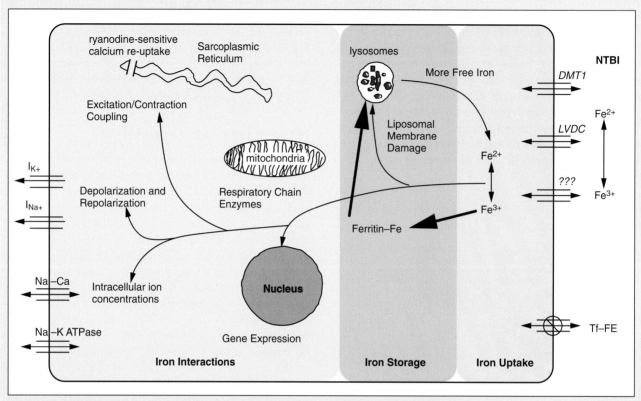

■ **Figure 12-3** Schematic of iron entry and toxicity in the heart. *(From Wood JC, Enriquez C, Ghugre N, et al: Physiology and pathophysiology of iron cardiomyopathy in thalassemia. Ann NY Acad Sci 2005;1054:386-395, with permission.)*

IRON ENTRY AND TOXICITY IN THE HEART

Iron enters the myocyte through divalent channels; both L-type voltage dependent channels and DMT1 have been implicated in different animal models (Figure 12-3). Transferrin-mediated uptake appears to be several orders of magnitude less important. Within the myocyte, ferritin quickly binds free iron and begins shuttling it to lysosomes for degradation and long-term storage. Iron stored with the lysosome is CMR-visible and forms the basis of noninvasive monitoring. If ferritin capacity is sufficient to maintain low labile iron stores, the heart has normal function despite CMR-detectable iron. However, when this capacity is overwhelmed, free-iron interacts with cardiac iron channels as well as catalyzing oxidative stress. Lipid peroxidation weakens lysosomal membranes, leading to rupture and further iron release in a catastrophic cascade. Iron impairs mitochondrial electron transduction and energy production. Ferrous iron noncompetitively inhibits the ryanodine calcium release channel, causing profound systolic dysfunction. Iron also compromises conduction through the fast sodium and delayed rectifier potassium channels, blunted conduction velocity and delaying repolarization. Last labile iron interacts with iron response elements to modify genetic transcription, promoting release of fibrinogenic factors.

CLINICAL FEATURES OF IRON CARDIOMYOPATHY

Often the earliest changes are nonspecific repolarization abnormalities on the electrocardiogram including QT prolongation, subtle leftward shift of the T-axis, as well as flattening or inversion of the T-waves in the inferior and lateral leads (Figure 12-4). First-degree heart block and cardiac arrhythmias are specific but insensitive findings, occurring in roughly 20% of heavily iron loaded patients. Arrhythmias can be either reentrant or triggered in nature and readily change morphology, consistent with a toxic myopathy. Cardiac iron deposition is greatest in working myocardium but can also be found in the atria and conduction system. Ablation is ineffective. Amiodarone can be effective for short-term stabilization, but aggressive iron chelation therapy is curative.

USE OF CARDIAC MAGNETIC RESONANCE TO DETECT IRON CARDIOMYOPATHY

Volumetric assessment of ventricular function by CMR provides more sensitive and robust detection of preclinical ventricular dysfunction than echocardiography (Figure 12-5). Stored cardiac iron is magnetically active and produces characteristic tissue darkening with length-

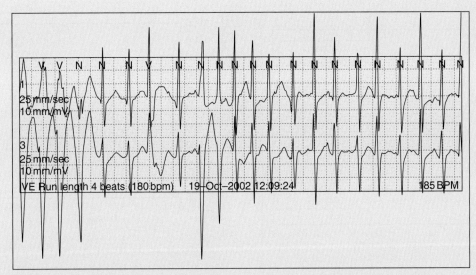

■ **Figure 12-4** Holter monitor recording of a patient with iron cardiomyopathy. Note the frequent atrial and ventricular premature beats and the four-beat run of nonsustained ventricular tachycardia.

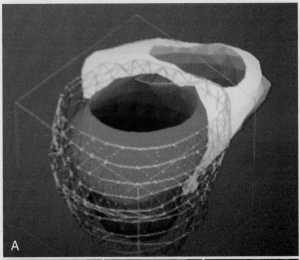

■ **Figure 12-5 A,** Volumetric assessment of ventricular function by CMR provides more sensitive and robust detection of preclinical ventricular dysfunction than echocardiography. More importantly, though, stored cardiac iron is magnetically active and produces characteristic tissue darkening with lengthening echo times (**B**). In a normal subject (**Bottom**), the heart muscle darkens at the same rate (from left to right) as chest wall muscle. In a patient with severe cardiac iron (**Top**), heart muscle darkens abruptly with increasing echo time. The half-life of tissue darkening is called T2* and the rate of darkening, R2*, is the reciprocal of T2*.

ening echo times. The half-life of tissue darkening is called T2* and the rate of darkening, R2*, is the reciprocal of T2*. Calculation of T2* is shown in Figure 12-6.

USE OF CARDIAC MAGNETIC RESONANCE TO MEASURE LIVER IRON

Liver R2* rises linearly with hepatic iron concentration (Figure 12-7). Liver R2, a similar relaxation parameter calculated from spin-echo instead of gradient-echo images, has a curvilinear relationship. Both have sufficient clinical accuracy for clinical use and have excellent interstudy reproducibility (5% to 7%). The liver represents the first organ where CMR iron quantitation was attempted because it is stationary. Liver is also the dominant iron storage organ in the body and accurately reflects total body iron balance. Experimental and clinical studies validating cardiac and liver CMR parameters are shown in Figures 12-8 to 12-10.

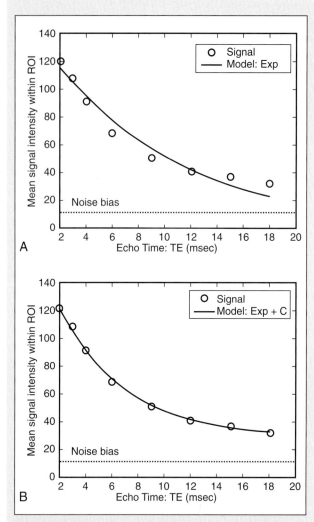

■ **Figure 12-6** Calculation of T2*. Average signal intensity is calculated from a region of interest encompassing the entire ventricular septum and plotted versus image echo time. In the presence of iron, there is initial rapid signal decay from the iron-rich myocardium. At late echo times, however, the signal is buoyed slightly by contributions from iron-poor tissues such as the blood volume. This extra contribution can confound simple monoexponential fits to the data, causing values to be inappropriately high (**Top**). This effect can be minimized by discarding the late echoes, fitting to two exponential functions, or by fitting to a monoexponential plus a constant offset (**Bottom**). All three techniques give reasonable answers if properly constrained. Newer black-blood T2* imaging methods have also reduced this problem. *(From Ghugre NR, Enriquez CM, Coates TD, et al: Improved R2* measurements in myocardial iron overload. J Magn Reson Imaging 2006;23:9-16, with permission.)*

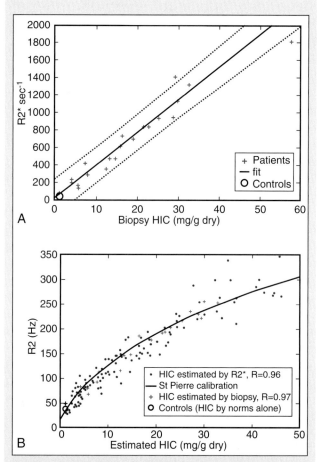

■ **Figure 12-7** Liver R2 and liver R2* are plotted as functions of hepatic iron concentration. Liver R2* (reciprocal of T2*) rises linearly with hepatic iron concentration. Liver R2, a similar relaxation parameter calculated from spin-echo instead of gradient-echo images, has a curvilinear relationship. *(From Wood JC, Enriquez C, Ghugre N, et al: MRI R2 and R2* mapping accurately estimates hepatic iron concentration in transfusion-dependent thalassemia and sickle cell disease patients. Blood 2005;106:1460-1465, with permission.)*

diac and liver iron burdens are nearly uncorrelated with one another. This disparity arises because the kinetics and mechanisms of iron uptake are organ specific. Although trends in serum ferritin as well as hepatic iron concentrations provide useful guidance for iron chelation, they provide inadequate information regarding cardiac risk to serve as the sole monitoring technique in iron overloaded patients.

RELATIONSHIP BETWEEN TOTAL BODY IRON STORES AND CARDIAC IRON

Figure 12-11 provides a graphical demonstration of the disparity between hepatic and cardiac iron loading. Multiple cross-sectional studies have demonstrated that car-

SLOW ELIMINATION OF CARDIAC IRON

Figure 12-12 highlights a patient who presented with a 48% ejection fraction, liver iron of 20 mg/g (normal, ≈1), and a cardiac T2* of 4.1 ms (normal, greater than 20 ms). Continuous deferoxamine administration completely de-

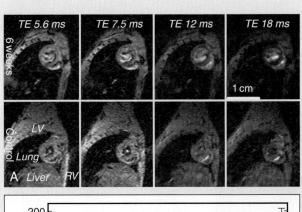

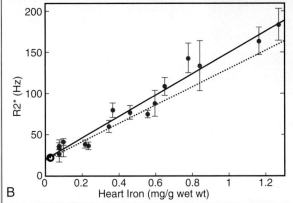

Figure 12-8 Experimental validation of cardiac T2*/R2* in the gerbil. Cardiac T2* imaging performed on a 1.5 Tesla clinical CMR machine in an iron overloaded (**Top**) and non iron overloaded (**Bottom**) gerbil. Cardiac R2* rises proportionally to cardiac iron concentration with a slope similar to that seen in gerbil liver tissue. *(From Wood JC, Otto-Duessel M, Aguilar M, et al: Cardiac iron determines cardiac T2*, T2, and T1 in the gerbil model of iron cardiomyopathy. Circulation 2005;112:535-543, with permission.)*

pleted his liver iron and improved his ejection fraction in 1 year; however, there was only a 50% improvement in his cardiac T2*. In fact, in a study by Anderson et al. (2004), the predicted "half-life" of cardiac iron clearance was roughly 20 months compared with 2.5 months for liver iron clearance. Terminating the chelation therapy after 1 year would have left the patient at high risk for recurrence. Low-dose continuous therapy was continued for 18 months with complete resolution of detectable cardiac iron.

TEMPORAL RELATIONSHIPS BETWEEN CARDIAC AND LIVER IRON

Longitudinal trajectories of heart and liver iron provide more information than cross-sectional studies. Figure 12-13 demonstrates cardiac R2* (a surrogate for cardiac iron) versus hepatic iron concentration in some instructive cases. Some patients exhibit fairly large fluctuations

in liver iron without accumulation of cardiac iron. However, persistent, severe elevations in liver iron often result in fairly precipitous cardiac iron accumulation. Thus high liver iron should be considered a negative prognostic sign and appropriately treated. However, Figure 12-13 (right panel) also demonstrates two patients who prospectively developed detectable cardiac iron despite having relatively modest liver iron levels. Therefore there is really no "safe" liver iron or ferritin level where cardiac iron will definitely not occur. These observations reinforce the necessity of routine cardiac iron screening in these patients.

CARDIAC IRON RISK IN NON-THALASSEMIC IRON OVERLOAD

Figure 12-14 compares cardiac T2* values versus ejection fraction in patients with both transfusional and nontransfusional sideroses. Thalassemia major and the other transfusional anemias demonstrate significant cardiac iron loading. The nontransfusional anemias do not demonstrate cardiac iron loading, although some ventricular dysfunction is noted. Although the sickle cell disease patients have similar total body iron burden to the other chronically transfused patients, their prevalence of cardiac iron is quite low. However, mild cardiac dysfunction is relatively common in this population, independent of cardiac iron, suggesting a different mechanism of cardiotoxicity. The explanation for the lower prevalence of cardiac iron and the noniron cardiotoxicity are areas of active research. Some studies suggest that NTBI levels are lower in sickle cell disease for any given somatic iron burden and may be related to a higher inflammatory tone in these patients. Taken together, these data indicate that cardiac risk depends upon the underlying disease in addition to the iron exposure.

WHEN SHOULD CARDIAC IRON SCREENING BE INITIATED?

Figure 12-15 demonstrates cardiac T2* as a function of age in 77 pediatric patients. No child under the age of 9.5 years old had detectable iron. There was a steep increase through the teenage years with an odds ratio of 1.28 per year. Thus in patients who have been well transfused and chelated since birth, routine CMR screening can be safely deferred until 8 years of age when they can be studied without anesthesia (approximately 175 units packed red blood cell [PRBC] exposure). In unchelated adult patients this threshold is lower (70 to 100 units) and can occur as quickly as 2 to 4 years.

SUMMARY OF IRON CHELATION THERAPY

The goal of iron chelation in acute heart failure is clearance of labile iron species. This is best achieved by continuous (24/7) administration of deferoxamine at doses of

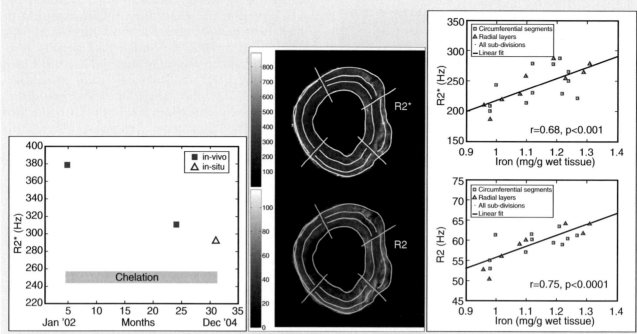

■ **Figure 12-9** Experimental validation of cardiac R2, R2* in humans. A thalassemia major patient was diagnosed with iron cardiomyopathy and placed on continuous deferoxamine therapy. Her symptoms resolved and cardiac iron levels slowly improved over a 2.5-year period (**Left**). She was immunosuppressed because of severe alloimmunization and she subsequently succumbed to overwhelming sepsis. Permission for limited autopsy and in vitro CMR measurements were obtained. Regional variation in CMR parameters and iron concentrations was compared with one another, generating a heart-specific iron calibration curve (**Right**). Both R2 and R2* rose proportionally to cardiac iron concentration with slopes comparable to those observed in liver. *(From Ghugre NR, Enriquez CM, Gonzalez I, et al: MRI detects myocardial iron in the human heart. Magn Reson Med 2006;56:681-686, with permission.)*

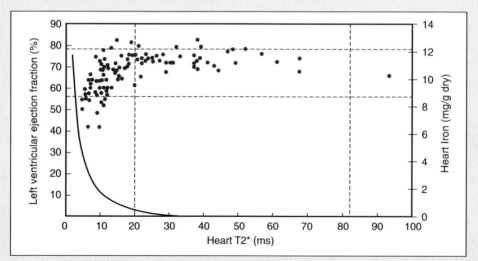

■ **Figure 12-10** Clinical Validation of Cardiac T2*/R2*. The relationship between left ventricular ejection fraction (LVEF) and cardiac T2* in thalassemia major patients is demonstrated. Normal T2* is greater than 20 ms; all patients with normal T2* have a normal ejection fraction. As T2* decreases (indicating more cardiac iron), the probability of left ventricular dysfunction increases. The solid line represents the predicted absolute cardiac iron concentration for a given T2* value. Note the sharp increase in predicted iron for T2* less than 10 ms, corresponding with an equally precipitous increased prevalence of left ventricular dysfunction. In clinical practice, the T2* value itself is used to grade the severity of cardiac iron deposition rather than a predicted iron level. Patients with T2* values less than 8 to 10 ms are at exceptionally high risk of cardiac complications and are increasingly being treated with intensive chelation even if their cardiac function is currently normal. Cardiac T2* has also proved to be an excellent biomarker for monitoring cardiac response to chelator therapies. *(From Wood JC, Otto-Duessel M, Aguilar M, et al: Cardiac iron determines cardiac T2*, T2, and T1 in the gerbil model of iron cardiomyopathy. Circulation 2005;112:535-543, with permission.)*

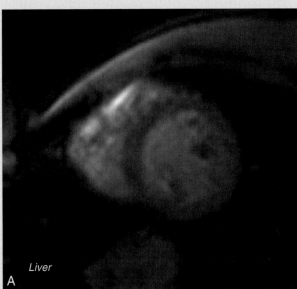

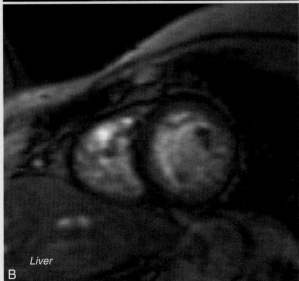

Figure 12-11 A graphical demonstration of the disparity between hepatic and cardiac iron loading. *(From Wood JC: Magnetic resonance imaging measurement of iron overload. Curr Opin Hematol 2007;14:183-190, with permission.)*

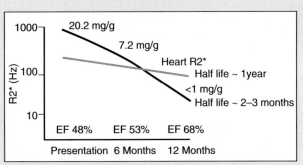

Figure 12-12 This patient who presented with a 48% ejection fraction, liver iron of 20 mg/g (normal, ≈1), and a cardiac T2* of 4.1 ms (normal, greater than 20 ms). Continuous deferoxamine administration completely depleted his liver iron and improved his ejection fraction in 1 year; however, there was only a 50% improvement in his cardiac T2*.

50 to 75 mg/kg/day. Deferoxamine is renally excreted, so kidney function must be supported by medication or dialysis if depressed. Continuous deferoxamine therapy removes between 4% and 5% of stored cardiac iron per month, but its benefits to cardiac rhythm and functional stabilization often occur on a time scale of 3 to 6 months or sooner. Iron cardiomyopathy is completely reversible, regardless of the initial ejection fraction, as long as organ perfusion can be adequately supported. Addition of the oral iron chelator deferiprone, to facilitate intramyocyte iron stabilization and chelation, can be considered in countries where the drug is licensed. It can also be used in the United States on compassionate use protocols approved by the FDA. Deferasirox, although the leading chelator for asymptomatic iron overload, remains unproven in acute iron cardiomyopathy. Table 12-3 presents a summary of iron chelation medications.

COMORBID DEFICIENCIES IN IRON CARDIOMYOPATHY

Patients with heart disease universally have panendocrine dysfunction (Table 12-4). As a result we place pressor-dependent patients on stress-dose steroids, empirically, while evaluating all of the other endocrine axes. Thiamine, vitamin D, carnitine, zinc, and selenium can also be profoundly deficient in these patients and empiric replacement therapy should be considered.

ROLE OF STANDARD CARDIOMYOPATHY THERAPIES

Digoxin and furosemide (Lasix) are well tolerated in TM patients (Table 12-5). Titration of afterload reduction can be complicated by orthostasis because chronically anemic patients already have low systemic vascular resistance. Arrhythmias are generally best treated with amiodarone because of its broad spectrum of action and patient tolerability; long-term therapy is rarely required if patients are being appropriately chelated. Given the disease reversibility, the use of implantable cardiac defibrillators (ICD) should be discouraged unless the short-term sudden death risk is unacceptably high. ICD placement precludes future CMR analysis that is critical for proper chelation management. Similarly, cardiac transplantation should be reserved for patients in whom organ support cannot be maintained long enough for iron chelation therapy to be effective.

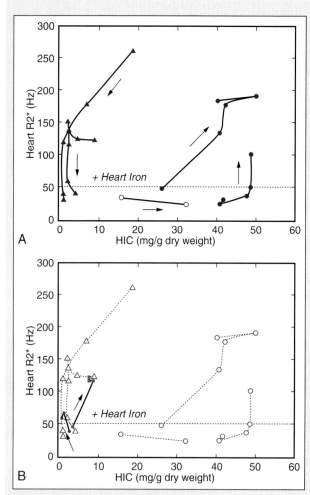

■ **Figure 12-13** Comparison of cardiac R2* (a surrogate for cardiac iron) versus hepatic iron concentration in some instructive cases. *(From Wood JC: Magnetic resonance imaging measurement of iron overload. Curr Opin Hematol 2007;14:183-190, with permission.)*

■ **Figure 12-14** Comparison of cardiac T2* values versus ejection fraction in patients with thalassemia major (TM), chronically transfused sickle cell disease (SCD), other transfusional sideroses (Tx), including Blackfan-Diamond syndrome, congenital dyserythropoietic anemia and pyruvate kinase deficiency, and nontransfusional iron overload (NTx), including hereditary hemochromatosis and thalassemia intermedia. Thalassemia major and the other transfusional anemias demonstrate significant cardiac iron loading; there is also markedly increased prevalence of cardiac dysfunction when T2* is less than 10 ms (*blue vertical line*). The nontransfusional anemias do not demonstrate cardiac iron loading, although some ventricular dysfunction is noted.

TABLE 12-4 Endocrine and Nutritional Deficiencies in Iron Cardiomyopathy

ENDOCRINE	NUTRITIONAL
Thyroid hormone	Thiamine
Parathyroid hormone	Vitamin D
Growth hormone	Carnitine
Insulin	Zinc
Mineralocorticoids	Selenium

TABLE 12-3 Iron Chelation Therapy

CHELATOR	DOSE	COMMENTS
Deferoxamine	50-75 mg/kg/D, subQ/IV	Must be given 8-12 hours per day for routine chelation and 24/7 for heart failure
Deferiprone	75-100 mg/kg/day, PO	Can be used alone or in combination with deferoxamine. Risk of agranulocytosis
Deferasirox	20-30 mg/kg/day, PO	Unproven in heart failure

TABLE 12-5 Conventional Heart Failure Strategies in Thalassemia

THERAPY	COMMENTS
Diuretics	First-line therapy. Well tolerated
ACE inhibition	First-line therapy. Associated with significant orthostasis
Digoxin	First-line therapy. Well tolerated
Beta blockade	Effective and generally well-tolerated. Watch glucose control.
Amiodarone	Very effective. Prolonged therapy (greater than 1 year) rarely required
RF ablation	Ineffective
Implantable cardioverter-defibrillator therapy	Relatively contraindicated in a reversible cardiomyopathy
Cardiac transplantation	Relatively contraindicated in a reversible cardiomyopathy

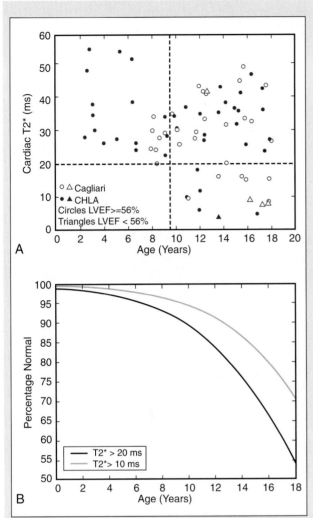

Figure 12-15 Cardiac T2* is shown as a function of age in 77 pediatric patients. Open symbols reflect data from Cagliari, Italy, and the filled symbols reflect data from Children's Hospital Los Angeles (CHLA). Circles represent patients with normal function and triangles represent patients with left ventricular dysfunction. Right panel demonstrates logistic regression for heavy cardiac iron (T2* less than 10 ms) and detectable cardiac iron (T2* less than 20 ms), respectively. *(From Wood JC, Origa R, Agus A, et al: Onset of cardiac iron loading in pediatric patients with thalassemia major. Haematologica 2008;93:917-920, with permission.)*

SUGGESTED READING

Adams PC, Barton JC: Haemochromatosis. Lancet 2007;370(9602):1855-1860.

Aessopos A, Berdoukas V, Tsironi M: The heart in transfusion dependent homozygous thalassaemia today—prediction, prevention and management. Eur J Haematol 2008;80(2):93-106.

Aessopos A, Farmakis D, Hatziliami A, et al: Cardiac status in well-treated patients with thalassemia major. Eur J Haematol 2004;73(5):359-366.

Anderson LJ, Holden S, Davis B, et al: Cardiovascular T2-star (T2*) magnetic resonance for the early diagnosis of myocardial iron overload. Eur Heart J 2001;22(23):2171-2179.

Anderson LJ, Westwood MA, Holden S, et al: Myocardial iron clearance during reversal of siderotic cardiomyopathy with intravenous desferrioxamine: a prospective study using T2* cardiovascular magnetic resonance. Br J Haematol 2004;127(3):348-355.

Borgna-Pignatti C, Rugolotto S, De Stefano P, et al: Survival and complications in patients with thalassemia major treated with transfusion and deferoxamine. Haematologica 2004;89(10):1187-1193.

Cabantchik, ZI, Breuer W, Zanninelli G, et al: LPI-labile plasma iron in iron overload. Best Pract Res Clin Haematol 2005;18(2):277-287.

Ganz, T: Molecular control of iron transport. J Am Soc Nephrol 2007;18(2):394-400.

Ghugre N, Enriquez C, Coates TD, et al: Improved R2* measurements in myocardial iron overload. J Magn Reson Imaging 2006;23(1):9-16.

Ghugre NR, Enriquez CM, Gonzalez I, et al: MRI detects myocardial iron in the human heart. Magn Reson Med 2006;56(3): 681-686.

Pennell DJ, Berdoukas V, Karagiorga M, et al: Randomized controlled trial of deferiprone or deferoxamine in beta-thalassemia major patients with asymptomatic myocardial siderosis. Blood 2006;107(9):3738-3744.

St Pierre TG, Clark PR, Chua-anusorn W, et al: Noninvasive measurement and imaging of liver iron concentrations using proton magnetic resonance. Blood 2005;1105(2):855-861.

Tanner MA, Galanello R, Dessi C, et al: A randomized, placebo-controlled, double-blind trial of the effect of combined therapy with deferoxamine and deferiprone on myocardial iron in thalassemia major using cardiovascular magnetic resonance. Circulation 2007;115(14):1876-1884.

Tanner MA, He T, Westwood MA, et al: Multi-center validation of the transferability of the magnetic resonance T2* technique for the quantification of tissue iron. Haematologica 2006;91(10):1388-1391.

Westwood MA, Anderson LJ, Maceira AM, et al: Normalized left ventricular volumes and function in thalassemia major patients with normal myocardial iron. J Magn Reson Imaging 2007;25(6):1147-1151.

Wood JC: Diagnosis and management of transfusion iron overload: the role of imaging. Am J Hematol 2007;82(12 Suppl):1132-1135.

Wood JC, Enriquez C, Ghugre N, et al: Physiology and pathophysiology of iron cardiomyopathy in thalassemia. Ann N Y Acad Sci 2005;1054: 386-395.

Wood JC, Origa R, Agus A, et al: Onset of cardiac iron loading in pediatric patients with thalassemia major. Haematologica 2008;93(6):917-920.

Wood JC, Otto-Duessel M, Aguilar M, et al: Cardiac iron determines cardiac T2*, T2, and T1 in the gerbil model of iron cardiomyopathy. Circulation 2005;112(4):535-543.

Wood JC, Tyszka JM, Carson S, et al. Myocardial iron loading in transfusion-dependent thalassemia and sickle-cell disease. Blood 2004;103(5):1934-1936.

Chapter 13

Myocarditis

Matthias G. Friedrich and Oliver Strohm

KEY POINTS

- Cardiovascular magnetic resonance (CMR) can be used to assess myocardial inflammation.

- A single CMR study provides comprehensive information on ventricular size, morphology, function, pericardial involvement, and inflammatory activity.

- Inflammatory activity of the myocardium can be assessed by:

  - T2-weighted CMR (identifies global or regional edema)

  - T1-weighted, gadolinium (Gd)-enhanced CMR shortly after contrast injection (hyperemia and capillary leakage caused by inflammatory activity)

  - T1-weighted, Gd-enhanced CMR late after contrast injection ("late Gd enhancement" identifies inflammation-induced irreversible injury)

- A combination of these sequences and derived criteria increases the diagnostic accuracy of CMR.

- CMR is useful for the follow-up of patients with complicated or ongoing myocarditis.

- CMR is useful for identifying patients suitable for endomyocardial biopsy.

Case 1   **Acute Myocarditis**

A 42-year-old man, previously healthy and active, presented with new-onset severe chest pain at rest, shortness of breath, and generalized weakness after a GI infection with severe diarrhea 2 weeks before. CMR was performed (Figures 13-1 to 13-5).

Comments

Myocardial inflammation may be caused by a variety of diseases such as viral infection, toxic agents, or autoimmune processes. The incidence has been underrated because of a lack of specific clinical findings and more importantly sensitive tools to detect myocarditis in clinical settings. Although usually of benign prognosis, more severe cases of myocarditis come with a substantial mortality. Endomyocardial biopsy with immunohistology is considered by many the gold standard. Its utility as a first line diagnostic tool, however, is significantly hampered by its limited sensitivity and invasiveness.

Cardiovascular MR (CMR) is being increasingly used in various clinical scenarios of myocarditis. The contribution of CMR in suspected myocarditis includes:

- Regional and/or global ventricular dysfunction
- Inflammatory activity in the myocardium
- Inflammation-induced irreversible tissue damage
- Pericardial involvement

For quantitatively assessing function, steady-state free precession techniques provide a very robust image quality and also allow for looking at pericardial effusion. It should be emphasized that the accurate quantification of ventricular size and ejection fraction/stroke volume are of specific use in the follow-up of patients with myocarditis, who may have only minor functional abnormalities.

The versatile MR technology is (as in other organ systems) especially helpful to identify inflammatory tissue characteristics. Three different criteria are being used:

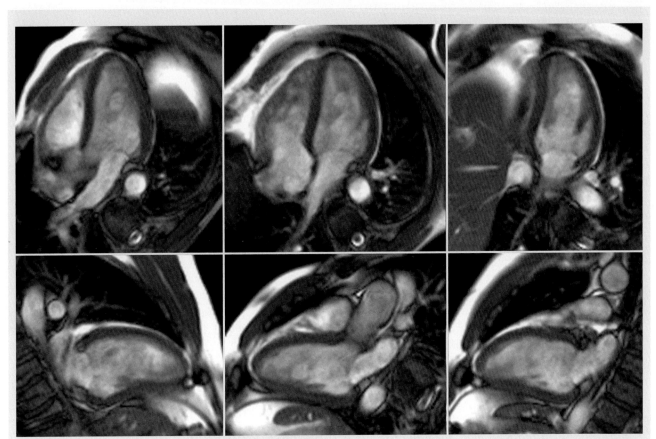

■ **Figure 13-1** End-diastolic frames, six long-axis views, obtained during two breath-holds using a multi-element coil and parallel acquisition: Normal end-diastolic left ventricular dimensions (LVEDV 168 ml = 100 ml/m height), normal mass (LVM 149 g, 89 g/m height).

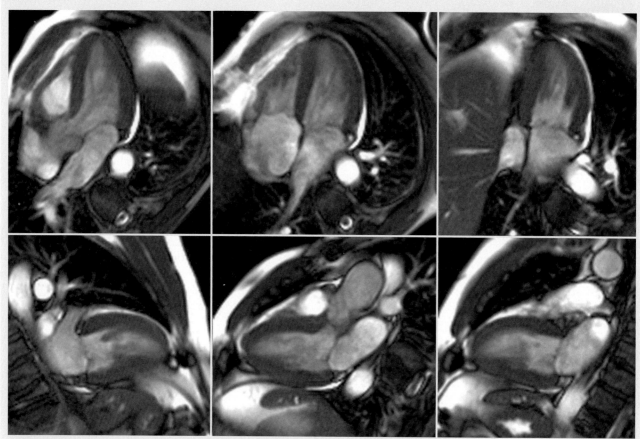

■ **Figure 13-2** End-systolic frames of the same cine set: Mild global systolic dysfunction (LVESV 84 ml; LVEF 50%).

- Globally or regionally increased water content in T2-weighted images (inflammatory edema)
- Globally increased blood volume (inflammatory hyperemia) and increased early distribution of interstitial Gd compounds (capillary leakage) in T1-weighted images pre- and early post-contrast administration (early enhancement). This is calculated using the following formula:

$$\frac{SI_{myo}(postcontrast) - SI_{myo}(precontrast)/SI_{myo}(precontrast)}{SI_{skeletal}(postcontrast) - SI_{skeletal}(precontrast)/SI_{skeletal}(precontrast)}$$

Alternatively, a myocardial enhancement (SI_{myo}(postcontrast) $-$ SI_{myo}(pre contrast)/SI_{myo}(precontrast) $\times 100\%$) of 45% indicates myocarditis.

- Necrosis and/or fibrosis as markers for irreversible inflammatory tissue damage of the myocardium and the pericardium in T1-weighted images later after contrast administration (late Gd enhancement)

Using two positive out of three criteria yields a diagnostic accuracy of at least 80% to detect or rule out myocarditis.

Case 2   **Acute Myocarditis**

A 40-year-old man presented with new-onset palpitations and mild shortness of breath during exercise. His recent medical history is empty; he does not remember any infection. CMR was performed in this patient (Figures 13-6 to 13-9).

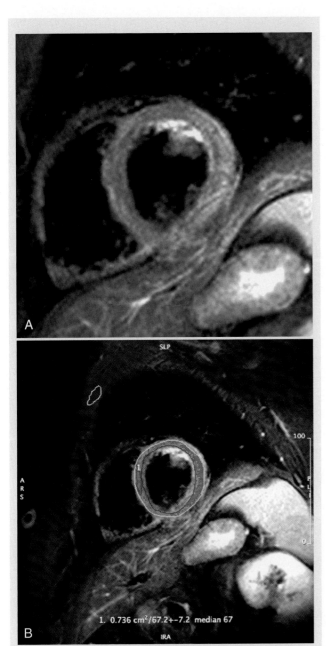

■ **Figure 13-3 A,** Short-axis T2-weighted spin echo image (breath-hold, slice thickness 15 mm, body coil): Increased normalized signal intensity (SI myocardium/SI skeletal muscle) of 2.2 (normal, less than 2.0) with higher values of the lateral and inferolateral segments (visually not apparent). **B,** Semiautomatic evaluation of the same image showing increased signal intensity of the lateral and inferolateral segment indicating regional edema, color-coded in red, reflecting pixels with signal intensity of greater than 2SD above mean of remote myocardium.

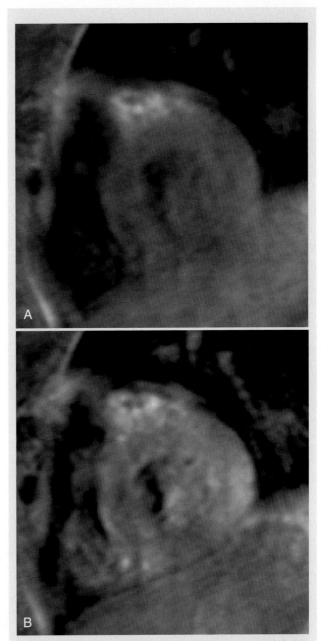

■ **Figure 13-4 A,** Short-axis T1-weighted image (non–breath-hold) before contrast administration. **B,** Repeated T1-weighted image (non–breath-hold) through the first 3 minutes after contrast administration ("early enhancement"). Although a strong signal intensity increase is visually apparent in the lateral region, the diagnostic criterion acquired in this sequence is the quantitative global myocardial signal enhancement normalized to that of skeletal muscle (8.1; normal, less than 4.0).

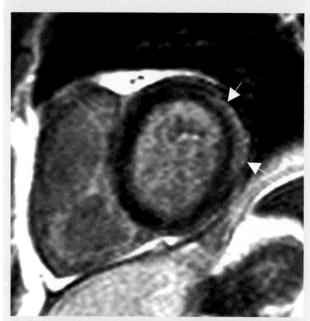

■ **Figure 13-5** Short-axis T1-weighted image ("late enhancement") shows mainly epicardial area with high signal intensity in the lateral and inferolateral segments, indicating nonischemic necrosis/fibrosis (*arrows*). The regional distribution allows for excluding an ischemic origin of tissue damage, which generally would include the subendocardial layers.

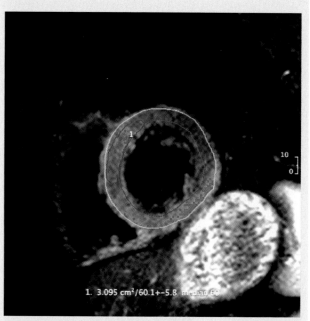

■ **Figure 13-7** Short-axis T2-weighted STIR image; the semiautomatic evaluation reveals inferolateral epicardial edema, color-coded in red, reflecting pixels with signal intensity of greater than 2SD above mean of remote myocardium.

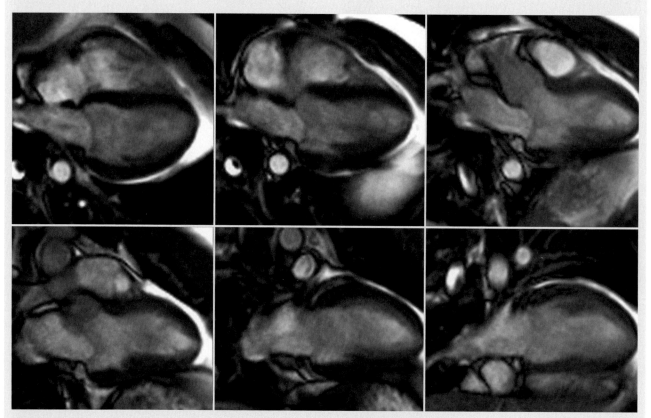

■ **Figure 13-6** End-diastolic frames, six long axis views, obtained during two breath-holds using a multielement coil and parallel acquisition: Normal LV size (LVEDV 133 ml, 73 ml/m height), LVEF low normal with 55%, normal LV mass of 133 g, 73 g/m height.

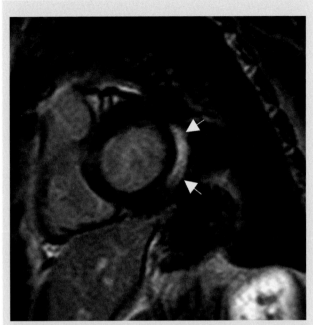

■ **Figure 13-8** Basal short view/late enhancement: Epicardial enhancement in the lateral and inferolateral segment, sparing the subendocardial layer (*arrows*).

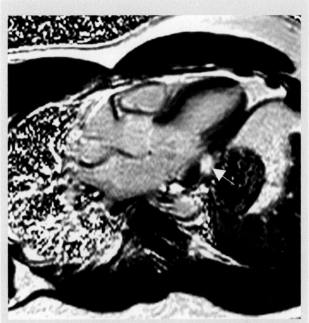

■ **Figure 13-9** Three-chamber view/late enhancement: Localized enhancement in the basal inferolateral segment (*arrow*), cross-referenced to Figure 13-7.

Comments

T2-weighted images may have a limited signal-to-noise ratio. A slice thickness of more than 10 mm typically increases the signal-to-noise ratio sufficiently. Edematous myocardium may visually appear normal, thus additional signal intensity quantification may be useful.

Such a comprehensive CMR protocol can be performed by experienced centers in less than 25 minutes and provides all the necessary information for diagnostic and therapeutic decision making. As previously proposed by others, CMR should be considered as the first-line diagnostic tool in patients with suspected myocarditis. Its safety is of special importance in patients with myocarditis, who often are young and may need follow-up studies. Similar considerations render CMR also a role in other forms of myocardial inflammation such as transplant rejection and cardiotoxicity. Pertinent data in these areas, however, are yet limited.

Recent technical advances allow for a more robust image quality of T2-weighted CMR and early enhancement images, shorter acquisition times, and even higher spatial and temporal resolution.

Case 3   **Postinflammatory Dilated Cardiomyopathy**

A 52-year-old patient with known dilated cardiomyopathy after severe myocarditis approximately 5 years before with worsening shortness of breath. He recently suffered an upper respiratory tract infection and developed ankle edema. CMR was performed (Figures 13-10 to 13-12).

Comments

This case illustrates the utility of late enhancement imaging for detecting persisting damage (scar) in patients with chronic disease. The presence of scar in combination with the lack of detectable inflammatory activity is consistent with a remote, irreversible injury (fibrosis/scar).

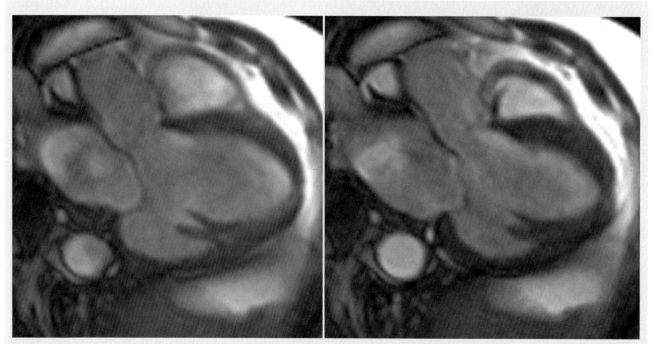

■ **Figure 13-10** Three-chamber view cine frames at end-diastole (**left**) and end-systole (**right**): Massive LV dilatation (LVEDV 368 ml, 213 ml /m height), severe reduction of systolic; function (EF 26%) and mild LV hypertrophy (185 g = 107 g/m height). Left atrium is normal in size, aortic and mitral valves are competent and are of normal appearance.

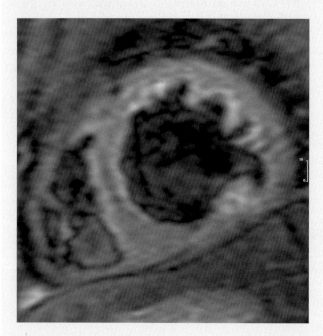

■ **Figure 13-11** Short-axis T2-weighted STIR image with homogenous signal intensity in the myocardium. Normal normalized signal intensity. This strongly indicates a lack of acute edema in the tissue.

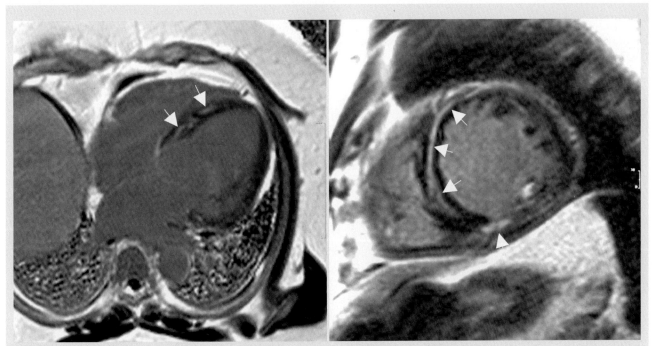

■ **Figure 13-12** Late enhancement images in four-chamber view (**left**) and mid ventricular short-axis (**right**) orientation: Midwall enhancement in the septum and in a single region of the inferior segment, consistent with nonischemic damage (*arrows*).

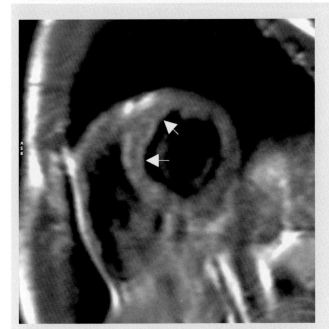

■ **Figure 13-13** Short-axis T2-weighted image: Evidence for myocardial edema of the anterior and anteroseptal segments with increased wall thickness and high signal intensity (*arrows*).

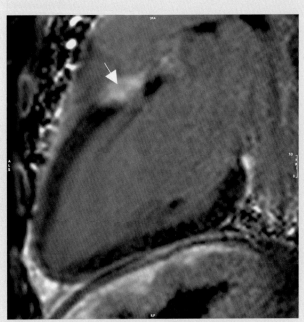

■ **Figure 13-14** Long-axis (two-chamber) view/late enhancement: Wedge-shaped area of late enhancement in the basal anterior segment. The damage is mainly subendocardial, clearly indicative of non-ischemic damage.

Case 4   **Myocarditis with Regional Edema**

A 34-year-old man presented with recent fatigue and atypical chest discomfort. He had a minor cold 4 weeks ago. There is ST elevation, but coronary arteries are normal on an invasive angiogram. CMR showed myocardial edema and subendocardial nonischemic damage (Figures 13-13 and 13-14).

Comments

Myocarditis can mimic acute myocardial infarction, including clinical presentation, enzyme release, and ST elevation. This case illustrates that focal inflammation may have an almost or even entirely transmural extent and thus come with pertinent ECG changes. The regional distribution allows for ruling out a primarily coronary event.

Case 5 **Healthy Volunteer**

CMR findings in a healthy volunteer are shown in Figures 13-15 to 13-17.

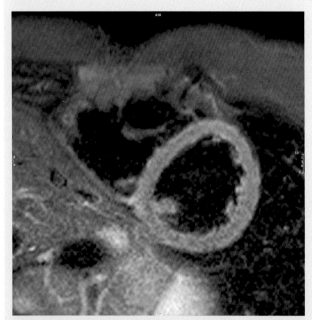

■ **Figure 13-15** Short-axis T2-weighted image: Homogenous myocardial signal, normal wall thickness. Normal signal intensity ratio myocardium : skeletal muscle (1.5; normal, less than 2.0).

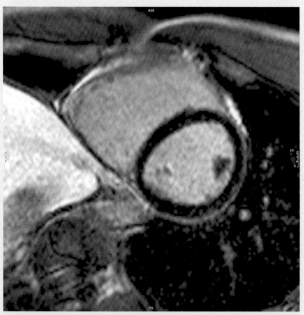

■ **Figure 13-17** Short-axis view/late enhancement: Homogenous myocardial signal suppression. The pericardium can easily be distinguished from the myocardium and shows normal thickness.

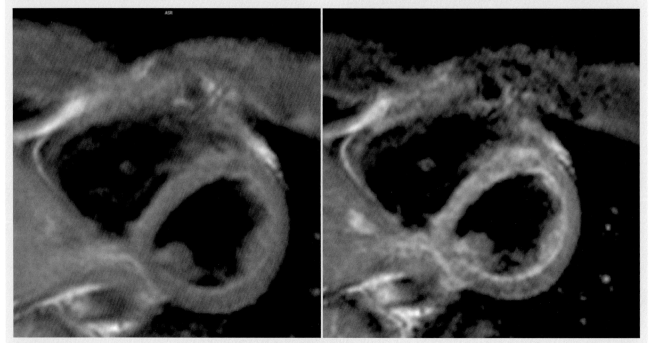

■ **Figure 13-16** Early enhancement in short axis before (**left**) and after (**right**) contrast application. Quantitative normalized enhancement (3.4; normal, less than 4.0).

SUGGESTED READING

Abdel-Aty H, Boye P, Zagrosek A, et al: Diagnostic performance of cardiovascular magnetic resonance in patients with suspected acute myocarditis: Comparison of different approaches. J Am Coll Cardiol 2005;45:1815-1822.

Assomull RG, Lyne JC, Keenan N, et al: The role of cardiovascular magnetic resonance in patients presenting with chest pain, raised troponin, and unobstructed coronary arteries. Eur Heart J 2007;28:1242-1249.

Friedrich MG, Strohm O, Schulz Menger J, et al: Contrast media-enhanced magnetic resonance imaging visualizes myocardial changes in the course of viral myocarditis. Circulation 1998;97:1802-1809.

Gutberlet M, Spors B, Thoma T, et al: Suspected chronic myocarditis at cardiac MR: Diagnostic accuracy and association with immunohistologically detected inflammation and viral persistence. Radiology 2008;246:401-409.

Ingkanisorn WP, Paterson DI, Calvo KR, et al: Cardiac magnetic resonance appearance of myocarditis caused by high dose IL-2: Similarities to community-acquired myocarditis. J Cardiovasc Magn Reson 2006;8:353-360.

Laissy JP, Hyafil F, Feldman LJ, et al: Differentiating acute myocardial infarction from myocarditis: Diagnostic value of early- and delayed-perfusion cardiac MR imaging. Radiology 2005;237:75-82.

Liu PP, Yan AT: Cardiovascular magnetic resonance for the diagnosis of acute myocarditis: Prospects for detecting myocardial inflammation. J Am Coll Cardiol 2005;45:1823-1825.

Magnani JW, Dec GW: Myocarditis: Current trends in diagnosis and treatment. Circulation 2006;113:876-890.

Mahrholdt H, Goedecke C, Wagner A, et al: Cardiovascular magnetic resonance assessment of human myocarditis: A comparison to histology and molecular pathology. Circulation 2004;109:1250-1258.

Mahrholdt H, Wagner A, Deluigi CC, et al: Presentation, patterns of myocardial damage, and clinical course of viral myocarditis. Circulation 2006;114:1581-1590.

Sarda L, Colin P, Boccara F, et al: Myocarditis in patients with clinical presentation of myocardial infarction and normal coronary angiograms. J Am Coll Cardiol 2001;37:786-792.

Skouri HN, Dec GW, Friedrich MG, Cooper LT: Noninvasive imaging in myocarditis. J Am Coll Cardiol 2006;48:2085-2093.

Wagner A, Schulz-Menger J, Dietz R, Friedrich MG: Long-term follow-up of patients with acute myocarditis by magnetic resonance imaging. Magma 2003;16:17-20.

Chapter 14

Simple Congenital Heart Disease

Rebecca S. Beroukhim and Tal Geva

KEY POINTS

- The distinction between "simple" and "complex" congenital heart disease is not well defined. In this chapter, simple congenital heart disease describes uncomplicated anatomic defects or shunt lesions that are not associated with other cardiovascular anomalies.

- This chapter describes cardiovascular magnetic resonance (CMR) findings in the following congenital cardiac anomalies:

  - Interatrial communications

  - Ventricular septal defect

  - Patent ductus arteriosus

  - Partially anomalous pulmonary venous connection

  - Coarctation of the aorta and bicommissural aortic valve

- CMR is usually used in concert with other imaging modalities for assessment of cardiovascular anatomy and function, measurements of blood flow, tissue characterization, and for evaluation of myocardial perfusion and viability.

- CMR is particularly helpful in adolescent and adult patients with congenital heart disease because it overcomes many of the limitations associated with echocardiography (e.g., restricted acoustic windows), cardiac catheterization (e.g., invasive, expensive, radiation exposure), computed tomography (e.g., radiation exposure, predominantly static anatomic information), and nuclear scintigraphy (e.g., low spatial resolution, lack of anatomic information, radiation exposure).

INTERATRIAL COMMUNCATIONS

Types of Interatrial Communications

Types of interatrial communications are shown in Figure 14-1. Patent foramen ovale (PFO) is the most common type of interatrial communication. Anatomically, it is located between normally formed septum primum and septum secundum. The second most common type of interatrial communication is secundum atrial septal defect, followed by primum atrial septal defect.

Secundum atrial septal defect (Figures 14-2 and 14-3) is a defect within the fossa ovalis, usually caused by a single or multiple defects within septum primum. Septum secundum is usually well formed. Most secundum atrial septal defects (ASDs) are not confluent with the vena cavae, right pulmonary veins, coronary sinus, or the atrioventricular (AV) valves. Primum atrial septal defect (Figures 14-4 to 14-6) is an endocardial cushion (AV canal) defect with an interatrial communication located between the anterior-inferior margin of the fossa ovalis and the AV valves. It is considered a form of partial AV canal defect with two separate AV valve annuli and no ventricular septal defect of the AV canal type. Sinus venosus defect is a communication between one or more of the right pulmonary veins and the cardiac end of the superior vena cava (SVC) and/or the posterior wall of the right atrium. Sinus venosus defect (Figures 14-7 to 14-9) comprises approximately 4% to 11% of interatrial communications. Although anatomically not a true atrial septal defect, sinus venosus defect results in an interatrial communication and is hemodynamically similar to an atrial septal defect.

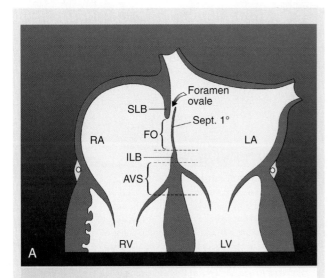

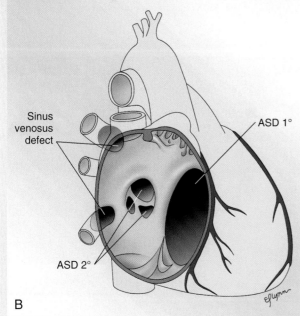

■ **Figure 14-1** Types of interatrial communications. **A,** Cross-section of the atria demonstrating the atrial septal components. Patent foramen ovale (PFO) is the most common type of interatrial communication. Anatomically, it is located between normally formed septum primum and septum secundum (*arrow*). AVS, atrioventricular septum; FO, fossa ovalis; ILB, inferior limbic band; LA, left atrium; LV, left ventricle; RA, right atrium; RV, right ventricle; Sept. 1⁰, septum primum; SLB, superior limbic band (septum secundum). **B,** The second most common type of interatrial communication is secundum atrial septal defect (ASD 2⁰), followed by primum atrial septal defect (ASD 1⁰). ASD 1⁰, primum atrial septal defect; ASD 2⁰, secundum atrial septal defect.

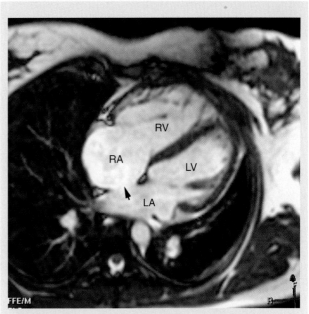

■ **Figure 14-2** ECG-gated steady-state free precession (SSFP) cine magnetic resonance (MR) image in the four-chamber plane showing a large secundum atrial septal defect. The defect results from a deficiency of septum primum. The hemodynamic consequence is a left-to-right shunt across the fossa ovalis. Note the dilated right atrium (RA) and right ventricle (RV). By velocity encoded cine MR measurements in the main pulmonary artery and ascending aorta, the pulmonary-to-systemic flow ratio measured 1.6. The defect was subsequently closed in the cardiac catheterization laboratory with an Amplatzer septal occluder.

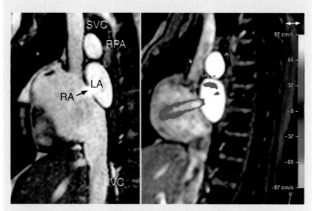

■ **Figure 14-3** Secundum atrial septal defect. **Left panel:** ECG-gated SSFP cine MR image in an oblique sagittal plane of the atrial septum, demonstrating a small secundum atrial septal defect. **Right panel:** ECG-gated velocity encoded cine MR in the same plane. Flow velocity is encoded in the anterior-posterior direction (in-plane; see *arrow* above color scale). Flow velocity and direction are color-encoded. Blue indicates flow from posterior (left atrium; LA) to anterior (right atrium; RA). Note the left-to-right flow jet through the secundum atrial septal defect.

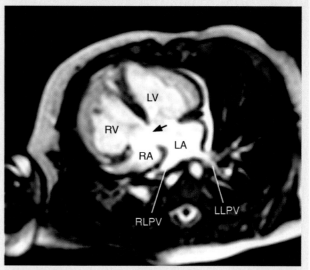

■ **Figure 14-4** ECG-gated SSFP cine MR image in the axial plane in an infant with heterotaxy syndrome and polysplenia. Note the dextrocardia and the large primum atrial septal defect (*arrow*). CMR was performed to evaluate the anatomy of the pulmonary veins to exclude stenosis as a potential cause of severe pulmonary hypertension. Note two unobstructed pulmonary venous connections into the left atrium. LA, left atrium; LV, left ventricle; RA, right atrium; RV, right ventricle; LLPV, left lower pulmonary vein; RLPV, right lower pulmonary vein.

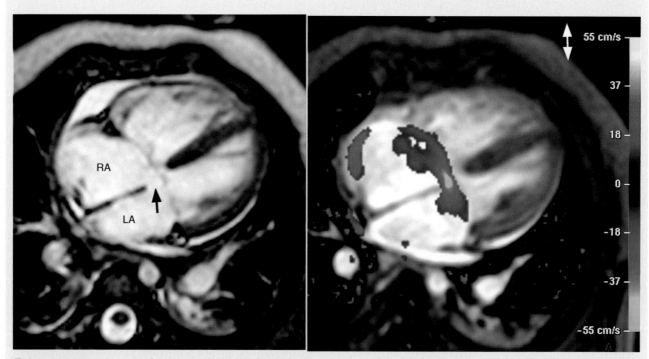

■ **Figure 14-5** CMR imaging of primum atrial septal defect. **Left panel:** ECG-gated, breath-hold cine SSFP MR image in the four-chamber plane. The primum atrial septal defect is located between the inferior rim of the fossa ovalis and the attachments of the AV valves to the ventricular septal crest (*arrow*). Note the intact fossa ovalis. **Right panel:** ECG-gated velocity encoded cine MR in the same plane. Flow velocity is encoded in the anterior-posterior direction (in-plane; see *arrow* next to color scale). Flow velocity and direction are color-encoded. Blue indicates flow from posterior (left atrium; LA) to anterior (right atrium; RA) through the primum atrial septal defect. Note the absence of flow at the ventricular level indicating absence of a ventricular septal defect component. By velocity encoded cine MR measurements in the main pulmonary artery and ascending aorta, the pulmonary-to-systemic flow ratio measured 1.7. The primum atrial septal defect was subsequently surgically closed with a pericardial patch.

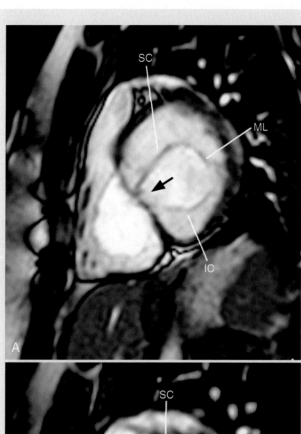

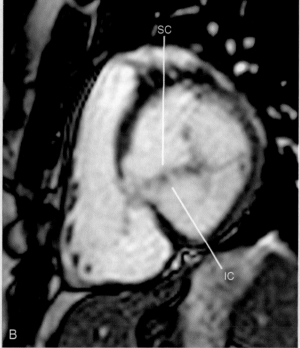

■ **Figure 14-6** Cleft anterior mitral valve leaflet in a patient with primum atrial septal defect. The anatomy of the AV valves is clearly seen on ECG-gated breath-hold cine SSFP MR images acquired in the short axis plane at the base of the ventricles. **A,** Diastolic frame showing the cleft between the superior and inferior components of the anterior mitral leaflet. The cleft is pointing toward the ventricular septal crest (*arrow*). **B,** Systolic frame showing the plane of coaptation between the superior and inferior components of the anterior mitral leaflet. IC, inferior component of the anterior mitral valve leaflet; SC, superior component of the anterior mitral valve leaflet; ML, mural (posterior) mitral valve leaflet.

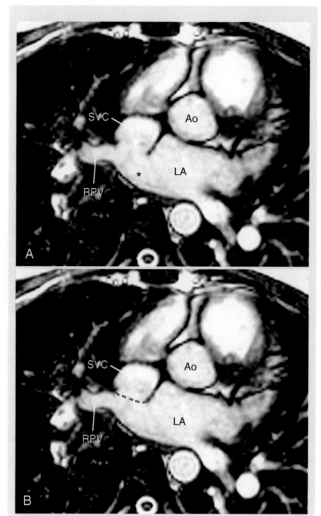

■ **Figure 14-7** Superior vena cava (SVC)-type sinus venosus defect. **A,** Axial plane ECG-gated breath-hold cine SSFP MR image depicting a defect between the posterior wall of the superior vena cava (SVC) and the anterior wall of the right pulmonary vein (RPV) (*arrow*). The communication between the left atrium (LA) and the superior vena cava is through the left atrial termination of the right pulmonary vein (*). **B,** The sinus venosus septum is depicted by the dashed line. Note the "normal" drainage of the right pulmonary vein once the sinus venosus septum is "restored." Ao, aorta.

Measurement of Pulmonary-to-Systemic Flow Ratio in Patients with Interatrial Communications

In the absence of associated cardiovascular anomalies and with normal pulmonary vascular resistance, interatrial communications result in a left-to-right shunt proximal to the AV valves. The volume of the left-to-right shunt depends on the size of the defect and the relative compliance of the right and left ventricles. Most patients are asymptomatic during childhood and adolescence. Some patients with unrepaired interatrial communications will develop complications during adult life, including pulmonary vascular disease, atrial arrhythmias, heart failure, and paradoxical emboli. Indications for closure of

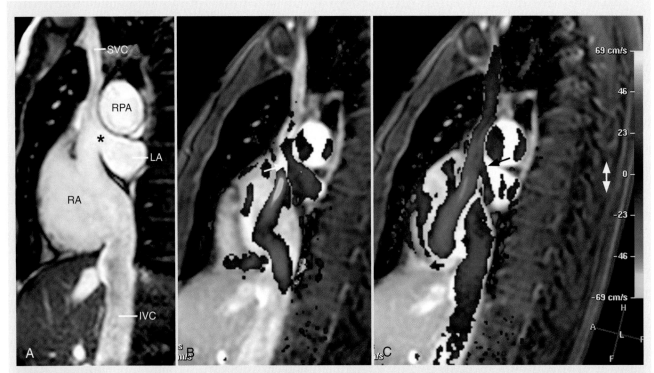

■ **Figure 14-8** Superior vena cava (SVC)-type sinus venosus defect. **A,** ECG-gated breath-hold cine SSFP
MR images acquired in an oblique sagittal plane, demonstrating a large defect between the posterior
wall of the superior vena cava (SVC) and the anterior wall of the right upper pulmonary vein (*). Note
that the resultant defect allows a communication between the left atrium (LA) and the superior vena
cava. Therefore this defect is not considered an atrial septal defect (ASD) because there is no direct
communication between the left and right atria. **B and C,** Systolic and diastolic frames from ECG-
gated velocity encoded cine MR in the same plane as **A.** Flow velocity is encoded in the superior-inferior
direction (in-plane; see *arrow* next to color scale in panel **C**). Flow velocity and direction are color
encoded. Blue indicates flow from superior to inferior and red indicates flow from inferior to superior.
Note the bidirectional flow through the sinus venosus defect. The net pulmonary-to-systemic flow ratio,
evaluated by through-plane velocity encoded cine MR perpendicular to the ascending aorta and main
pulmonary artery, measured 2.3.

interatrial communications in children include symptoms
(e.g., exercise intolerance, dyspnea, slow weight gain),
left-to-right shunt greater than 1.5 to 2.0 associated
with right ventricular volume overload, and paradoxical emboli. Although a patent foramen ovale or a small
secundum atrial septal defect may decrease in size or even
close spontaneously during infancy and early childhood,
larger secundum atrial septal defects can increase in size
during adulthood. Primum atrial septal defects and sinus
venosus defects almost never decrease in size over time.
CMR allows evaluation of the location and size of the
interatrial communication as well as quantitative assessment of the hemodynamic burden from the defect(s),
such as pulmonary-to-systemic flow ratio, right ventricular size and function, etc. (Figures 14-10 and 14-11).

VENTRICULAR SEPTAL DEFECTS

Different types of ventricular septal defects (VSDs) are
shown in Figure 14-12.

Conoventricular septal defect (Figure 14-13) results from
malalignment between the conal (outlet) septum superiorly and the muscular ventricular septum inferiorly. A
conoventricular septal defect may be membranous if its
posterior-inferior border is confluent with the tricuspid
valve or may be muscular if the inferior limb of septal
band forms its inferior-posterior border.

Membranous VSD (Figure 14-14) is located under the
commissure between the septal and anterior tricuspid
valve leaflets, at the site of the membranous septum.
It is bordered by fibrous tissue, which is contiguous
with tricuspid valve tissue. Anatomically, the membranous septum is located at the junction of the following
anatomic-embryologic segments of the interventricular
septum: atrioventricular canal (inlet) septum; the muscular septum between the left and right ventricular sinuses;
and the conal or infundibular (outlet) septum. Membranous VSDs vary in size and may involve adjacent septal
segments because of deficient myocardium in those segments. For example, membranous VSD with deficient

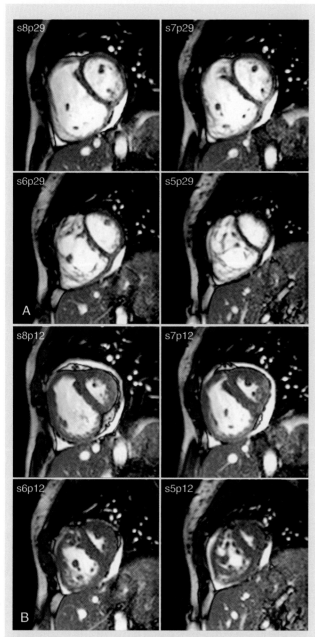

■ **Figure 14-9** Right ventricular volume load in a patient with SVC-type sinus venosus defect and a large left-to-right shunt with pulmonary-to-systemic flow ratio of 2.3. Ventricular short-axis ECG-gated breath-hold SSFP cine MR images in diastole (**A**) and systole (**B**). Note the dilated right ventricle and the flat systolic configuration of the interventricular septum in diastole (**A**) indicating volume overload. In systole (**B**), the interventricular septum maintains its flat configuration, indicating right ventricular hypertension. This patient was treated for pulmonary hypertension prior to successful surgical closure of her sinus venosus defect.

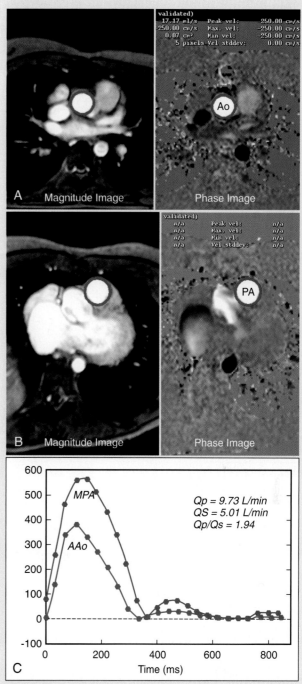

■ **Figure 14-10** ECG-gated, breathe-through velocity encoded cine MR perpendicular to the ascending aorta (**A**) and main pulmonary artery (**B**). **C,** Graph showing flow rate (Y axis) versus time (X axis) during the cardiac cycle. Stroke volume is the area under the flow rate-time curve. Multiplying the stroke volume by the heart rate yields the flow per minute (L/min) through the blood vessel. In this example, flow through the ascending aorta equals systemic blood flow (Qs) and flow through the main pulmonary artery equals pulmonary blood flow (Qp).

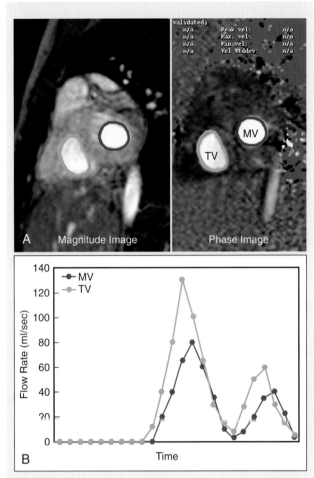

■ **Figure 14-11** ECG-gated, breathe-through velocity encoded cine MR perpendicular to the mitral (*red contour*) and tricuspid (*green contour*) valves (**A**). **B**, Graph showing flow rate (Y axis) versus time (X axis) during diastole. Stroke volume is the area under the flow rate-time curve. Multiplying the stroke volume by the heart rate yields the flow per minute (L/min). In patients with interatrial communications, flow through the mitral valve (MV) equals systemic flow (Qs) and flow through the tricuspid valve (TV) equals pulmonary blood flow (Qp). See Figure 14-19 for other examples of shunt calculations.

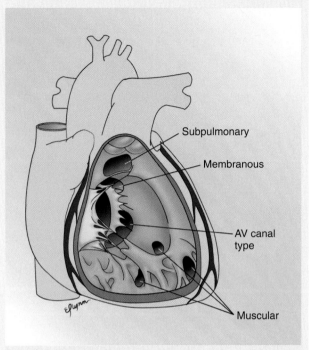

■ **Figure 14-12** Schematic diagram illustrating different types of ventricular septal defects (VSDs).

infundibular (outlet) septum is often described as "membranous VSD with outlet extension."

Atrioventricular canal-type VSD (also known as inlet VSD) results from deficiency within the ventricular aspect of the atrioventricular septum. The posterior border of the defect comprises the fibrous annulus of the AV valves. Other features of common AV canal defect (e.g., cleft mitral valve) may or may not be present.

Muscular VSD (Figure 14-15) results from a defect within the myocardium separating the left and right ventricular sinuses or between the left ventricle and the proximal infundibulum. The defect is entirely surrounded by myocardium, and does not involve the membranous septum or the AV or semilunar valves. Malalignment between embryologic-anatomic septal segments may be a contributing factor and multiple muscular VSDs are common.

Subpulmonary VSD (also called conal or infundibular, outlet, doubly committed, subarterial, and supracristal defects) is located within the infundibular septum, which separates the left and right ventricular outflow tracts. The pulmonary valve annulus often forms the superior border of the defect, but in some patients the defect is surrounded by myocardium. A prolapsing right coronary cusp of the aortic valve often restricts the left-to-right flow through the VSD.

Ventricular septal defect is the most common congenital heart disease diagnosed in infants and children with a median incidence of ≈2.8 per 1000 live births. Although VSD is often encountered as an isolated defect, it frequently accompanies many forms of congenital heart disease. The natural history of VSD relates to the size and location of the defect. The size of membranous and muscular defects often decreases during infancy and early childhood reaching spontaneous closure in many patients with a small or moderate initial defect size. In contrast, conoventricular, AV canal-type, and large subpulmonary VSDs usually do not decrease in size. The clinical course of patients with VSD is determined by the defect size, the resistances of the systemic and the pulmonary vascular beds, and presence of associated cardiovascular anomalies. When the resistance in the pulmonary vascular bed is lower than that of the systemic vascular bed, flow through the VSD is left-to-right, resulting in increased pulmonary blood flow and volume load on the left side of the heart. A small VSD rarely causes symptoms. Moderate or large VSDs are often associated with clinically significant pulmonary overcirculation, which leads to shortness

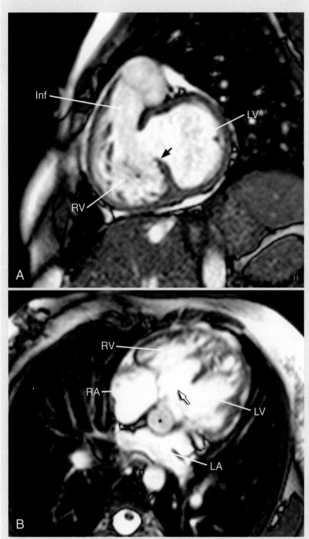

■ **Figure 14-13** ECG-gated breath-hold SSFP cine MR images showing a conoventricular VSD in a 49-year-old woman with pulmonary vascular disease and cyanosis. **A,** Ventricular short-axis diastolic image demonstrating the defect between the conal septum superiorly (*white arrow*) and muscular interventricular septum inferiorly (*black arrow*). Note mild anterior malalignment of the conal septum and an unobstructed infundibulum (Inf). **B,** Four-chamber view showing the subaortic (*) location of the conoventricular septal defect (*arrow*). Pulmonary-to-systemic flow ratio measured 0.68. LA, left atrium; LV, left ventricle; RA, right atrium; RV, right ventricle.

■ **Figure 14-14** ECG-gated breath-hold SSFP cine MR images showing a membranous VSD. **A,** Four-chamber view showing a large aneurysm of the membranous septum nearly completely covering the ventricular septal defect (*white arrow*). Note the small signal void on the right ventricular side of the membranous tissue corresponding to a small left-to-right flow jet (*black arrowhead*). **B,** Ventricular short-axis image showing the large aneurysm of the membranous septum (*white arrows*) and the tricuspid valve (*black arrowhead*). LA, left atrium; LV, left ventricle; RA, right atrium; RV, right ventricle.

of breath, diaphoresis, recurrent respiratory infections, and slow weight gain in infants and exercise intolerance in older patients. The pulmonary arteries and veins, left atrium, and left ventricle are typically enlarged because of increased blood flow. Symptomatic patients with a moderate or large VSD, in whom the likelihood of spontaneous decrease in defect size is deemed unlikely, are referred for VSD closure. Membranous, conoventricular, AV canal-type, and subpulmonary VSDs are almost always closed surgically. Some muscular defects can be closed in the catheterization laboratory using

septal occluders. Patients with untreated large VSDs may develop irreversible pulmonary vascular disease (Eisenmenger syndrome). Other complications include bacterial endocarditis, aortic valve prolapse and regurgitation, and left ventricular dysfunction. CMR allows evaluation of the location and size of VSDs and assessment of the hemodynamic burden from the defect(s) (e.g., measurements of the pulmonary-to-systemic flow ratio, left ventricular size and function, and qualitative assessment of right ventricular systolic pressure based on the systolic configuration of the interventricular septum).

PATENT DUCTUS ARTERIOSUS

The ductus arteriosus is derived from the embryonic distal left sixth aortic arch and normally closes within several hours after birth. It connects the aortic isthmus to the pulmonary artery bifurcation at the origin of the left pulmonary artery. Rarely the ductus arteriosus can be right-sided or bilateral (persistence of the embryonic distal right sixth aortic arch). Patent ductus arteriosus (PDA) is common in premature infants but is abnormal in full-term infants beyond the first week of life. The primary hemodynamic burden is caused by flow from the aorta to the pulmonary arteries throughout the cardiac cycle, which occurs when the pulmonary vascular resistance is lower than that of systemic vascular bed. The left-to-right shunt leads to volume load on the left side of the heart with dilatation of the pulmonary veins, left atrium, and left ventricle. Patients with a small PDA are usually asymptomatic. Persistence of a large PDA can lead to pulmonary vascular disease. Other complications include bacterial endocarditis, aneurysm formation and dissection, heart failure, and pulmonary hypertension. Treatment options include surgical ligation and/or division, which in many cases can be performed using either a video-assisted thoracoscopic approach or transcatheter coil occlusion. CMR is seldom used for assessment of an isolated PDA in infants and children because the clinically relevant information can usually be gleaned from echocardiography. When CMR is performed in a patient with PDA (Figure 14-16), the hemodynamic burden should be evaluated by measuring the pulmonary-to-systemic flow

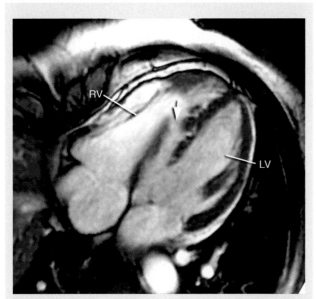

■ **Figure 14-15** ECG-gated breath-hold SSFP cine MR images in the four-chamber plane showing a muscular VSD (*arrow*). Note the malalignment between the basal and apical segments of the muscular septal components.

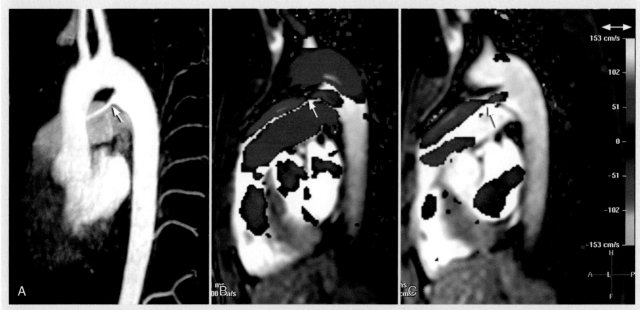

■ **Figure 14-16** Patent ductus arteriosus (PDA). **A,** Subvolume maximal intensity projection of gadolinium-enhanced three-dimensional magnetic resonance angiogram showing a small PDA (*arrow*). Note the ductal diverticulum at the inner curvature of the aortic isthmus. **B and C,** Systolic (**B**) and diastolic (**C**) frames from ECG-gated velocity encoded cine MR in the same plane as **A**. Flow velocity is encoded in the posterior-anterior direction (in-plane; see *arrow* next to color scale in panel **C**). Flow velocity and direction are color-encoded. Blue indicates flow from posterior to anterior and red indicates flow from anterior to posterior. Note the flow from the aorta to the main pulmonary artery through the PDA in systole and diastole.

ratio and by quantitative assessment of left ventricular size and function.

PARTIALLY ANOMALOUS PULMONARY VENOUS CONNECTION

Partially anomalous pulmonary venous connection (PAPVC) is defined as connection of one or more (but not all) of the pulmonary veins to a systemic vein (Figure 14-17). It is important to distinguish between anomalous *connection* and anomalous *drainage* of the pulmonary veins. The former is present when one or more pulmonary veins connect to a systemic vein via persistence of an embryonic connection between the splanchnic and the cardinal venous systems. In contrast, anomalous pulmonary venous drainage occurs when a normally positioned pulmonary vein(s) drains anomalously because of malposition of septum primum or unroofing of the sinus venosus septum, which separates the right pulmonary veins from the superior vena cava and/or right atrium. PAPVC results in an obligatory left-to-right shunt with

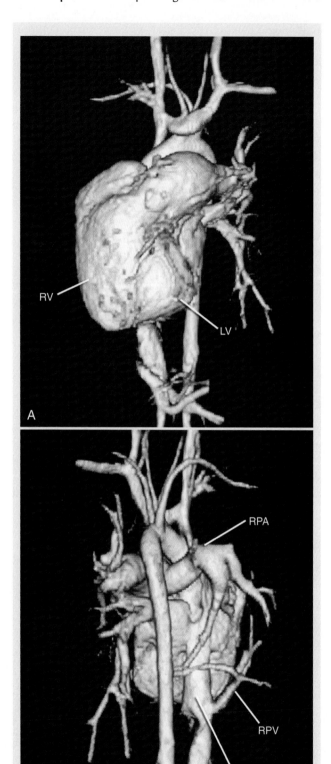

A

B

Figure 14-18 Scimitar syndrome. **A,** Anterior view of a volume rendered image of gadolinium-enhanced three-dimensional magnetic resonance angiogram showing dextrocardia and a dilated right ventricle (RV) and main pulmonary artery. **B,** Posterior view showing the right pulmonary veins (RPV) connecting to the inferior vena cava (IVC) as well as abnormal morphology of the right pulmonary artery (RPA).

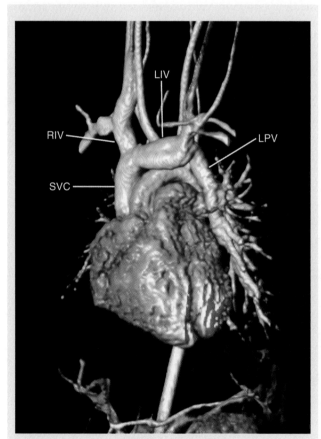

Figure 14-17 Anterior view of a volume-rendered image of gadolinium-enhanced three-dimensional magnetic resonance angiogram demonstrating partially anomalous pulmonary venous connection (PAPVC) of the left pulmonary veins (LPV) to the left innominate vein (LIV). Note the dilated left pulmonary veins that converge into a large ascending vertical vein, which connects to the left innominate vein with subsequent drainage to the superior vena cava (SVC). RIV, right innominate vein.

physiologic consequences similar to interatrial communications. The majority of children with a single PAPVC are asymptomatic, the degree of volume load on the right side of the heart is modest, and development of pulmonary vascular disease is rare.

Scimitar syndrome with anomalous connection of the right pulmonary veins to the inferior vena cava is an uncommon form of PAVC (Figure 14-18). Scimitar syndrome can be associated with hypoplasia of the right lung and right pulmonary artery, dextrocardia, collateral arterial blood supply to segments of the right lung from the descending aorta, and pulmonary sequestration. Some patients with scimitar syndrome present in early infancy with severe pulmonary hypertension, cyanosis, and heart failure. Other patients remain asymptomatic or minimally symptomatic well into adulthood. CMR is ideally suited for comprehensive evaluation of the pulmonary venous anatomy and assessment of the hemodynamic consequences, obviating the need for diagnostic cardiac catheterization in most patients.

EVALUATION OF PULMONARY-TO-SYSTEMIC FLOW RATIO BY CARDIOVASCULAR MAGNETIC RESONANCE

Abnormal communications between the left and right sides of the heart and between the systemic and the pulmonary circulations are common in patients with congenital heart disease. Cardiovascular magnetic resonance (CMR) allows accurate measurements of blood flow and evaluation of the pulmonary-to-systemic flow ratio. Figure 14-19 illustrates three examples of assessment of the pulmonary-to-systemic flow ratio (Qp/Qs)-atrial septal defect, ventricular septal defect, and patent ductus arteriosus. Pulmonary and systemic blood flow is measured by ECG-gated velocity-encoded cine MR perpendicular to the main pulmonary artery, ascending aorta, and AV valves. Additionally, left and right ventricular stroke volumes are measured using ECG-gated steady state free precession cine MR in the ventricular short-axis. Our practice is to evaluate the pulmonary-to-systemic flow ratio by velocity-coded cine MR and by volumetric stroke volume analysis, using the redundant data for internal confirmation.

COARCTATION OF THE AORTA

Coarctation of the aorta refers to narrowing of the aortic isthmus either with or without hypoplasia of the aortic arch. An atypical location may involve stenosis of other segments of the thoracic and abdominal aorta. Elongation and hypoplasia of the distal transverse arch between the left common carotid and left subclavian arteries are frequently associated with coarctation of the aorta. Bicommissural aortic valve is present in ≈22% to 42% of patients with coarctation of the aorta. In infancy, patients with severe coarctation present with symptoms of heart failure, systemic hypoperfusion, and shock. In the most severe cases survival depends on patency of the ductus arteriosus, and immediate intravenous administration of

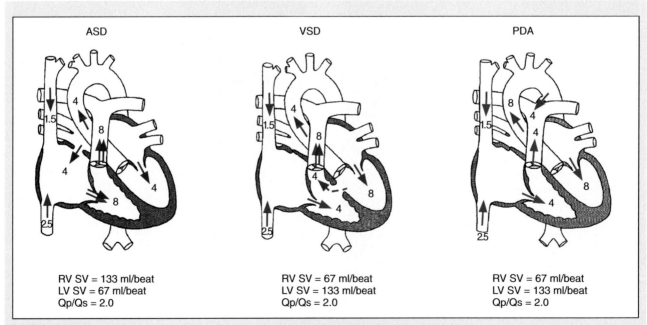

■ **Figure 14-19** Examples of flow measurements across the aortic, pulmonary, mitral, and tricuspid valves and left and right ventricular stroke volumes in hypothetical patients with atrial septal defect, ventricular septal defect, and patent ductus arteriosus. The arrows and numbers within the hearts represent direction and volume of flow (L/min). In all three examples, the pulmonary-to-systemic flow ratio is 2.

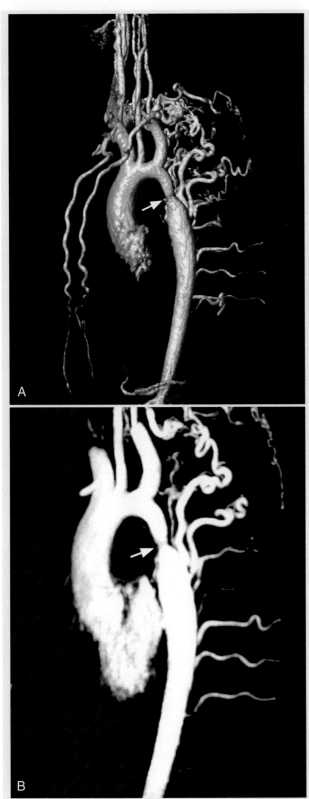

■ **Figure 14-20** Coarctation of the aorta. **A,** Lateral view of a volume rendered image of gadolinium-enhanced three-dimensional magnetic resonance angiogram demonstrating severe coarctation of the aorta (*arrow*) and multiple tortuous collateral vessels to the descending aorta. Note the dilated left and right internal mammary arteries. **B,** Maximum intensity projection of the same image dataset. Blood pressure measurements in the four extremities showed that the systolic pressure in the arms was 50 mm Hg higher than those measured in the legs. At cardiac catheterization, a stent was placed across the coarctation site with elimination of the pressure gradient.

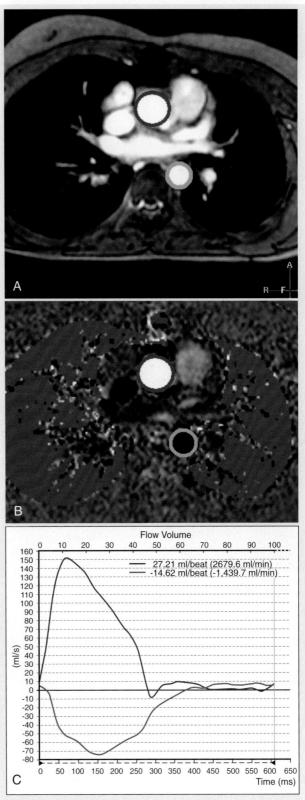

■ **Figure 14-21** ECG-gated velocity-encoded cine MR images perpendicular to the ascending and descending aorta in a patient with mild coarctation of the aorta. **A,** Magnitude image. **B,** Phase velocity image. **C,** Flow rate versus time in the ascending aorta (*red*) and descending aorta (*green*). Note the normal flow profile in the ascending aorta (*red*), and the abnormal flow profile in the descending aorta (*green*) characterized by blunting of the upstroke and a prolonged deceleration phase.

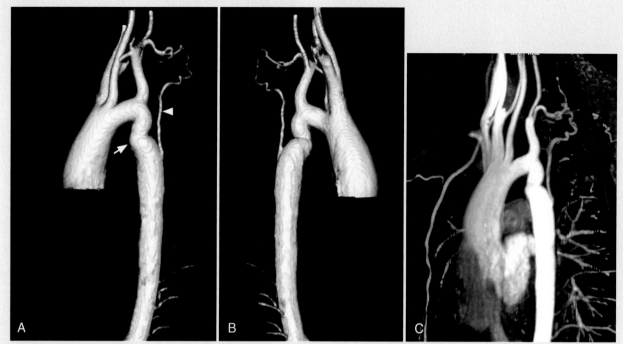

■ **Figure 14-22** Mild coarctation of the aorta. **A and B,** Left and right views of volume rendered image of gadolinium-enhanced three-dimensional magnetic resonance angiogram demonstrating elongation and tortuosity of the aortic isthmus (*arrow*). Note the increased distance between the left common carotid and left subclavian arteries and the small collateral vessel to the descending aorta (arrowhead). **C,** Maximum intensity projection image showing mild luminal narrowing at the coarctation site.

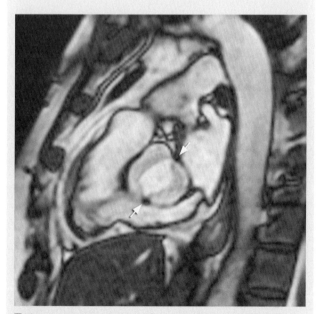

■ **Figure 14-23** Bicommissural aortic valve. Systolic frame of ECG-gated steady-state free precession (SSFP) cine MR image orthogonal to the aortic root showing underdevelopment and fusion of the intercoronary commissure and two large aortic valve leaflets. The well-developed left-noncoronary and right-noncoronary commissures are clearly seen (*arrows*). Bicommissural aortic valve is often associated with coarctation of the aorta.

prostaglandin E can be life-saving. Older children and adults with coarctation of the aorta are often asymptomatic and may present with systemic hypertension, diminished femoral pulses, and a continuous murmur heard best over the back related to collateral vessels. Without treatment, a hemodynamically important coarctation is associated with high morbidity, including heart failure, aortic aneurysm, premature coronary artery disease, cerebral aneurysms, and endocarditis. CMR plays an important role in the diagnosis and follow-up before and after repair of aortic coarctation, especially in older children and adults in whom echocardiography is limited by restricted acoustic windows. The goals of the CMR examination include anatomic assessment of the coarctation site, evaluation of collateral vessels, exclusion of associated anomalies (e.g., bicommissural aortic valve), and quantitative evaluation of left ventricular size and function (Figures 14-20 to 14-23).

SUGGESTED READING

Geva T, Powell AJ: Pediatric heart disease. In Edelman RR, Hesselink JR, Zlatkin MB, Crues JV (eds): Clinical Magnetic Resonance Imaging. Philadelphia, Saunders, 2006, pp 1041-1069.

Geva T, Powell AJ: Magnetic resonance imaging. In Allen HD, Driscoll DJ, Feltes T, Shaddy R (eds): Moss & Adams' Heart Disease in Infants, Children, and Adolescents, 7th Edition. Philadelphia, Lippincott Williams & Wilkins, 2008, pp 163-199.

Geva T, Van Praagh S: Anomalies of the pulmonary veins. In Allen HD, Driscoll DJ, Feltes T, Shaddy R (eds): Moss & Adams' Heart

Disease in Infants, Children, and Adolescents, 7th Edition. Philadelphia, Lippincott Williams & Wilkins, 2008, pp 761-792.

Greil GF, Powell AJ, Gildein HP, Geva T: Gadolinium-enhanced three-dimensional magnetic resonance angiography of pulmonary and systemic venous anomalies. J Am Coll Cardiol 2002;39:335-341.

Grosse-Wortmann L, Al-Otay A, Goo HW, et al: Anatomical and functional evaluation of pulmonary veins in children by magnetic resonance imaging. J Am Coll Cardiol 2007;49:993-1002.

Nielsen JC, Powell AJ, Gauvreau K, et al: Magnetic resonance imaging predictors of coarctation severity. Circulation 2005;111:622-628.

Powell AJ, Tsai-Goodman B, Prakash A, et al: Comparison between phase-velocity cine magnetic resonance imaging and invasive oximetry for quantification of atrial shunts. Am J Cardiol 2003;91:1523-1525.

Tsai-Goodman B, Geva T, Odegard KC, et al: Clinical role, accuracy, and technical aspects of cardiovascular magnetic resonance imaging in infants. Am J Cardiol 2004;94:69-74.

Valente AM, Sena L, Powell AJ, et al: Cardiac magnetic resonance imaging evaluation of sinus venosus defects: comparison to surgical findings. Pediatr Cardiol 2007;28:51-56.

Wald RM, Powell AJ: Simple congenital heart lesions. J Cardiovasc Magn Reson 2006;8:619-631.

Chapter 15

Complex Congenital Heart Disease

Mark A. Fogel

KEY POINTS

- Anatomic delineation of complex CHD is just that—complex. No assumptions should be made regarding anatomy; segments (atria, ventricles, and great vessels), intersegmental connections (atria-to-ventricle and ventricle-to-great vessel), and venous structures (systemic and pulmonary) must clearly be defined. The CMR imager needs to be aware of the spectrum of complex CHD along with the myriad of surgical reconstructions that can be performed to accomplish this successfully.

- As with anatomy, the physiologic and functional correlates of complex CHD are intricate. Delineation of which way blood is flowing and quantification of flow along with evaluation of ventricular and valve function are crucial to successful medical and surgical management. Understanding complex physiologic and functional principles to sort out the most intricate details is expected, even if the CMR imager has never had the opportunity to study a particular case before.

- Spatial relationships, both among the various cardiovascular structures and between cardiovascular structures and other thoracic and abdominal organs, are important to define. This not only aids in diagnosis but also helps the cardiovascular surgeon and pediatric cardiologist plan out repairs. As such, the CMR imager should have a good grasp of how to reconstruct the heart and other organs in three-dimensions in his or her mind and how to convey this information to other health care providers.

- The old cliché "the devil is in the details" is very appropriate to CMR imaging of complex CHD. This is especially true when imaging neonates, infants, and children. Spatial as well as temporal resolution details, for example, can make a huge difference between accurate diagnosis and misdiagnosis. Signal to noise and contrast to noise concerns are critical to successful imaging. The CMR imager must be familiar with the technical details of imaging and convey to others involved in the patient's care both the differential diagnosis of the images as well as the potential for artifact.

- Knowing the limitations of CMR and the advantages and disadvantages of other modalities is vital in the evaluation of complex CHD. In general a combination of CMR and other techniques are necessary for the complete care of the patient.

In 1971 Mitchell et al. defined congenital heart disease (CHD) as a "gross structural abnormality of the heart or intrathoracic great vessels that is actually or potentially of functional significance." Although this definition is problematic in simple CHD (e.g., patients with persistent fifth aortic arch or persistent left superior vena cava, both of which are not functionally significant), it fits complex CHD very well. Therefore this definition can include D-looped transposition of the great arteries (TGA) (i.e., segments [S,D,D]) as well as corrected TGA (i.e., segments [S,L,L]) without other lesions such as ventricular septal defect; patients with corrected TGA may not have any "actual" functional significance, but the potential for systemic right ventricular failure is always present. For this chapter on complex CHD, the Mitchell et al. definition will be used.

CHD itself is fairly common and complex CHD, although not as common as simple CHD, makes up a significant portion of young patients who present to the physician for care. In 2002, Hoffman and Kaplan reported the results of a survey of the literature on the incidence of CHD and found the average incidence of all these studies to be 9596 of one million live births (excluding nonstenotic bicuspid aortic valve, silent patent ductus arteriosus, and isolated partial anomalous pulmonary venous connections). Although complex CHD does not equate to cyanotic CHD, this literature review estimated the incidence of cyanotic CHD at 1391 per million live births (14.5% of all CHD). The New England Regional Infant Care Program (NERICP), however, estimated the incidence of "severe" CHD at 2033 per million live births with 888 being cyanotic. Clinicians, however, report that their patient population with these types of lesions requires a disproportionate share of their time (at least 50%). In addition, because of advances in medical care, more and more patients with complex CHD are living to adulthood and will need the care of adult and pediatric cardiologists; from 1985 to 2000, the prevalence of "severe" CHD increased significantly to such a degree that in 2000, there were equal number of children and adults alive with this type of heart disease.

Cardiac magnetic resonance (CMR) can play an important role in the medical and surgical management of complex CHD. Besides being a noninvasive technique without ionizing radiation, with regard to complex CHD, it has a wide field of view, which is important in determining the myriad of abnormal connections and anomalous structures that may be present both intracardiac and extracardiac. Because imaging extracardiac structures with CMR is routine (e.g., trachea, liver, etc.), the intricate relationship between cardiovascular structures and extracardiac structures can be evaluated to aid in surgical reconstruction. Along these lines, three-dimensional CMR imaging also is used in both the preoperative and postoperative surgical evaluation of these patients.

Another major strength of CMR as it relates to complex CHD is the ability to assess ventricular function and physiology. Ventricular volumes, mass, and ejection phase parameters of function, for example, can be very precisely calculated by CMR using cine techniques independent of geometric assumptions; this is clinically important in cases of complex CHD with the bizarre ventricular shapes as occurs in such as lesions as single ventricles, heterotaxy, or L-looped ventricles. Since these patients generally undergo surgery with cardiopulmonary bypass and deep hypothermic circulatory arrest (in some cases, multiple times), ventricular function is important to follow serially and accurately. In most instances, these images are the result of many heartbeats averaged together, which better reflect the true nature of ventricular function (as opposed to measurements that average three to four heartbeats such as in echocardiography). This "average" is embedded in the image, whereas the echocardiographer would need to examine many heartbeats and "average" these in his or her mind and come to a conclusion. CMR has been the gold standard in this area for nearly 20 years.

Because complex CHD can have complex flow patterns, CMR phase encoded velocity mapping can measure flows in any vessel to yield clinically important information such as shunt flow (e.g., Qp/Qs) or pulmonary flow in, for example, a patient with tricuspid atresia (S,D,S) with ventricular septal defect and pulmonic stenosis. This technique is also an average of many heartbeats, which is advantageous for the reasons stated above. Regurgitant fractions in lesions with valve insufficiency (e.g., pulmonary insufficiency after transannular patch for tetralogy of Fallot) can also be calculated in this manner.

Other CMR-based techniques are useful in the assessment of ventricular function and physiology of complex CHD. Time resolved, maximum intensity projection dimensional gadolinium sequence yields a set of three-dimensional images with temporal information and is useful to track the flow of blood from the venous side of the circulation onward. It can provide physiologic information on shunts; for example, in a case of a superior vena cava overriding the atrial septum with a sinus venosus atrial septal defect, both right and left atria would become signal intense. If there is a question of severe stenosis or discontinuity between branch pulmonary arteries, a small amount of gadolinium may be seen entering both right and left branches, confirming patency. Myocardial tagging, which noninvasively "labels" tissue, is useful in identifying regional ventricular wall dysfunction, which may be present in patients with coronary manipulations such as after arterial switch operation for TGA or after a Ross procedure for aortic stenosis. Myocardial perfusion imaging, performed by injecting gadolinium and observing the signal intensity in the myocardium, can be used for the assessment of these coronary lesions as well. Viability imaging, used by injecting gadolinium and waiting to image the myocardium (delayed enhancement technique), can identify regions of myocardial scar tissue (e.g., after surgery or after coronary manipulation) and foreign bodies (e.g., patch repair of an endocardial cushion defect). Finally, coronary imaging using the navigator technique can be used to determine coronary anomalies that can occur with complex CHD as well as to assess the coronaries after their manipulation.

Case 1   The Fontan Baffle

A 19-year-old patient presents for routine follow-up of her single ventricle lesion (Figure 15-1). The anatomy is TGA (S,L,L) with dextrocardia, tricuspid atresia and a right ventricular outflow chamber who is after Fontan. Systemic blood flow enters the pulmonary arteries passively from the superior vena cava and inferior vena cava via the Fontan baffle. Pulmonary venous blood enters the left atrium followed by the right-sided left ventricle, across ventricular septal defects into the left-sided right ventricular outflow chamber and then the aorta. CMR found obstruction to flow across the ventricular septal defects with a peak instantaneous gradient of 85 mm Hg; at cardiac catheterization, the peak to peak gradient was found to be 50 mm Hg (left ventricular systolic pressure of 170 mm Hg and the right ventricular outflow chamber of 120 mm Hg).

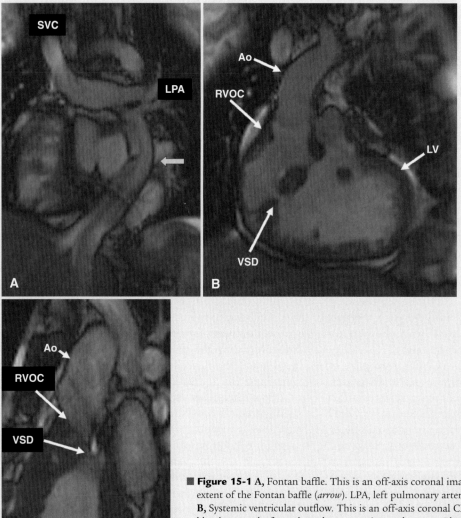

■ **Figure 15-1 A,** Fontan baffle. This is an off-axis coronal image demonstrating the long axis extent of the Fontan baffle (*arrow*). LPA, left pulmonary artery; SVC, superior vena cava. **B,** Systemic ventricular outflow. This is an off-axis coronal CMR image demonstrating the path blood must take from the pulmonary veins to the aorta. Blood enters the left ventricle (LV) from the left atrium and then must traverse two small ventricular septal defects (VSD) to enter the right ventricular outflow chamber (RVOC) and then the aorta (Ao). **C,** Assessment of ventricular outflow obstruction. The image is a cine through the superior ventricular septal defect (VSD) demonstrating turbulence as blood flows from the left ventricle (LV) to the right ventricular outflow chamber (RVOC).

Case 2 **Pulmonary Venous Pathway Obstruction after Senning Procedure for TGA**

A 32-year-old man who had transposition of the great arteries (S,D,D) after Senning procedure (baffling of systemic venous blood to the mitral valve and pulmonary venous blood to the tricuspid valve) presented in atrial flutter. A cardiac catheterization with angiography demonstrated an abnormal structure apparently connected to the right superior vena cava, which dye entered during a right superior vena cava injection. CMR was performed to evaluate this abnormal structure (Figure 15-2). An anomalous right upper pulmonary vein was seen to connect to the right superior vena cava; a saccular aneurysmal mass originated from this right upper pulmonary vein and formed a fistulous communication with the pulmonary venous pathway as visualized with gradient echo cine with saturation tagging. The upper limb of the systemic venous pathway also appeared severely narrowed. The patient was brought back to the catheterization lab where a covered stent was placed to completely cover the os of the right upper pulmonary vein and to dilate the upper limb of the systemic venous pathway. With the covered stent placement, blood from the right upper pulmonary vein cannot enter the superior vena cava (or cannot flow retrograde from the superior vena cava and enter the right upper pulmonary vein and enter the pulmonary venous pathway via the fistulous communication) and is forced via the fistulous communication to the pulmonary venous pathway.

Case 3 **RVOT Obstruction in TGA after Arterial Switch Operation**

A 2-year-old boy with TGA (S,D,D) who is after arterial switch procedure was found to have a gradient across the right ventricular outflow tract by echocardiography with high right ventricular pressures estimated by the tricuspid regurgitation jet. It was decided that a stent should be placed in the right ventricular outflow tract; however, the transplanted coronaries may be compressed by the stent if they coursed behind it. CMR was performed to better visualize the right ventricular outflow tract narrowing along with identifying the coronary arteries and evaluating whether the coronary arteries would be compromised when the right ventricular outflow tract was dilated with a stent (Figure 15-3). CMR confirmed the moderate to severely narrowed right ventricular outflow tract in the anteroposterior dimension; the coronary arteries arose to either side of the right ventricular outflow tract and would not be compressed by the stent. Stent placement proceeded without incident and the high right ventricular pressures and gradient decreased significantly.

Case 4 **TGA with Ventricular Septal Defect and Pulmonic Stenosis after Rastelli Procedure**

A 17-year-old young man had TGA (S,D,D) with a ventricular septal defect (VSD) and pulmonic stenosis (PS) is after a Rastelli procedure, where the VSD is closed to the aorta creating a new left ventricular outflow tract and a right ventricle (RV) to pulmonary artery conduit is placed. There was Doppler evidence of right ventricular outflow tract obstruction; however, because the RV to pulmonary artery conduit is so anterior, anatomic visualization by echocardiography was difficult. On CMR, significant narrowing was noted of the RV to pulmonary artery conduit at the exit from the RV as well as near the pulmonary bifurcation (Figure 15-4). Velocity mapping demonstrated moderate conduit insufficiency with a conduit regurgitant fraction of 42% and a peak instantaneous velocity of 3.8 m/s.

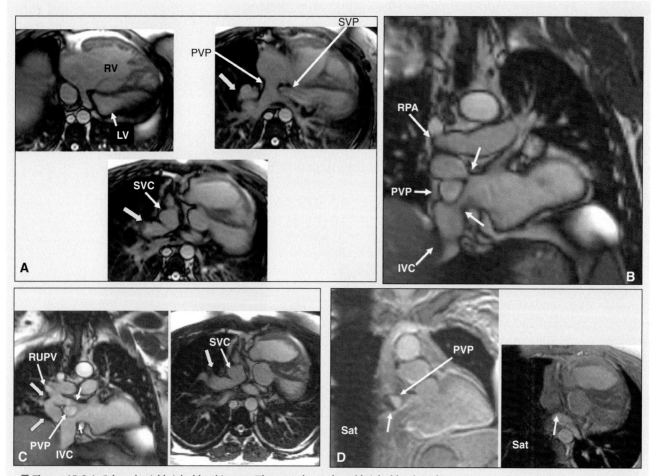

■ **Figure 15-2 A,** Selected axial bright blood images. These are three selected bright blood axial images demonstrating the anatomy. The progression of the images are from inferior to superior as the images progress from left to right and then bottom. Note how dilated and hypertrophied the right ventricle (RV) is and how thin walled the left ventricle (LV) is. The systemic venous pathway (SVP) and pulmonary venous pathway (PVP) can be easily seen. The abnormal structure, which was identified as an abnormally dilated and fistulous anomalous right upper pulmonary vein, is shown by the light blue arrow. Ao, aorta; RPA, right pulmonary artery; SVC, superior vena cava. **B,** Baffle obstruction. This is an off-axis image demonstrates baffle obstruction of the upper limb of the systemic venous pathway (SVP). The SVP consists of a lower limb bringing inferior vena cava (IVC) blood to the mitral valve and an upper limb bringing superior vena cava blood to the mitral valve. *Arrows* point to the upper and lower limbs of the SVP. The top *arrow* shows how narrow the upper limb is. The pulmonary venous pathway (PVP) is seen in cross-section in this image. **C,** Abnormal structure. Both images demonstrate the abnormal structure which was identified as an abnormally dilated and fistulous anomalous right upper pulmonary vein (*light blue arrows*). The images are an off-axis coronal cine (left) and an off-axis axial cine (right). Note on the left the aneurysmal saccular dilation originating from the right upper pulmonary vein (RUPV). The pulmonary venous pathway (PVP) can be visualized in cross-section. *White arrows* on the left point to the upper and lower limbs of the systemic venous pathway (SVP). The image on the right clearly shows the RUPV attaching to the superior vena cava. IVC, inferior vena cava. **D,** Fistula between aneurysmal saccular dilation originating from the right upper pulmonary vein and the pulmonary venous pathway (PVP). The images are gradient echo cines which utilized a saturation band (*dark band on the image*) to label blood flowing from the aneurysmal saccular dilation as well as the right upper pulmonary vein; the saturation band makes the blood appear dark on the image. Care was taken so that the saturation band did not label any other structures. The image on the left is an off-axis coronal image; the *arrow* points to dark blood seen in the pulmonary venous pathway, indicating a fistulous communication between the aneurysmal saccular dilation originating from the right upper pulmonary vein and the PVP. The right image is a still frame from a cine; *arrows* point to labeled blood from the right upper pulmonary vein washing in and out of the superior vena cava (SVC). Sat, saturation band.

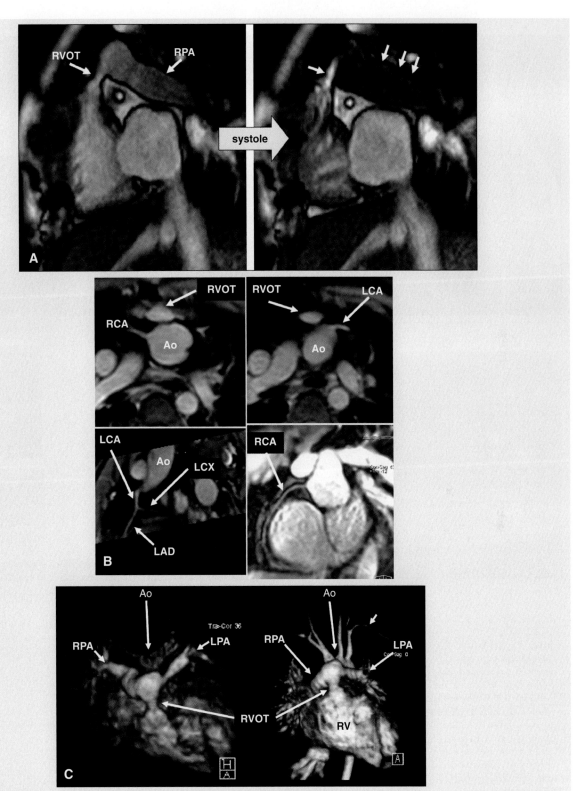

■ **Figure 15-3 A,** Right ventricular outflow tract (RVOT) obstruction in TGA (S,D,D} after arterial switch operation. The left panel is a single frame from a cine at end diastole demonstrating the long axis of the right ventricular outflow tract (RVOT) with the long axis of the right pulmonary artery (RPA). The right panel is a single frame from the same cine but at mid systole, demonstrating the turbulence and loss of signal (*arrows*) because of the obstruction. **B,** Coronary arteries. Both right (RCA) and left main coronary arteries (LCA) are visualized to originate from the right and left facing sinuses of the aorta (Ao) to either side of the right ventricular outflow tract (RVOT) in the upper left and upper right panels, respectively; if a stent was expanded in the RVOT, it would not impinge upon either coronary. The lower left panel demonstrates the left coronary system in long axis including the left anterior descending (LAD) and left circumflex (LCx) coronary arteries. The right lower panel demonstrates the RCA in long axis. **C,** Three-dimensional volume rendered images. These images demonstrate the LeCompte maneuver as well as the right ventricular outflow tract narrowing. Both images in this panel are of the same heart, just rotated into different positions. The right image is an anterior view and the left image is also an anterior view except tipped upward to obtain a better view of the right ventricular outflow tract and branch pulmonary arteries. Ao, aorta; LPA, left pulmonary artery; RPA, right pulmonary artery; RV, right ventricle; RVOT, right ventricular outflow tract.

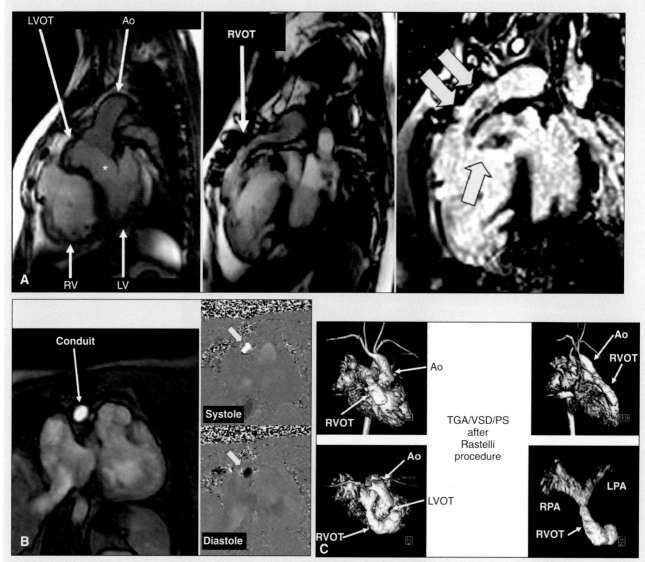

■ **Figure 15-4 A,** Right ventricular (RV) outflow tract (RVOT) and left ventricular (LV) outflow tract
(LVOT). The image on the left demonstrates the LVOT created by closure of the ventricular septal
defect (*) from the LV to the aorta (Ao). The middle image is a static steady-state free precession image
profiling the RVOT; note the compression of the conduit in the anteroposterior dimension. The right
panel is a phase-sensitive steady-state free precession viability image with the *arrows* demonstrating
delayed enhancement of the conduit (*two arrows*) and part of the ventricular septal defect patch (*single
arrow*). **B,** Velocity mapping across the right ventricular to pulmonary artery conduit. To quantify both
degree of obstruction as well as insufficiency, through-plane phase-encoded velocity mapping was
performed. This measured flow into and out of the plane of the image. Directionality is encoded by
signal enhancement (*white on the image*) in one direction or decreased signal intensity (*black on the image*)
in another direction. The panel on the left is the magnitude (anatomic) image of the cross-section of
the conduit where the velocity and flow measurements were made. The phase image (where flow is
actually measured) in systole and diastole are in the upper and lower panels just to the right of the
magnitude image respectively and anatomically correspond to the magnitude image on the left. Note
the increased signal intensity in the upper image in systole and how black that same cross-sectional area
of the conduit is in diastole in the lower right image (*arrows* point to the cross-section of the conduit
on the phase images). **C,** Three-dimensional volume rendering of the Rastelli procedure: The two upper
panels are views from anterior and right lateral aspects of the heart left and right respectively. Note
how easy it is to tell the relationship of the aorta (Ao) to the pulmonary arteries and the conduit. The
narrowing of the conduit is easily seen. The left lower panel is a "tipped up view" (i.e., a transverse view,
looking down from above) to visualize the pulmonary arteries better and to demonstrate the right
ventricular outflow tract (RVOT) from a different plane. The lower right panel isolates the RVOT and
pulmonary arteries viewed from above. LPA, left pulmonary artery; LVOT, left ventricular outflow tract;
RPA, right pulmonary artery.

Case 5   **Truncus Arteriosus**

A 3-day-old male infant with the diagnosis of truncus arteriosus was intubated and mechanically ventilated in the intensive care unit. Echocardiography demonstrated a large truncal artery and a ventricular septal defect; however, arch imaging and the status of the branch pulmonary arteries could not be discerned. The patient underwent CMR, which demonstrated truncus arteriosus A4, where the transverse aortic arch was hypoplastic (Figure 15-5). The left pulmonary artery originated extremely superiorly near a patent ductus arteriosus, which made an acute 90-degree bend from the superior aspect of the main pulmonary artery. The right pulmonary artery was hypoplastic and originated inferiorly.

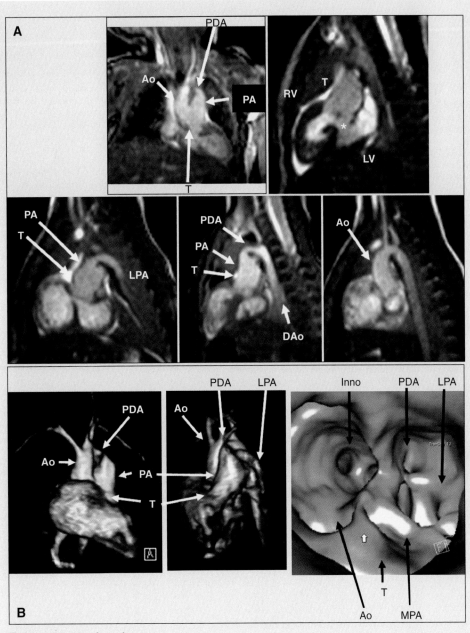

■ **Figure 15-5** For legend see next page.

■ **Figure 15-5 A,** Selected off-axis images: These images demonstrate the major parts of the anatomy. The upper left panel is an off-axis static coronal image demonstrating the bifurcation of the truncus (T) into the aorta (Ao) and main pulmonary artery (MPA) and the origin of the patent ductus arteriosus. The lower panels are single frames from cines demonstrating the long axis of the T, PA (left and middle), the left pulmonary artery (LPA) (left), the patent ductus arteriosus (PDA), and the aortic arch (Ao). The upper right image is a ventricular outflow tract view demonstrating the ventricular septal defect (*) in between right (RV) and left ventricles (LV). **B,** Three-dimensional gadolinium imaging: The set of two images on the left and middle are selected views from anterior and left lateral views. These images clearly demonstrate the truncus (T, upper images), aorta (Ao, all images), main pulmonary artery (PA), patent ductus arteriosus (PDA), and left pulmonary arteries (LPA). The image on the right is an "endoscopic" view of the interior of the truncus arteriosus (T) of the three-dimensional image as viewed from the truncal valve looking toward the head. The os and the endovascular surface of vessels can be visualized in this fashion. The bifurcation of the T into Ao (on the left) and PA (on the right) is clearly seen. The innominate artery (Inno) os originating from the superior aspect of the Ao as well as the os of the PDA (most superior), the LPA (os to the viewer's right), and RPA (not labeled but to the viewer's left of the LPA and underneath the PDA) originating from the PA are clearly visualized.

SUGGESTED READING

Beerbaum P, Korperich H, Barth P, et al: Noninvasive quantification of left-to-right shunt in pediatric patients. Phase-contrast cine magnetic resonance imaging compared with invasive oximetry. Circulation 2001;103:2476-2482.

Brown DW, Gauvreau K, Powell AJ, et al: Cardiac magnetic resonance versus routine cardiac catheterization before bidirectional Glenn anastomosis in infants with functional single ventricle: a prospective randomized trial. Circulation 2007;116:2718-2725.

Dorfman AL, Geva T: Magnetic resonance imaging evaluation of congenital heart disease: conotruncal anomalies. J Cardiovasc Mag Resonan 2006;8:645-659.

Finn JP, Baskaran V, Carr JC, et al: Low-dose contrast-enhanced three-dimensional MR angiography with subsecond temporal resolution: Initial results. Radiology 2002;224:896-904.

Fogel MA: Cardiac magnetic resonance of single ventricles. J Cardiovasc Mag Resonan 2006;8:661-670.

Fogel MA, Baxter B, Weinberg PM, et al: Midterm follow-up of patients with transposition of the great arteries after atrial inversion operation using two- and three-dimensional magnetic resonance imaging. Pediatr Radiol 2002;32:440-446.

Fogel MA, Hubbard A, Weinberg PM: A simplified approach for assessment of intracardiac baffles and extracardiac conduits in congenital heart surgery with two- and three-dimensional magnetic resonance imaging. Am Heart J 2001;142:1028-1036.

Fogel MA, Weinberg PM, Chin AJ, et al: Late ventricular geometry and performance changes of functional single ventricle throughout staged Fontan reconstruction assessed by magnetic resonance imaging. J Am Coll Cardiol 1996;28:212-221.

Fogel MA, Weinberg PM, Hubbard A, et al: Diastolic biomechanics in normal infants utilizing MRI tissue tagging. Circulation 2000;102:218-224.

Fogel MA, Weinberg PM, Rychik J, et al: Caval contribution to flow in the branch pulmonary arteries of Fontan patients using a novel application of magnetic resonance presaturation pulse. Circulation 1999;99:1215-1221.

Grotenhuis HB, Kroft LJ, van Elderen SG, et al: Right ventricular hypertrophy and diastolic dysfunction in arterial switch patients without pulmonary artery stenosis. Heart 2007;93:1604-1608.

Harris M, Johnson T, Weinberg P, Fogel M: Delayed enhancement cardiovascular magnetic resonance identifies fibrous tissue in children after congenital heart surgery. J Thorac Cardiovasc Surg 2007;133:676-681.

Hong YK, Park YW, Ryu SJ, et al: Efficacy of MRI in complicated congenital heart disease with visceral heterotaxy syndrome. J Comp Assist Tomography 2000;24:671-682.

Kang IS, Redington AN, Benson LN, et al: Differential regurgitation in branch pulmonary arteries after repair of tetralogy of Fallot: A phase-contrast cine magnetic resonance study. Circulation 2003;107:2938-2943.

Knauth AL, Gauvreau , Powell AJ, et al: Ventricular size and function assessed by cardiac MRI predict major adverse clinical outcomes late after tetralogy of Fallot repair. Heart 2008;94:211-216.

Menteer J, Weinberg PM, Fogel MA: Quantifying Regional Right Ventricular Function in tetralogy of Fallot. J Cardiovasc Mag Reson 2005;7:753-761.

Muthurangu V, Taylor AM, Hegde SR, et al: Cardiac magnetic resonance imaging after stage I Norwood operation for hypoplastic left heart syndrome. Circulation 2005;112:3256-3263.

Oosterhof T, van Straten A, Vliegen HW, et al: Preoperative thresholds for pulmonary valve replacement in patients with corrected tetralogy of Fallot using cardiovascular magnetic resonance. Circulation 2007;116:545-551.

Rebergen SA, Chin JGJ, Ottenkamp J, et al: Pulmonary regurgitation in the late postoperative follow-up of tetralogy of Fallot: Volumetric quantification by MR velocity mapping. Circulation 1993;88:2257-2266.

Taylor AM, Dymarkowski S, Hamaekers P, et al: MR coronary angiography and late-enhancement myocardial MR in children who underwent arterial switch surgery for transposition of great arteries. Radiology 2005;234:542-547.

Chapter 16

Postoperative Evaluation of Congenital Heart Disease

Karen G. Ordovas and Charles B. Higgins

KEY POINTS

- Cardiac magnetic resonance (CMR) can be used to detect and quantify the most common complications after repair of tetralogy of Fallot. CMR can accurately measure pulmonary regurgitant fraction (phase-contrast CMR) and assess right ventricular function (cine CMR) and morphology in these patients.

- CMR can assess hemodynamic significance of recurrent or residual coarctation of the aorta.

- After surgical correction for transposition of great arteries, CMR can be used to evaluate for possible complications of atrial switch and arterial switch procedures.

- CMR can identify and estimated the severity of conduit stenosis and regurgitation after the Rastelli operation.

- CMR can be used to assess for the most common complications associated with the Fontan procedure, which are conduit stenosis or thrombosis and dysfunction of the single functioning ventricle.

Case 1 Pulmonary Regurgitation after Correction of Tetralogy of Fallot

A 28-year-old man presents with a recent history of shortness of breath and palpitation during exercise. Clinical examination is unremarkable, except for a diastolic cardiac murmur. Past medical history is significant for surgical correction of tetralogy of Fallot at the age of 4.

Comments

Pulmonary regurgitation is the most common complication observed after correction of tetralogy of Fallot, usually presenting clinically as intolerance to exercise. It is nearly always present in patients who underwent a transannular patch repair for correction of the right ventricular outflow tract stenosis and is often associated with dyskinesis or aneurysm on the patch area. Chronic pulmonary regurgitation eventually causes right ventricular dilatation and dysfunction. The CMR study can accurately measure pulmonary regurgitant fraction (phase-contrast CMR) and assess right ventricular function (cine CMR) and morphology in these patients (Figure 16-1).

Case 2 Residual Pulmonary Stenosis after Correction of Tetralogy of Fallot

A 30-year-old woman presents with intolerance to exercise and shortness of breath. Clinical examination is noticeable for both systolic and diastolic murmurs. Patient underwent correction of tetralogy of Fallot with infundibulectomy and pulmonary valvotomy at the age of 2.

Comments

A common complication after correction of tetralogy of Fallot with infundibulectomy is residual infundibular and/or valvular pulmonary stenosis, which is usually associated with a mild to moderate degree of pulmonary regurgitation. Branch pulmonary artery stenosis is a common coabnormality seen in patients with tetralogy of Fallot and is often diagnosed later in life, after the initial surgical correction has been performed. A comprehensive CMR study allows for evaluation of morphology of stenosis and quantification of stenotic pressure gradient and ventricular function (Figure 16-2).

Case 3 Coarctation of the Aorta after Surgical Correction of CHD

A 35-year-old woman presents for clinical evaluation 1 year after coarctation of the aorta angioplasty because blood pressure levels remain higher in the upper extremities (BP: 160/100 mm Hg) than in the lower extremities (BP: 126/80 mm Hg). Clinical examination is unremarkable.

Comments

Residual or recurrent coarctation of the aorta is a common complication after either angioplasty or surgical intervention. CMR can not only assess the morphology of the coarctation site but also determine if the lesion is hemodynamically significant, based on the presence of collateral circulation (Figure 16-3).

Case 4 Baffle Stenosis after Mustard TGA Procedure

A 30-year-old woman with history of complete transposition of great arteries (TGA) corrected at the age of 1. Patient presents with swelling and venous distension in the neck and arms.

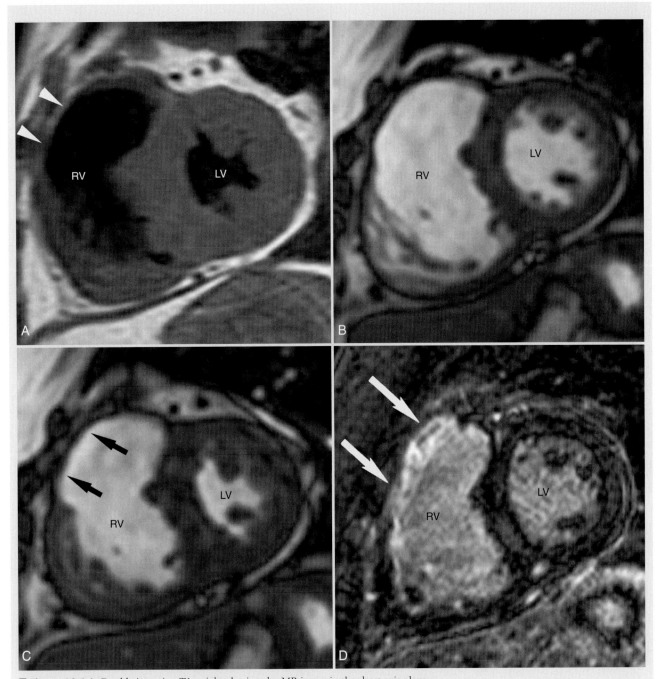

■ **Figure 16-1 A,** Double-inversion T1-weighted spin-echo MR image in the short-axis plane
demonstrates the right ventricular outflow tract denuded of normal myocardium (*arrowheads*),
consistent with status post a transannular patch repair for correction of tetralogy of Fallot. RV,
right ventricle; LV, left ventricle. **B-C,** Short-axis steady-state free-precession (SSFP) cine images at
end-diastole (**B**) and end-systole (**C**) show dyskinesis of the right ventricular outflow tract (*arrows*),
a common complication after transannular patch repair. RV, right ventricle; LV, left ventricle. **D,**
Inversion-recovery turbo spin-echo image in the short-axis plane obtained 10 minutes after the
administration of gadolinium chelate. Note the area of delayed contrast enhancement in the right
ventricular outflow tract (arrows), corresponding to the area of dyskinesis. The enhancement indicates
the presence of fibrosis at the site of the surgical patch and/or adjacent nonviable myocardium. RV,
right ventricle; LV, left ventricle.

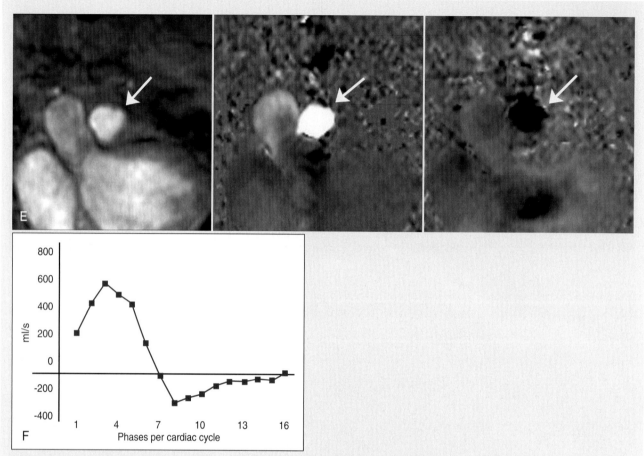

■ Figure 16-1, cont'd E, Velocity-encoded cine images obtained to quantify pulmonary regurgitant fraction in a plane perpendicular to the direction of blood flow in the main pulmonary artery. Oblique axial magnitude image (left), and phase images in systole (middle) and diastole (right) are shown. Phase contrast images show forward flow in systole (*dark voxels*) and retrograde flow in diastole (*bright voxels*) (*arrow*). **F,** Flow versus time curve displays the forward and retrograde flow in the pulmonary artery. Area under negative component of the curve yields a direct quantification of the volume of regurgitation. Pulmonary regurgitant fraction was calculated as 40%.

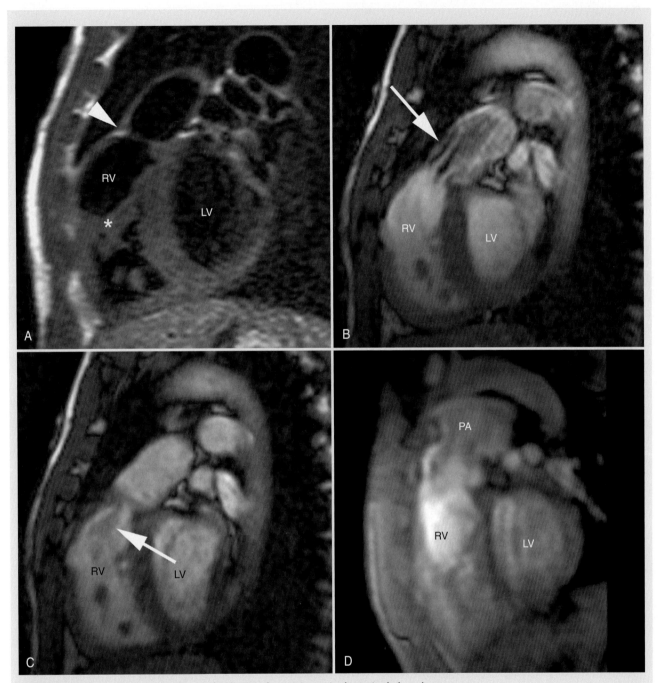

■ **Figure 16-2 A,** Double-inversion T1-weighted spin-echo MR image in the sagittal plane demonstrates residual valvular pulmonic stenosis (*arrowhead*), a common complication after infundibulectomy and valvotomy to correct tetralogy of Fallot. Note the thick right ventricular myocardium and trabeculations (*asterisk*) consistent with chronic pressure overload. RV, right ventricle; LV, left ventricle. **B-C,** SSFP cine images in the right ventricular outflow tract plane were obtained during systole (**B**) and diastole (**C**). A flow void is identified distal to the pulmonary valve in systole, indicating a high velocity jet caused by pulmonary stenosis (*arrow*). During diastole, a high velocity jet is seen below the level of the pulmonary valve (*arrow*), consistent with associated pulmonary regurgitation. RV, right ventricle; LV, left ventricle.

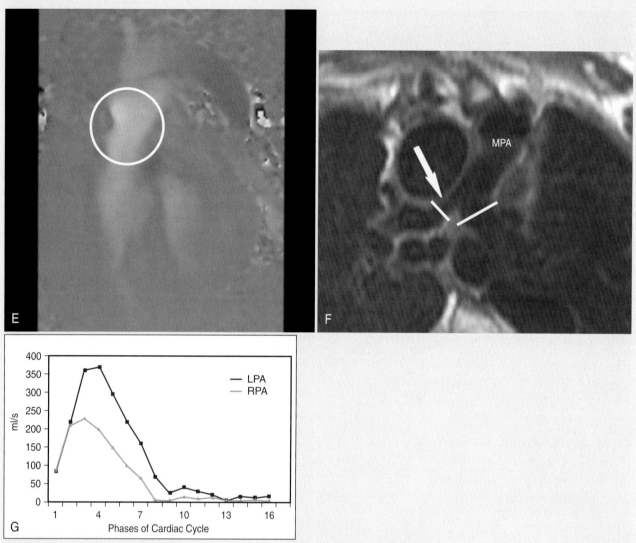

■ **Figure 16-2, cont'd D-E,** VEC-MR images were obtained parallel to the direction of blood flow in the main pulmonary artery. Magnitude (d) and phase (e) images are shown. A region of interest was placed in the phase image to interrogate the peak velocity distal to the pulmonary valvular stenosis, which was measured as 5 m/s. Using the modified Bernoulli equation ($\Delta P = 4 \times PV^2$, where P = pressure in mm Hg and PV = peak velocity in m/s) a pressure gradient of 100 mm Hg was estimated across the stenosis. RV, right ventricle; LV, left ventricle; PA, pulmonary artery. **F-G,** Double-inversion T1-weighted spin-echo MR image in the axial plane (**F**) shows a long segment stenosis of the right pulmonary artery (*arrow*). VEC-MR images were obtained perpendicular to the direction of blood flow in the branch pulmonary arteries (*white lines*) for calculation of differential pulmonary blood flow. Flow versus time graphic (**G**) displays substantially higher blood flow to the left pulmonary artery compared to the right pulmonary artery, with a right to left flow ratio of 0.5. MPA, main pulmonary artery.

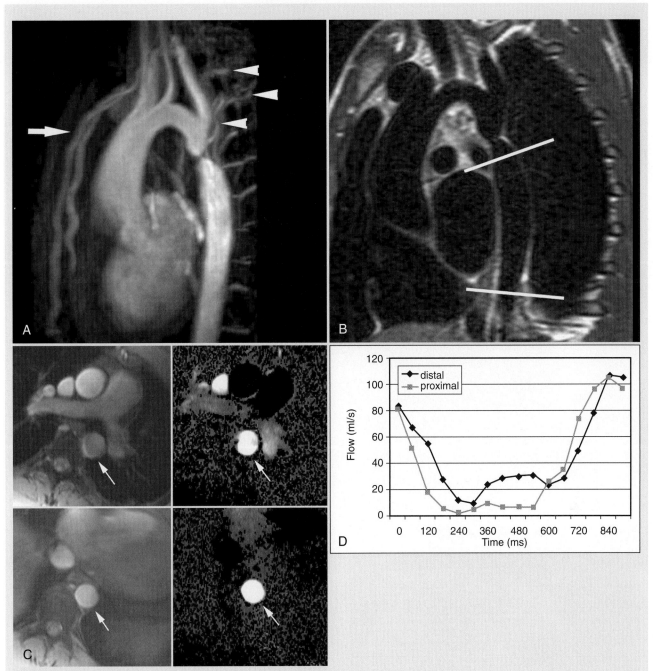

■ **Figure 16-3 A**, Sagittal display of a three-dimensional MRA demonstrates a severe juxtaductal aortic coarctation. Note the prominent internal mammary (*arrow*) and superior intercostal arteries (*arrowheads*), which indicate the presence of collateral circulation. **B,** Double-inversion T1-weighted spin-echo MR image in an oblique sagittal plane (B) confirms the presence of a severe stenosis at the proximal descending aorta. To assess for hemodynamic significance of the stenosis, measurement of collateral circulation was performed using VEC-CMR at two sites in the descending aorta (*white lines*). **C-D,** Magnitude (left) and phase (right) images (**C**) were obtained in a plane perpendicular to the direction of blood flow in the descending (*arrows*) approximately 1 cm bellow the coarctation site (upper row) and at the level of the diaphragm (lower row). Flow versus time curve (**D**) displays a higher flow in the distal compared to the proximal descending aorta during diastole, consistent with the presence of collateral circulation indicating a hemodynamically significant residual or recurrent coarctation.

Comments

Most adults with surgically corrected TGA have had an atrial switch procedure (Mustard or Senning), which is now frequently evaluated by CMR. The Mustard procedure, the most common, consist of excising the atrial septum and creating a pericardial or synthetic baffle encompassing the ostia of the superior vena cava (SVC), inferior vena cava (IVC), and the mitral valve. In this way systemic venous blood is redirected into the left ventricle.

The blood arriving into the reconstructed atria from pulmonary veins is excluded from the baffle, and flows to the RV. Baffle stenosis, particularly of the upper limb near the anastomosis with the SVC, is sometimes seen after Mustard procedure. Other complications include SVC stenosis, baffle leak, pulmonary venous obstruction, tricuspid regurgitation, and right ventricular dysfunction. CMR can demonstrate the complex postoperative cardiac morphology and assess the severity of a baffle leak or ventricular dysfunction (Figure 16-4).

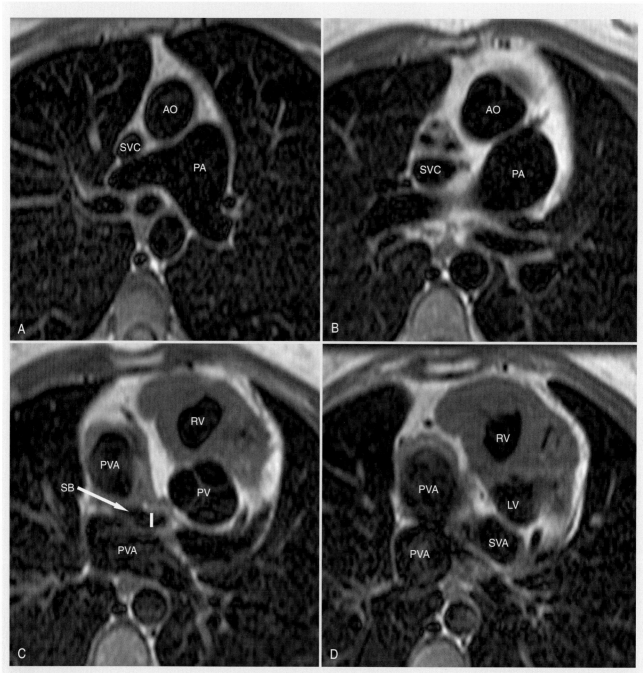

■ **Figure 16-4** For legend see opposite page.

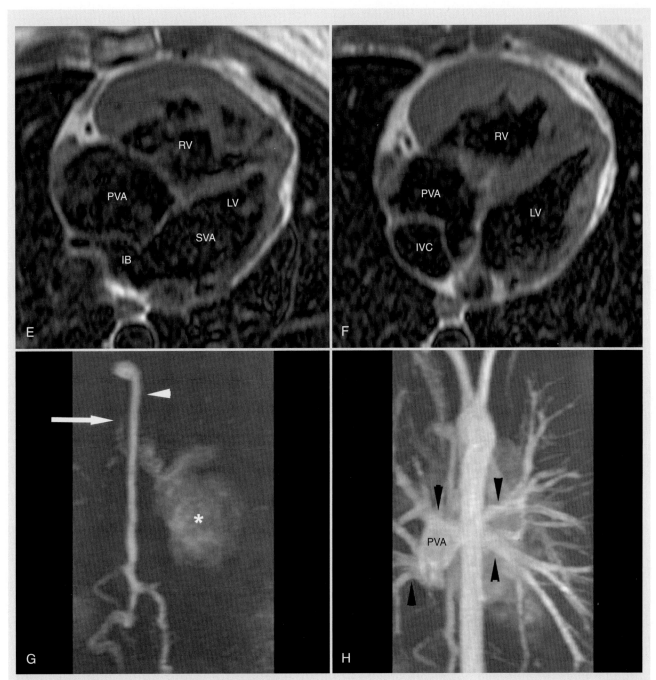

■ **Figure 16-4 A-F,** Axial double-inversion T1-weighted spin-echo MR images from base (upper left) to apex (lower right) demonstrate the cardiac anatomy after Mustard procedure. Note the presence of a baffle connecting SVC, IVC, and mitral valve. Superior (SB) and inferior (IB) portions of the baffle arrive to the systemic venous atrium (SVA). A stenosis is seen in the superior baffle, which measures approximately 10 mm in the anteroposterior diameter (*white line*) near the junction with the SVC (*arrow*). The pulmonary veins drain to the pulmonary venous atrium (PVA). AO, aorta; PA, pulmonary artery; SVC, superior vena cava; IVC, inferior vena cava; PV, pulmonary valve; PVA, pulmonary venous atrium; RV, right ventricle; LV, left ventricle. **G-H,** Gadolinium-enhanced MRA in the coronal plane was obtained in a early venous (**G**) and arterial phase (**H**), with a left arm injection. On the venous phase, the narrowing of the superior baffle can be seen (*arrow*) followed by poor opacification of the left ventricle (*asterisk*). Note the intense opacification of the azygous vein caused by preferential retrograde flow through this vessel (*arrowhead*). On the arterial phase, overlying enhancement of four pulmonary veins (*arrowheads*) connecting to the pulmonary venous atrium (PVA), can be seen.

Case 5 **Pulmonary Artery Stenosis after Arterial Switch Procedure**

A 9-year-old girl presents with dyspnea and wheezing. Patient is status post correction of complete transposition of great arteries as an infant.

Comments

Jatene procedure (arterial switch) is the current method of choice for correction of complete TGA, consisting of disconnecting the pulmonary artery and aorta from their respective outflow tracts, valves and roots, and reanastomosing these vessels in switched positions. Coronary arteries are also disconnected from the native aortic root (still connected to right ventricle) and anastomosed to the neo-aorta (now connected to the left ventricle). Most common complications are stenoses of the branch pulmonary arteries as they course around the repositioned ascending aorta. Stenoses at the coronary arteries anastomosis can also occur. CMR can depict the anatomy of the great arteries and estimate severity of a pulmonary artery stenosis by quantification of differential pulmonary flow (Figure 16-5).

Case 6 **Conduit Stenosis after Rastelli Procedure**

A 13-year-old boy presents with ascites and edema of inferior extremities. At age 2, he underwent cardiac surgery for correction of pulmonary atresia and ventricular septal defect.

Comments

The Rastelli procedure is now performed for correction of any lesion characterized by two adequate size ventricles and severe right ventricular outflow tract stenosis or pulmonary atresia. The procedure consists of placing a nonvalved or valved conduit between the right ventricle and the pulmonary artery in the simplest circumstances. In some patients with multiple sources of blood supply to the lungs, those are connected to a central confluent structure in a preliminary operation. In a later operation a conduit is placed between the RV and the confluent vascular structure ("manifold").

The main complications of late postoperative Rastelli patients are related to lack of growth and degeneration of the pulmonary homograft (conduit) and its replacement may be required. Calcification and stenosis of the conduit as well as conduit valvular insufficiency are common complications that need to be corrected to protect the right ventricle from flow or pressure overload. Spin echo (SE) and cine-GRE images in a sagittal plane can demonstrate the dynamic characteristics of the right ventricular outflow tract and possible stenoses at the anastomoses (Figure 16-6). Three-dimensional MRA can effectively depict conduit stenosis. Cine-CMR short-axis imaging can evaluate right ventricular function. Velocity encoded cine (VEC)-CMR acquired perpendicular to the long axis of the conduit is used to quantify retrograde flow (pulmonary regurgitation). VEC-CMR parallel and perpendicular to the stenotic flow jet can be used to measure peak velocity and thereby estimate the pressure gradient ($\Delta P = 4 \times PV^2$, where P = pressure in mm Hg and PV = peak velocity in m/s).

Case 7 **Conduit Stenosis Following the Fontan Procedure**

A 5-year-old boy with history of tricuspid atresia was submitted to surgical correction as an infant. Patient presents with acute dyspnea. Physical examination is unremarkable.

Comments

Fontan procedure consists of connecting systemic venous blood flow to the pulmonary circulation. A baffle/tunnel through the right atrium or an extra cardiac conduit connects IVC to right pulmonary artery. SVC is separately anastomosed to the right pulmonary artery. CMR can be used to assess for the most common complications associated with the Fontan procedure, which are conduit stenosis or thrombosis and dysfunction of the single functioning ventricle (Figure 16-7). MRA, SE, and Cine-CMR images can display stenoses. VEC-CMR can be acquired on planes perpendicular or parallel to the blood flow in conduits or baffles to assess for the presence of thrombus or stenosis. Cine-CMR images in the short-axis plane can be used to monitor volumes and ejection fraction of the functioning single ventricle.

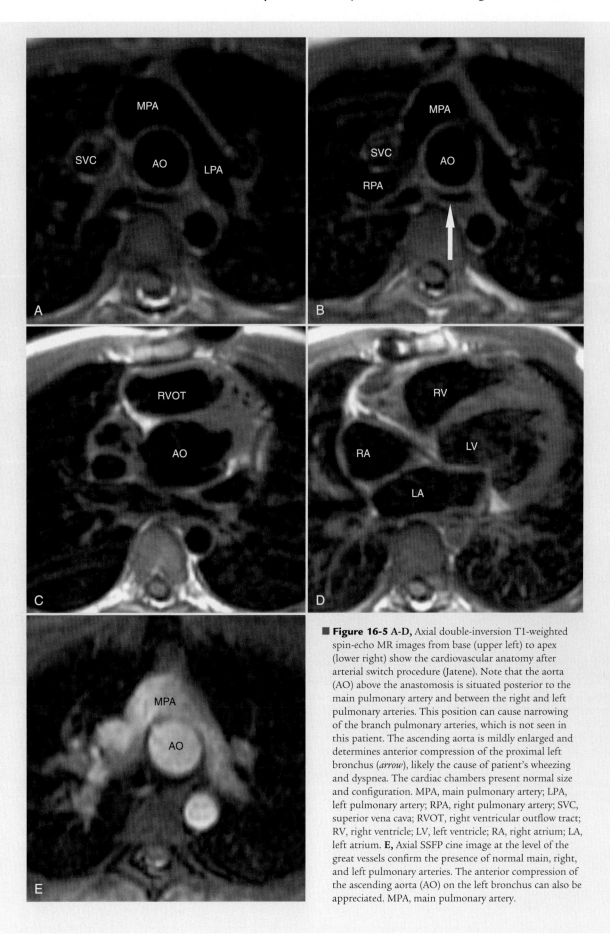

■ **Figure 16-5 A-D,** Axial double-inversion T1-weighted spin-echo MR images from base (upper left) to apex (lower right) show the cardiovascular anatomy after arterial switch procedure (Jatene). Note that the aorta (AO) above the anastomosis is situated posterior to the main pulmonary artery and between the right and left pulmonary arteries. This position can cause narrowing of the branch pulmonary arteries, which is not seen in this patient. The ascending aorta is mildly enlarged and determines anterior compression of the proximal left bronchus (*arrow*), likely the cause of patient's wheezing and dyspnea. The cardiac chambers present normal size and configuration. MPA, main pulmonary artery; LPA, left pulmonary artery; RPA, right pulmonary artery; SVC, superior vena cava; RVOT, right ventricular outflow tract; RV, right ventricle; LV, left ventricle; RA, right atrium; LA, left atrium. **E,** Axial SSFP cine image at the level of the great vessels confirm the presence of normal main, right, and left pulmonary arteries. The anterior compression of the ascending aorta (AO) on the left bronchus can also be appreciated. MPA, main pulmonary artery.

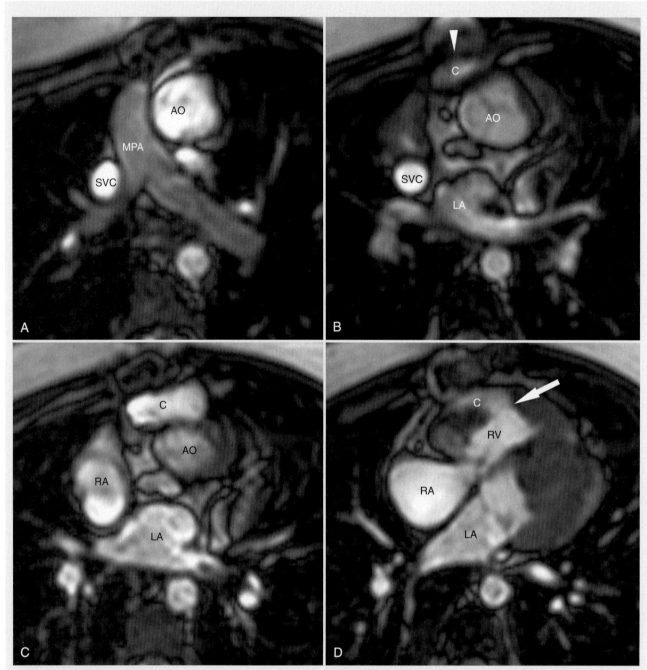

■ **Figure 16-6 A-D,** Axial SSFP cine images from base (upper left) to apex (lower right) demonstrate cardiac anatomy after Rastelli procedure. A right ventricle (RV) to main pulmonary artery (MPA) conduit (C) was placed. Note the conduit irregularity and stenosis (*arrowhead*) just below the anastomosis with the MPA, situated anterior to the ascending aorta (AO). The anastomosis with the RV free wall is normal in appearance (*arrow*). SVC, superior vena cava; LA, left atrium; RA, right atrium.

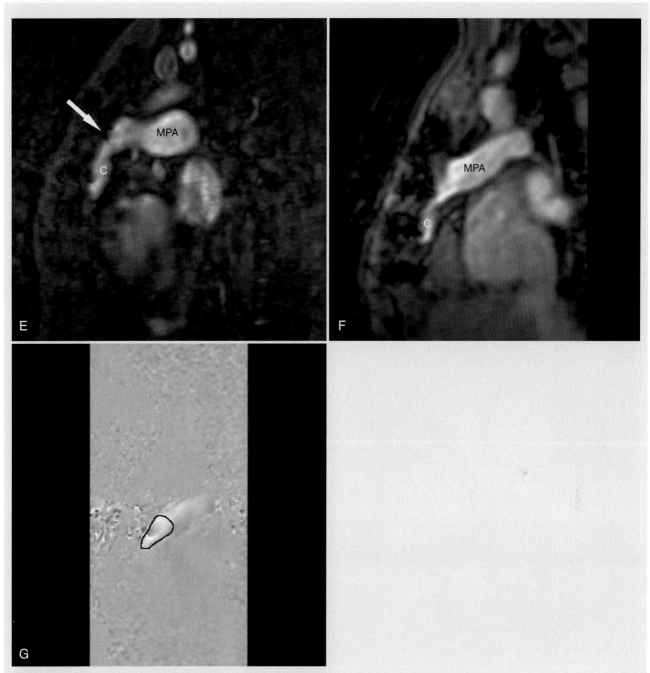

■ **Figure 16-6, cont'd E,** Gadolinium-enhanced MRA in the sagittal plane also shows the conduit (C) stenosis, which is narrowest (*arrow*) just bellow the anastomosis with the main pulmonary artery (MPA). **F-G,** Velocity-encoded cine CMR was obtained in a plane parallel to the direction of blood flow in the conduit (C) and main pulmonary artery (MPA) for assessment of the severity of the stenosis. Magnitude (**F**) and phase (**G**) images are shown. A region of interest was drawn above the point of maximum stenosis to interrogate the peak velocity. A peak velocity of 4 m/s was measured. Using the modified Bernoulli equation, a pressure gradient of 64 mm Hg was estimated across the stenosis.

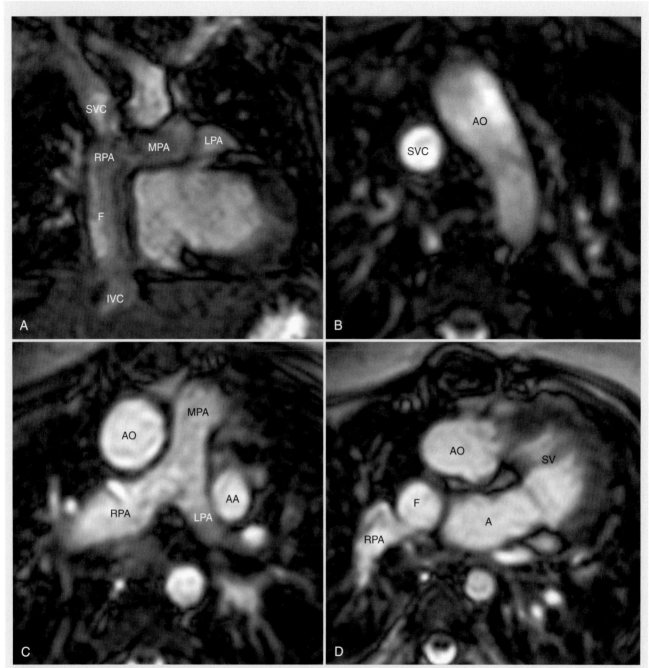

■ **Figure 16-7 A,** Gadolinium-enhanced MRA obtained in the coronal plane shows a Fontan conduit (F) adjacent to the right atrium connecting the right pulmonary artery (RPA) to both superior vena cava (SVC) and inferior vena cava (IVC), configuring a lateral tunnel type of Fontan operation. There is no evidence of conduit stenosis. MPA, main pulmonary artery; LPA, left pulmonary artery.

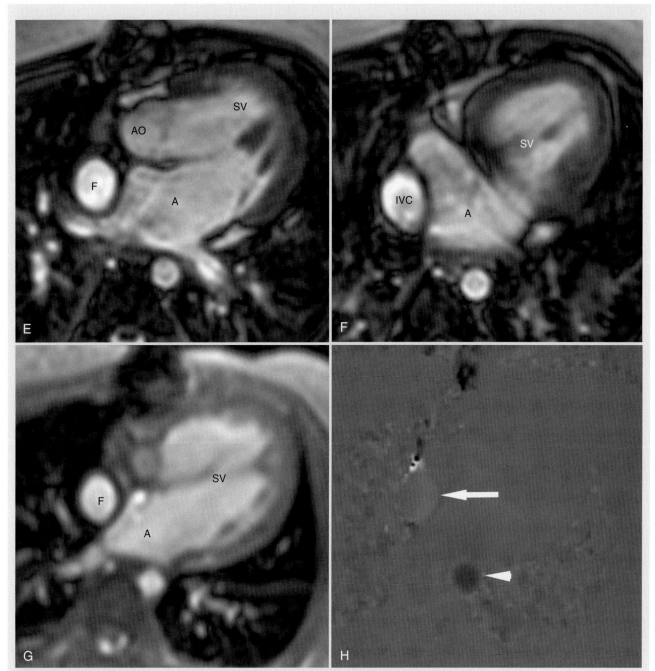

■ **Figure 16-7, cont'd B-F,** Axial SSFP cine images from base (upper left) to apex (lower right) demonstrate the cardiac anatomy after Fontan operation. One atrium (A) is identified, which connects to the pulmonary veins. A single atrioventricular valve connects the atrium to a single functional ventricle (SV). The ascending aorta (AO) originates from the single ventricle. There is no connection between the main pulmonary artery (MPA) and the single ventricle. The images also demonstrate normal high signal intensity within the Fontan conduit (F), inferior vena cava (IVC), superior vena cava (SVC), right (RPA), and left (LPA) pulmonary arteries, which indicate normal blood flow with no evidence for thrombus formation. AA, atrial appendage. **G-H,** Velocity-encoded cine CMR was obtained in a plane perpendicular to the direction of blood flow in the Fontan conduit (F). Magnitude (**G**) and phase (**H**) images show normal blood flow within the conduit with bright signal voxels (*arrow*) corresponding to blood flow in the opposite direction of the descending aorta, which presents voxels with dark signal (*arrowhead*). A, atrium; SV, single ventricle.

SUGGESTED READING

Araoz PA, Reddy GP, Tarnoff H, et al: MR findings of collateral circulation are more accurate measures of hemodynamic significance than arm-leg blood pressure gradient after repair of coarctation of the aorta. J Magn Reson Imaging 2003;17:177-183.

Eicken A, Fratz S, Gutfried C, et al: Hearts late after fontan operation have normal mass, normal volume and reduced systolic function: A magnetic resonance imaging study. J Am Coll Cardiol 2003;42(6):1061-1065.

Fogel MA: Cardiac magnetic resonance of single ventricles. J Cardiovasc Magn Reson 2006;8(4):661-670.

Fogel MA, Hubbard A, Weinberg PM: A simplified approach for assessment of intracardiac baffles and extracardiac conduits in congenital heart surgery with two- and three-dimensional magnetic resonance imaging. Am Heart J 2001;142(6):1028-1036.

Grotenhuis HB, Kroft LJM, Vliegen HW, et al: Magnetic resonance imaging of function and flow in postoperative congenital heart disease. In: Higgins CB, de Roos A, (eds): MRI and CT of the Cardiovascular System, 2nd Edition. Philadelphia: Lippincott Williams & Wilkins, 2006, pp 411-428.

Norton KI, Tong C, Glass RB, Nielsen JC: Cardiac MR imaging assessment following tetralogy of Fallot repair. Radiographics 2006;26(1):197-211.

Ordovás KG, Higgins CB: Postoperative evaluation in adult congenital heart diseases. In: Hundley WG (ed.). Cardiovascular Magnetic Resonance Self-Assessment Programs of the American College of Cardiology. Washington, DC: American College of Cardiology Foundation and Society for Cardiovascular Magnetic Resonance, September 2004.

Shih MC, Tholpady A, Kramer CM, et al: Surgical and endovascular repair of aortic coarctation: normal findings and appearance of complications on CT angiography and MR angiography. AJR Am J Roentgenol 2006;187(3):W302-W312.

Soler R, Rodriguez E, Alvarez M, Raposo I: Postoperative imaging in cyanotic congenital heart diseases: part 2, Complications. AJR Am J Roentgenol 2007;189(6):1361-1369.

Varaprasathan GA, Araoz PA, Higgins CB, Reddy GP: Quantification of flow dynamics in congenital heart disease: Applications of velocity-encoded cine MR imaging. Radiographics 2002; 22: 895-906.

Chapter 17

Perfusion Stress Magnetic Resonance

Amedeo Chiribiri, Sven Plein, and Eike Nagel

KEY POINTS

- Cardiovascular magnetic resonance (CMR) first-pass perfusion has developed considerably in recent years, showing good results in single- and multicenter trials.

- CMR first-pass perfusion provides high spatial resolution images of myocardial ischemia, allowing regional myocardial perfusion assessment and separate visualization of both subendocardial and subepicardial layers.

- CMR first-pass perfusion is more sensitive than dobutamine stress test in the detection of ischemia, as it is aimed toward the imaging of blood flow, which is first reduced in the progression of the ischemic cascade.

- Adenosine-stress CMR first-pass perfusion is safe; the side effects of adenosine are usually mild and fully reversible.

- The absence of ionizing radiation and noninvasive nature of the method make it the optimal clinical tool for repetitive evaluations of the patients during follow-up.

- First-pass perfusion imaging can be combined with detailed assessment of myocardial function and viability.

The basic principle of CMR perfusion imaging is that the first myocardial passage of a contrast agent is visualized rapidly (i.e., every heart beat). Consequently this technique is called *first-pass perfusion imaging*. The contrast agents used are based on gadolinium, which shortens the time magnetization required to recover to normal after being partially used for imaging. This is also called T1 relaxation. In the imaging sequences used, a shorter T1 leads to a stronger signal and thus a brighter image. Most of these gadolinium-based contrast agents are interstitial, because they diffuse rapidly from the vessels into the interstitium (but not into intact cells; thus, they are also called *extracellular agents*). The pharmacokinetic behavior of the contrast agent is based on its chelation, which also makes the contrast agent nontoxic (Figure 17-1). Imaging is performed during approximately 40 to 60 heartbeats after injection of the contrast agent (Figure 17-2). The contrast agent is administered into an antecubital vein at a speed of 3 to 5 ml/sec using an automatic MR compatible pump. Higher doses (e.g., 0.1 mmol/kg body weight) are preferred for visual assessment; lower doses (e.g., 0.025 mmol/kg body weight) are more suitable for quantitative and semiquantitative evaluation (Table 17-1). A full dataset (e.g., three to four short-axis views or a combination of short and long axis) is acquired every heartbeat to visualize the flow of the contrast agent through the left ventricular cavity and myocardium. Table 17-2 reports the instructions for patient preparation.

Different imaging sequences can be used. Unfortunately the faster the imaging sequence (which is advantageous for higher spatial resolution), the more artifacts occur. Most centers either use turbo-gradient echo imaging (TGrE, TFE, FLASH) or steady-state free precession (SSFP, BFFE, FIESTA). In addition to using an appropriate imaging sequence to visualize the data, a method to generate optimal T1 contrast has to be chosen. Most centers use saturation prepulse to null the signal and then wait for signal recovery (Figure 17-3). With such saturation recovery pulse sequences signal depends on the amount of the contrast agent: good perfusion = high concentration of contrast agent = rapid recovery of signal = bright image; reduced perfusion = low concentration = slow recovery of signal = dark image (see Figure 17-1). In comparison with inversion-recovery sequences that are used for late gadolinium enhancement, saturation recovery pulse sequences have the advantage that the contrast is independent of heartbeat variations during ECG-triggered image acquisition.

Imaging is usually performed first during adenosine stress (140 mcg/kg body weight/minute for up to 6 minutes) and repeated approximately 10 to 15 minutes later at rest. The time between the stress and the rest scan

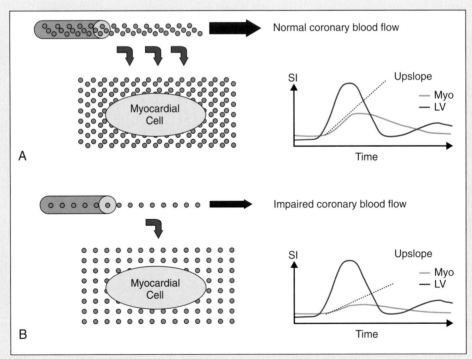

■ **Figure 17-1** The extracellular contrast agent reaches the myocardium and passes in the extracellular space with an amount and rate that is proportional to blood flow. In normal conditions (**A**), a certain amount of contrast agent diffuses into the interstitium, giving a strong myocardial signal (Myo) occurring later than the increment of signal in the left ventricle (LV). When regional coronary blood flow is impaired (**B**), the amount and rate of wash-in of the contrast agent is reduced (up slope), and peak signal intensity is lower.

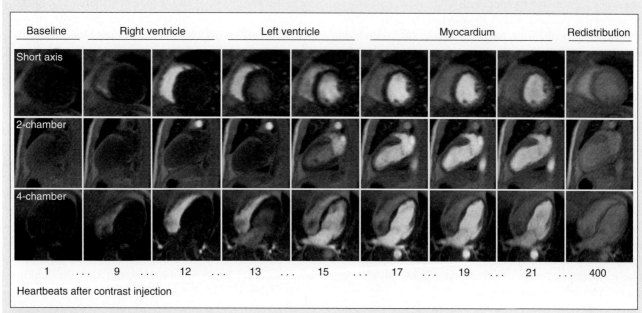

■ **Figure 17-2** Example of first-pass perfusion images in short axis, two-, and four-chamber view. The first image corresponds to the beginning of intravenous injection of the contrast agent (baseline). Then the contrast reaches the right ventricle (9-12 heartbeats), the left ventricle (13-15 heartbeats), and finally the myocardium (17-21 heartbeats). After 40 heartbeats the redistribution of the contrast agent is complete. After 15 minutes most of the contrast agent is washed out and a second scan (e.g., rest) can be performed.

TABLE 17-1 Contrast Medium

- Conventional extracellular Gadolinium-chelates at doses of 0.025-0.1 mmol/kg injected intravenously at 3-5 ml/sec (automatic injector).
- Contrast agent is followed by a flush of 20-25 ml of saline (at 3-5 ml/sec)
- Two separate IV lines (preferentially in the cubital fossa for adenosine and contrast agent)

TABLE 17-2 Patient Preparation

- Cessation of caffeine intake (beverages and food) and smoking 24 hours before the examination
- Cessation of medication (beta-blockers, calcium antagonists) typically the day before the examination, unless therapeutic success is to be documented

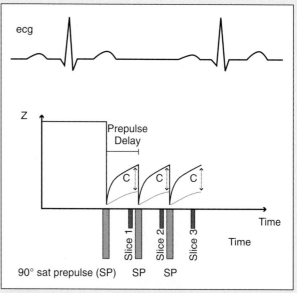

■ **Figure 17-3** Regardless of the type of image readout adopted (turbo-gradient echo imaging or steady-state free precession), perfusion sequences are usually built with a 90° saturation prepulse (SP) to generate the T1 contrast. Triggering on the QRS complex of the ECG, the scanner produces the SP, which nulls the longitudinal magnetization of tissues. Immediately after, magnetization starts to recover, at a speed that is proportional to the T1 of tissues. Left ventricular myocardium perfused by normal coronary arteries receives more blood than ischemic zones, resulting in a higher concentration of the contrast agent and shorter T1. Ischemic myocardium presents with less contrast agent and thus with a longer T1. After a delay (prepulse delay) that allows the magnetization to recover dependent on the contrast agent concentration, the scanner starts the image readout. The contrast (C) between normally perfused and ischemic myocardium is caused by the difference of T1.

can be used for cine imaging for function and flow. After the second perfusion scan some additional contrast agent is given (e.g., up to 0.4 ml Gd-DTPA or other chelates/kg body weight) to allow for late gadolinium enhancement imaging (Figure 17-4). The combination of images (stress, rest, late gadolinium enhancement) is used for visual interpretation (Figure 17-5).

Adenosine induces maximal vasodilatation in the arterial coronary vessels. Because the microvasculature distal to a coronary artery stenosis is fully dilated at rest, this area does not dilate further with adenosine and resistance to blood flow is higher in comparison with normal vessels. This mechanism, together with a mild reduction of the coronary perfusion pressure, is responsible for a differential distribution of coronary blood flow and thus of the gadolinium-based contrast agent during first-pass perfusion, making it possible to visualize areas of myocardium with reduced blood flow as darker areas (Figure 17-6).

SIDE EFFECTS

The vasodilator effect of adenosine may result in a mild-to-moderate reduction in systolic, diastolic, and mean arterial blood pressure (less than 10 mm Hg) with a reflex increase in heart rate. Most patients complain about chest pain, usually caused by the stimulation of nociceptors. These effects, however, are transient and usually do not require medical intervention.

Because adenosine exerts a direct depressant effect on the SA and AV nodes transient first-, second-, and third-degree AV block and sinus bradycardia were reported in a minority of patients. Also, adenosine can cause significant hypotension. Patients with intact baroreceptor reflex are able to maintain blood pressure in response to adenosine by increasing cardiac output and heart rate. Adenosine can also cause a paradoxic increase in systolic and diastolic blood pressure, which mostly develops in individuals with significant left ventricular hypertrophy. These

increases are transient and resolve spontaneously. Because adenosine is a respiratory stimulant primarily through activation of carotid body chemoreceptors, intravenous administration showed increases in minute ventilation, reduction in arterial Pco_2, and respiratory alkalosis. Approximately 14% of patients complain of dyspnea and an urge to breathe deeply during adenosine infusion.

Table 17-3 reports the monitoring requirements for adenosine stress MR imaging. Contraindications to adenosine administration are reported in Table 17-4.

Adenosine should be discontinued in patients who develop persistent or symptomatic high-grade block or significant drop in systolic blood pressure (greater than 20 mm Hg). The drug should be discontinued in case of persistent or symptomatic hypotension. If a patient develops severe respiratory difficulties, adenosine should be immediately discontinued and an antagonist of adenosine receptors (aminophylline) may be administered (Table 17-5).

VISUAL ASSESSMENT

Visual assessment is based on the identification of regions with lower signal in comparison with normal myocardial segments. The speed of the contrast agent wash in is the best parameter for visual assessment. Care needs to be taken to not interpret small subendocardial rimlike black areas as ischemia (Figure 17-7). They are usually caused by susceptibility artefacts (i.e., artefacts owing to strong

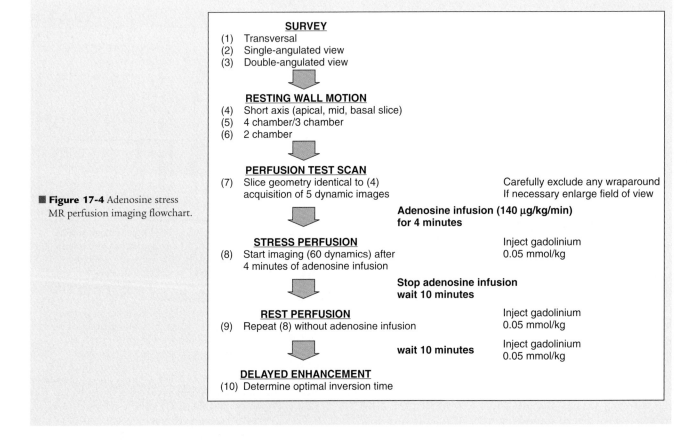

■ **Figure 17-4** Adenosine stress MR perfusion imaging flowchart.

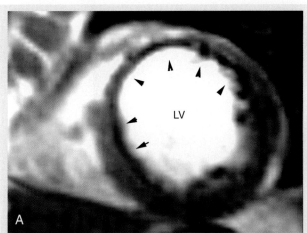

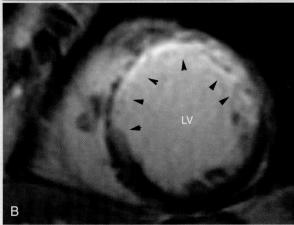

■ **Figure 17-5** Visual interpretation of stress and rest perfusion requires the integration of the information with late gadolinium enhancement. **A,** A subendocardial perfusion defect is present during adenosine administration and at rest (*arrows*). This suggests the presence of a previous chronic myocardial infarction, which is confirmed with the late enhancement images that show subendocardial late enhancement in the same segments (**B,** *arrows*).

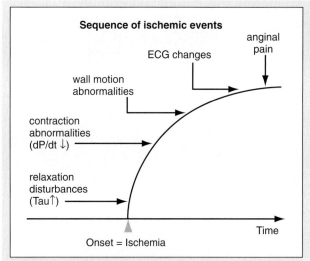

■ **Figure 17-6** The ischemic cascade. Adenosine stress first-pass perfusion is more sensitive than dobutamine stress test in the detection of ischemia, as it is aimed toward the imaging of blood flow itself, which is the first event in the progression of the ischemic cascade. Dobutamine stress visualizes the wall motion abnormalities, which occur later in the scheme. *(From Gould KL, Lipscomb K, Hamilton GW: Physiologic basis for assessing critical coronary stenosis. Instantaneous flow response and regional distribution during coronary hyperemia as measures of coronary flow reserve. Am J Cardiol 1974;33:87-94.)*

TABLE 17-3 Monitoring Requirements for Adenosine Stress Magnetic Resonance Imaging

- Heart rate and rhythm (vector-ECG): continuously*
- Blood pressure: every minute
- Optional pulse oximetry (for rhythm monitoring): continuously
- Symptoms monitoring: continuously

*Vector-ECG monitoring is needed to check heart rhythm but cannot be used to diagnose myocardial ischemia.

TABLE 17-4 Contraindications for Adenosine Stress First-Pass Perfusion Imaging

- Myocardial infarction less than 3 days
- Unstable angina pectoris
- Severe arterial hypertension
- Asthma or severe obstructive pulmonary disease requiring treatment (chronic obstructive pulmonary disease, COPD)
- AV-block > IIa, trifascicular block
- Allergy against vasodilator (in this case, consider, for example, dobutamine)
- Allergy against gadolinium-based contrast agents or renal insufficiency
- Other contraindications for adenosine or dipyridamole administration

Adenosine must be administered with caution in patients with:
- Autonomic nerve dysfunction
- Stenotic valvular disease
- Cerebrovascular insufficiency
- Any obstructive lung disease (COPD)
- Comedication with beta-blockers, Ca-antagonists, or cardiac glycosides (because of AV/sinus node depression)

Sternal wires/clips after cardiac surgery and coronary stents do not interfere with perfusion-CMR. The quality of adenosine stress first-pass perfusion can be limited in patients with frequent extrasystoles (greater than 10/min) or in atrial fibrillation, resulting in a lower diagnostic accuracy.

TABLE 17-5 Termination Criteria

- Persistent or symptomatic AV block
- Significant drop in systolic blood pressure (greater than 20 mm Hg)
- Persistent or symptomatic hypotension
- Severe respiratory difficulty

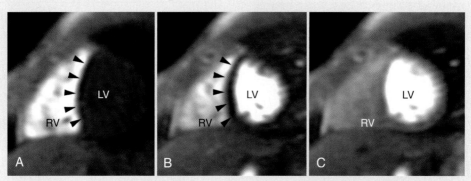

■ **Figure 17-7** Example of dark rim artifact. **A**, A black rim corresponding to the interventricular septum appears when the contrast agent enhances the right ventricle (*arrows*). **B**, The black rim is extended through the interventricular septum when the contrast agent reaches the left ventricle, and then rapidly vanishes (**C**) when some contrast agent has left the cavity and arrives in the myocardium (left ventricle, LV; right ventricle, RV).

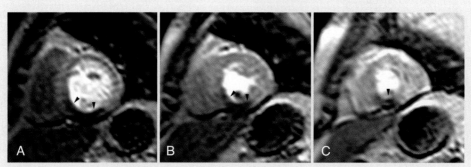

■ **Figure 17-8** Visual assessment of first-pass perfusion during adenosine administration in a patient with a 90% proximal lesion of the right coronary artery. The black arrow marks a transmural perfusion defect in the inferior and inferoseptal segments at basal (**A**), equatorial (**B**), and apical (**C**) level.

differences of magnetization within a small area; e.g., one voxel) and pose the greatest difficulty in interpreting the images. The artefact can be reduced by using smaller doses of contrast agent, TGrE rather than SSFP and higher spatial resolution. True ischemia is usually not black, not circumferential, lasts for several heartbeats after the contrast agent has left the left ventricle, and is more than one pixel in width (Table 17-6).

Visual assessment is usually performed comparing stress and rest images, and viability images obtained with late gadolinium-enhancement techniques (Figure 17-8).

SEMIQUANTIFICATION

Similarly to the visual assessment, the speed of the wash in of the contrast agent is the best parameter for semiquantification. The up slope of the contrast agent wash in is used as an index for blood flow. To correct for signal inhomogeneities caused by differences of the coils used for data acquisition, the change of the up slope with ade-

TABLE 17-6 Criteria for Visual Assessment of Regional Myocardial Perfusion Deficits during First-Pass of Contrast Agent

- Location
  Subendocardial location or transmural extent of a perfusion defect is suggestive of ischemia.
- Dynamic myocardial filling pattern
  "True" perfusion defects appear when the contrast begins to enhance myocardial signal. An artifact should be suspected if a defect appears during contrast arrival in the ventricular cavity and before contrast arrival in the myocardium.
  A dynamic change of the transmural extent of the defect with filling from the epicardium toward the endocardium over several heart beats is typical for regional perfusion abnormalities.
- Myocardial distribution of the defect
  Perfusion defects typically affect more than one slice. The mid-ventricular slice should be evaluated first and suspected defects sought in corresponding segments of adjacent slices.
- Comparison stress versus rest
  Perfusion defects present in the stress scan but not in the rest scan suggest inducible ischemia (dynamic lesion). Matching defects at stress and rest (static lesion) suggest artifact or scar and should be confirmed with late gadolinium enhanced CMR.

nosine stimulation, rather than the up slope itself is used. The simplest approach is a linear fit of the time curve of the myocardial signal. To correct for different arrival speeds of the bolus during rest and stress, the myocardial up slope is corrected for the up slope of the signal in the left ventricular cavity (Figure 17-9). Obviously such an approach is far away from full quantification and must yield relatively low values; that is, it is nearly impossible to achieve an alteration of the up slope by a factor of two, as would be expected when measuring true perfusion reserve. Consequently the parameters obtained from semiquantification are termed *myocardial perfusion reserve index*. Even though this approach is not fully quantitative and needs careful placement of the regions of interest, it has been shown to accurately discriminate between ischemic and normal territories and has been highly reproducible among different sites. However, each sequence requires its own set of normal values.

FULL QUANTIFICATION

Absolute quantification of myocardial perfusion in [ml/g/min] of tissue is feasible from first-pass myocardial perfusion CMR data. Several fitting models have been proposed to deconvolve the myocardial signal and account for the different compartments of contrast agent distribution (Figures 17-10 to 17-17). All quantification models have in common that they anticipate linearity between signal intensity and contrast concentration, so that relatively low doses of contrast (0.03 to 0.05 mmol/kg) have to be used for data acquisition. Absolute quantification of CMR perfusion data may have a role in the detection of balanced multivessel ischemia and in longitudinal studies of therapeutic interventions but is currently less used in clinical routine.

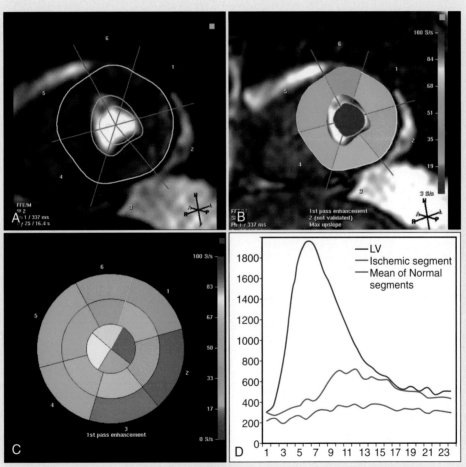

■ **Figure 17-9** Example of semiquantitative evaluation of first-pass perfusion during adenosine administration in a patient with a 90% proximal lesion of the first diagonal branch. **A,** A short-axis view is divided in six radial segments and the signal from the left ventricular blood is marked. The anterior segment presents a subendocardial reduction of the signal, the anterolateral segment shows a transmural defect. **B,** The software analyzes the signal from each segment, calculating the maximum up slope of signal. The reduction of signal in the antero and anterolateral segments is visualized using a color scale. **C,** This process is repeated for every segment of the left ventricle, and a map of the signal up slope is created. **D,** Signal intensity from the left ventricle (LV), compared with the signal intensity from normal and ischemic myocardial segments.

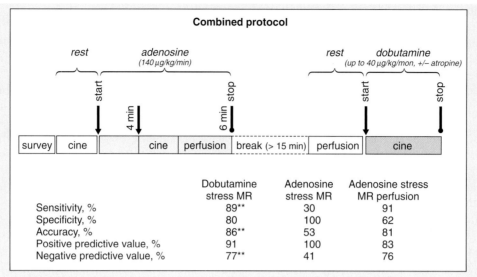

Combined protocol

	Dobutamine stress MR	Adenosine stress MR	Adenosine stress MR perfusion
Sensitivity, %	89**	30	91
Specificity, %	80	100	62
Accuracy, %	86**	53	81
Positive predictive value, %	91	100	83
Negative predictive value, %	77**	41	76

■ **Figure 17-10** Adenosine and dobutamine stress MR combined protocol. *(From Jahnke C, Nagel E, Gebker R, et al: Prognostic value of cardiac magnetic resonance stress tests: adenosine stress perfusion and dobutamine stress wall motion imaging. Circulation 2007;115:1769-1776, with permission.)*

■ **Figure 17-11** In a multicenter trial the performance of first-pass perfusion-cardiac magnetic resonance was determined and compared with the diagnostic accuracy of single photon emission computed tomography (SPECT). The receiver operating characteristic curve analyses show that first-pass perfusion magnetic resonance imaging is at least not inferior to SPECT for the detection of CAD. **A**, The efficacy of different contrast medium doses was tested. The best performance was achieved at the highest dose (0.10 mmol/kg of Gd-DTPA-BMA). Head to head comparison versus single-photon emission computed tomography in (**B**) did not show any significant difference in the area under the receiver operating characteristic curve. *(From Schwitter J, Wacker CM, van Rossum AC, et al: MR-IMPACT: Comparison of perfusion-cardiac magnetic resonance with single-photon emission computed tomography for the detection of coronary artery disease in a multicentre, multivendor, randomized trial. Eur Heart J 2008;29:480-489.)*

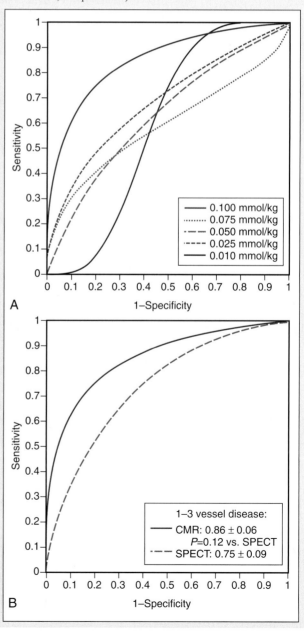

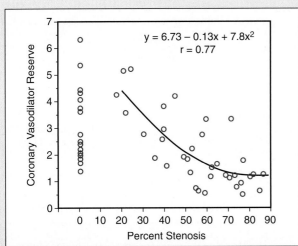

Figure 17-12 Over a wide range, myocardial blood flow in humans remains constant at rest regardless of the severity of a coronary artery stenosis. However, during hyperemia, flow progressively decreases when the degree of stenosis is about 40% or more, and does not differ significantly from basal flow when stenosis is 80% or greater. This figure shows the coronary vasodilator reserve (flow during hyperemia/flow at base line) in relation to a stenosis (as a percentage of vessel diameter). Coronary vasodilator reserve decreased significantly as stenosis increased. *(From Uren NG, Melin JA, De Bruyne B, et al: Relation between myocardial blood flow and the severity of coronary-artery stenosis. N Engl J Med 1994;330:1782-1788.)*

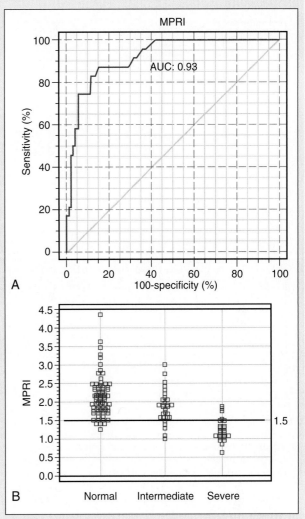

Figure 17-13 First-pass perfusion magnetic resonance during adenosine stress was validated in comparison with fractional flow reserve. It has a high sensitivity and specificity in the discrimination of relevant from nonrelevant coronary lesions (**A**). **B,** The individual first-pass perfusion magnetic resonance values for the perfusion territories with normal, intermediate, and severe coronary stenosis, as described by a myocardial perfusion reserve index (MPRI = stress up slope/rest up slope) cutoff of 1.5. *(From Rieber J, Huber A, Erhard I, et al: Cardiac magnetic resonance perfusion imaging for the functional assessment of coronary artery disease: A comparison with coronary angiography and fractional flow reserve. Eur Heart J 2006;27:1465-1471.)*

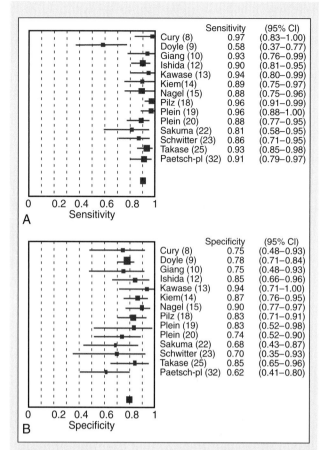

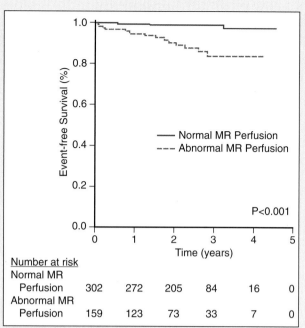

Figure 17-14 An evidence-based evaluation of adenosine first-pass perfusion magnetic resonance from 24 datasets (1516 patients). Perfusion imaging demonstrated a sensitivity (**A**) of 0.91 and specificity (**B**) of 0.81. (*From Nandalur KR, Dwamena BA, Choudhri AF, et al: Diagnostic performance of stress cardiac magnetic resonance imaging in the detection of coronary artery disease: A meta-analysis. J Am Coll Cardiol 2007;50:1343-1353, with permission.*)

Figure 17-15 In patients with known or suspected CAD, myocardial ischemia detected by adenosine first-pass magnetic resonance perfusion identifies patients at high risk for subsequent cardiac death or nonfatal myocardial infarction. Normal test results are associated with a very low event rate. This figure shows a Kaplan-Meyer curve for the composite endpoint of cardiac death and nonfatal myocardial infarction, stratifying the patients on the result of adenosine first-pass perfusion imaging. (*From Jahnke C, Nagel E, Gebker R, et al: Prognostic value of cardiac magnetic resonance stress tests: Adenosine stress perfusion and dobutamine stress wall motion imaging. Circulation 2007;115:1769-1776.*)

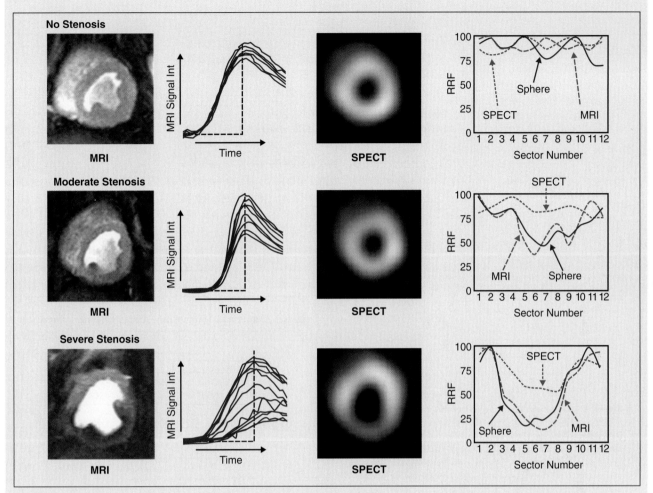

■ **Figure 17-16** Magnetic resonance first-pass perfusion can identify regional reduction in myocardial blood flow during global coronary vasodilatation over a wide range better than single photon emission computed tomography imaging (SPECT). It can also identify transmural flow gradients. Myocardial blood flow under pharmacologic vasodilatation was measured with microspheres in chronically instrumented dogs without and with a severe or moderate stenosis of the left circumflex artery. It was compared with magnetic resonance first-pass perfusion and with SPECT. **From left to right:** A single frame from the magnetic resonance short axis image stack; the magnetic resonance first pass perfusion signal-intensity curves for 12 myocardial segments; the corresponding 99mTc-sestamibi SPECT image; and relative magnetic resonance first-pass perfusion curve areas, 99mTc-sestamibi count rates, and microsphere concentrations in each sector. Magnetic resonance first-pass perfusion correctly identifies a moderate flow reduction as a mild reduction of enhancement, showing a markedly reduced enhancement in animals with severe stenosis. A transmural gradient in flow is visually evident in both cases. SPECT images show uniform signal intensity in the absence of flow reduction and the presence of moderate flow reduction, whereas it is capable of identifying severe stenosis as an apparent perfusion deficit. The performance magnetic resonance first-pass perfusion is confirmed by the close correspondence of the signal-intensity curve area with the microsphere concentration. *(From Lee DC, Simonetti OP, Harris KR, et al: Magnetic resonance versus radionuclide pharmacological stress perfusion imaging for flow-limiting stenoses of varying severity. Circulation 2004;110:58-65, with permission.)*

■ **Figure 17-17 A,** Indications for adenosine stress first-pass perfusion MR for the diagnosis of coronary artery disease were scored depending on the clinical symptoms as appropriate, uncertain, and inappropriate. **B,** Similarly adenosine stress first-pass perfusion MR is appropriate as post-test assessment in patients with previous coronary angiography showing stenosis of unclear significance.

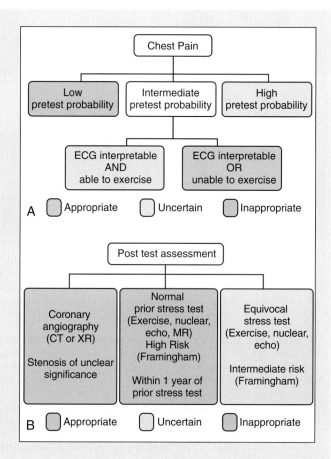

Case 1 **Subendocardial Perfusion Deficit**

A 63-year-old man with diabetes and past history of smoking complained about worsening dyspnea during exertion and was referred for adenosine stress first-pass perfusion magnetic resonance (Figure 17-18). The perfusion sequence was performed during adenosine infusion using a turbo-gradient echo sequence. After 20 minutes the adenosine infusion was repeated and a second perfusion study was made using a steady-state free precession sequence to demonstrate the differences of distinct imaging sequences.

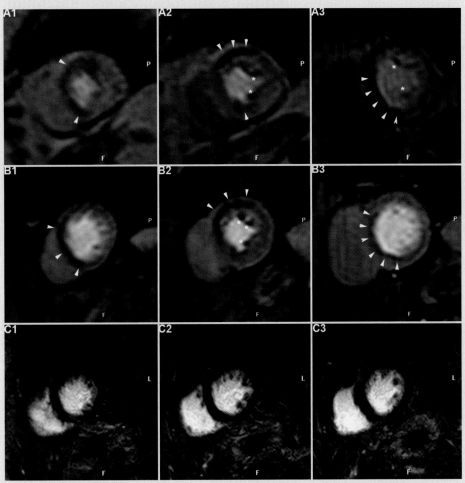

■ **Figure 17-18** Turbo-gradient echo sequence (A1, A2, A3) shows a subendocardial perfusion deficit (*arrows*) involving the apical septum, the anterior and the inferior wall in the equatorial slice, and the inferior and the inferoseptal segment in the basal slice. A dark rim artifact is also present in the equatorial image (*), because of susceptibility between the left ventricular blood and papillary muscle. The steady-state free precession sequence (B1, B2, B3) confirmed the findings. Note the higher definition and image sharpness (which depends on a better signal-to-noise ratio) obtained using this sequence. Unfortunately the dark rim artifact is usually with steady-state free precession in comparison with turbo-gradient echo imaging. The late gadolinium enhancement images (C1, C2, C3) confirms myocardial viability in the ischemic segments. Coronary angiography diagnosed a two-vessel coronary artery disease involving the right and left anterior descending coronary artery.

A 70-year-old man presented with systemic arterial hypertension and hypercholes-terolemia despite pharmacologic treatment with statins. His father died of myocardial infarction at the age of 59. He had no past history of heart diseases. He experienced chest discomfort during physical stress (while skiing, in the cold season), and was referred by his cardiologist for adenosine stress first-pass perfusion MR. There were no abnormal physical findings at rest. Adenosine stress first-pass perfusion magnetic resonance was performed following the procedure depicted in Figure 17-4 (Figure 17-19). During adenosine infusion he experienced the same chest discomfort (described as a feeling of pressure), as during physical exertion.

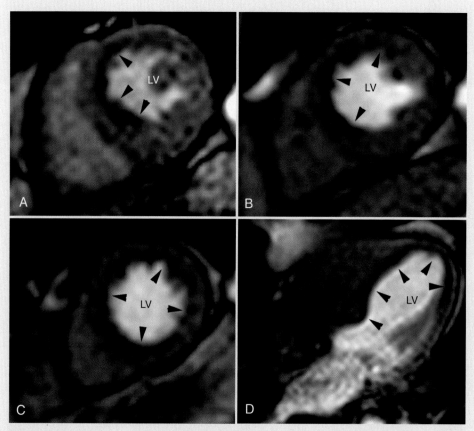

■ **Figure 17-19** Adenosine first-pass perfusion showed an inducible subendocardial perfusion defect, absent at rest, which was visible in all slices (*black arrows*). **A,** Short axis of the left ventricle, basal slice: The perfusion defect is seen in the anterior segment and the interventricular septum; **B,** short axis, equatorial slice: The perfusion deficit spreads from the lateral segment to the interventricular septum; **C,** short axis, apical slice: The subendocardial perfusion defect is present in all segments. The findings are confirmed in the four-chamber view **D.** Coronary angiography found a long lesion of the left main and left anterior descending, of about 80%, which was successfully treated with percutaneous coronary angioplasty.

Case 3   **Perfusion Deficit in the Lateral Wall**

A 68-year-old woman with a long-standing history of arterial hypertension complained about chest discomfort during physical effort and was referred for adenosine stress first-pass perfusion magnetic resonance because of persisting ECG repolarization alterations at rest. Imaging was performed according to the flowchart reported in Figure 17-4 (Figure 17-20). During adenosine administration she experienced the same symptoms.

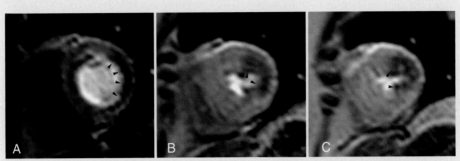

■ **Figure 17-20** Adenosine stress images show a perfusion deficit in the lateral wall, with a clear gradient from the subendocardium to the subepicardium. No scar was present in the late enhancement images. Coronary angiography found a single-vessel disease of the left circumflex artery, which was treated with percutaneous coronary angioplasty.

Case 4   **Subendocardial Perfusion Defect**

A 69-year-old man, a smoker, presented with previous anteroseptal myocardial infarction caused by a disease of the proximal anterior descending coronary artery and new onset of angina (Figure 17-21).

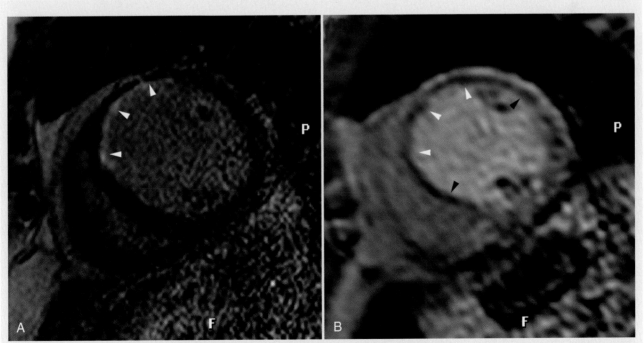

■ **Figure 17-21** The gadolinium late-enhancement image (**A**) shows an area of fibrosis extending from the anteroseptal to the anterior segment (*white arrows*). Adenosine stress first-pass perfusion (**B**) shows a subendocardial perfusion defect corresponding to the scar and present also at rest (*white arrows*), and a inducible perfusion defect extending up to the lateral wall in one direction and down to the inferoseptal segments in the other (*black arrows*). In the same segments the absence of gadolinium late enhancement demonstrated the viability of the myocardium.

Case 5   **Perfusion Defect of the Hypertrophic Septum and the Lateral Wall**

A 24-year-old man with known hypertrophic cardiomyopathy, diagnosed during a family screening, performed after sudden cardiac death of his father, which showed a form of asymmetric massive septal hypertrophy during autopsy. Screening for known risk factors for sudden death showed the following: massive septal hypertrophy (39 mm of maximum left ventricular thickness), no sustained episodes of ventricular arrhythmias in 24-hour ECG monitoring, no hypotension nor arrhythmias during treadmill exercise test. The patient was in NYHA functional class I (Figure 17-22).

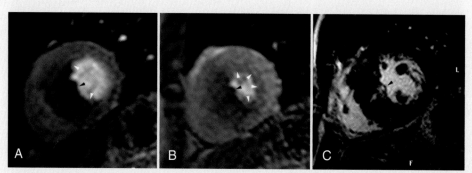

■ **Figure 17-22** Adenosine stress first-pass perfusion magnetic resonance showed a marked perfusion defect mainly involving the hypertrophic septum and also to a lesser degree the lateral wall, with a gradient of reduction of the perfusion from the subendocardium to the subepicardium (**A, B,** *white arrows*). The pathogenesis of this defect involves a microvascular dysfunction of the small intramyocardial coronary vessels, with a reduction of the coronary flow reserve. Late enhancement sequences (**C**) showed enhancement of the interventricular septum in correspondence with the insertion points of the right ventricular wall and the middle part of the septum (*black arrow*). This area of enhancement corresponds with the most pronounced perfusion defect. The first-pass perfusion defect can be explained by a reduced vascularization of the scarred myocardium.

Case 6   **Coronary Artery Stenosis**

A 70-year-old man was admitted for extracardiac surgery and evaluated with adenosine stress first-pass perfusion imaging because of suspected coronary artery disease during preoperative workup (Figure 17-23).

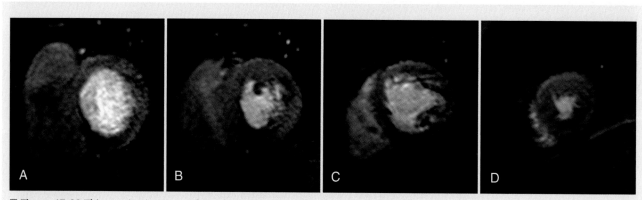

■ **Figure 17-23** This examination was performed using a 3 Tesla scanner and a turbo gradient echo sequence. Perfusion at 3 T has a high accuracy for the detection of hemodynamically relevant coronary artery stenosis in patients with suspected and known CAD. Note the high signal-to-noise ratio and image sharpness of the images.

Case 7   **Transmural Perfusion Defect**

This was a 55-year-old man who had been previously treated with percutaneous coronary angioplasty of the left anterior descending coronary artery and the distal right coronary artery for the onset of angina and dyspnea during physical exercise. Six months after the intervention, he complained about symptoms and was evaluated with adenosine stress first-pass perfusion magnetic resonance (Figure 17-24).

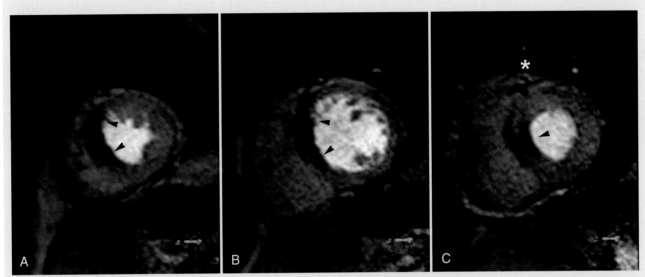

■ **Figure 17-24** Adenosine stress first-pass perfusion magnetic resonance (performed with a k-t SENSE sequence; note the high image quality and resolution), demonstrates a transmural perfusion defect (*arrows*) in the segments supplied by the left anterior descending (**A,** apical slice. **B,** equatorial slice). The coronary angiography confirmed an in-stent restenosis in the left anterior descending. In the basal slice (**C**) an epicardial artifact caused by the presence of a coronary stent is visible (*).

Case 8   **Subendocardial Necrosis and Perfusion Defect**

A 58-year-old male patient was scanned 4 days after an acute myocardial infarction (Figure 17-25).

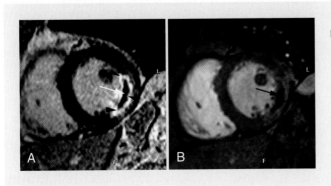

■ **Figure 17-25 A,** Late gadolinium enhancement showed a subendocardial necrosis (75% of transmurality), with peripheral white hyperenhanced area (*black arrows*) and black central not reperfused zone (microvascular obstruction, *white arrow*). Rest first-pass magnetic resonance perfusion has showed a perfusion defect in the same segments. **B,** Perfusion image is shown at peak contrast in the LV myocardium. Rest perfusion was performed with a k-t SENSE accelerated perfusion method at 1.5 T, with spatial resolution 1.5 × 1.5 mm. Note the high image quality and resolution.

SUGGESTED READING

Al-Saadi N, Nagel E, Gross M, et al: Noninvasive detection of myocardial ischemia from perfusion reserve based on cardiovascular magnetic resonance. Circulation 2000;101:1379-1383.

Cerqueira MD, Verani MS, Schwaiger M, et al: Safety profile of adenosine stress perfusion imaging: results from the Adenoscan Multicenter Trial Registry. J Am Coll Cardiol 1994;23:384-389.

Gebker R, Jahnke C, Paetsch I, et al: MR myocardial perfusion imaging with k-space and time broad-use linear acquisition speed-up technique: feasibility study. Radiology 2007;245:863-871.

Gebker R, Jahnke C, Paetsch I, et al: Diagnostic performance of myocardial perfusion MR at 3 T in patients with coronary artery disease. Radiology 2008;247:57-63.

Gebker R, Schwitter J, Fleck E, Nagel E: How we perform myocardial perfusion with cardiovascular magnetic resonance. J Cardiovasc Magn Reson 2007;9:539-547.

Giang TH, Nanz D, Coulden R, et al: Detection of coronary artery disease by magnetic resonance myocardial perfusion imaging with various contrast medium doses: First European multi-centre experience. Eur Heart J 2004;25:1657-1665.

Greenwood JP, Younger JF, Ridgway JP, et al: Safety and diagnostic accuracy of stress cardiac magnetic resonance imaging vs exercise tolerance testing early after acute ST elevation myocardial infarction. Heart 2007;93:1363-1368.

Hendel RC, Patel MR, Kramer CM, et al: ACCF/ACR/SCCT/SCMR/ASNC/NASCI/SCAI/SIR 2006 appropriateness criteria for cardiac computed tomography and cardiac magnetic resonance imaging: A report of the American College of Cardiology Foundation Quality Strategic Directions Committee Appropriateness Criteria Working Group, American College of Radiology, Society of Cardiovascular Computed Tomography, Society for Cardiovascular Magnetic Resonance, American Society of Nuclear Cardiology, North American Society for Cardiac Imaging, Society for Cardiovascular Angiography and Interventions, and Society of Interventional Radiology. J Am Coll Cardiol 2006;48:1475-1497.

Ibrahim T, Nekolla SG, Schreiber K, et al: Assessment of coronary flow reserve: comparison between contrast-enhanced magnetic resonance imaging and positron emission tomography. J Am Coll Cardiol 2002;39:864-870.

Jahnke C, Nagel E, Gebker R, et al: Prognostic value of cardiac magnetic resonance stress tests: adenosine stress perfusion and dobutamine stress wall motion imaging. Circulation 2007;115:1769-1776.

Kellman P, Arai AE: Imaging sequences for first pass perfusion: A review. J Cardiovasc Magn Reson 2007;9:525-537.

Lee DC, Simonetti OP, Harris KR, et al: Magnetic resonance versus radionuclide pharmacological stress perfusion imaging for flow-limiting stenoses of varying severity. Circulation 2004;110:58-65.

Nagel E, Klein C, Paetsch I, et al: Magnetic resonance perfusion measurements for the noninvasive detection of coronary artery disease. Circulation 2003;108:432-437.

Nandalur KR, Dwamena BA, Choudhri AF, et al: Diagnostic performance of stress cardiac magnetic resonance imaging in the detection of coronary artery disease: A meta-analysis. J Am Coll Cardiol 2007;50:1343-1353.

Paetsch I, Jahnke C, Wahl A, et al: Comparison of dobutamine stress magnetic resonance, adenosine stress magnetic resonance, and adenosine stress magnetic resonance perfusion. Circulation. 2004;110:835-842.

Petersen SE, Jerosch-Herold M, Hudsmith LE, et al: Evidence for microvascular dysfunction in hypertrophic cardiomyopathy: New insights from multiparametric magnetic resonance imaging. Circulation 2007;115:2418-2425.

Plein S, Greenwood JP, Ridgway JP, et al: Assessment of non-ST-segment elevation acute coronary syndromes with cardiac magnetic resonance imaging. J Am Coll Cardiol 2004;44:2173-2181.

Plein S, Radjenovic A, Ridgway JP, et al: Coronary artery disease: myocardial perfusion MR imaging with sensitivity encoding versus conventional angiography. Radiology 2005;235:423-430.

Plein S, Ridgway JP, Jones TR, et al: Coronary artery disease: assessment with a comprehensive MR imaging protocol: Initial results. Radiology 2002;225:300-307.

Plein S, Ryf S, Schwitter J, et al: Dynamic contrast-enhanced myocardial perfusion MRI accelerated with k-t sense. Magn Reson Med 2007;58:777-785.

Rieber J, Huber A, Erhard I, et al: Cardiac magnetic resonance perfusion imaging for the functional assessment of coronary artery disease: A comparison with coronary angiography and fractional flow reserve. Eur Heart J 2006;27:1465-1471.

Schwitter J, Nanz D, Kneifel S, et al: Assessment of myocardial perfusion in coronary artery disease by magnetic resonance: A comparison with positron emission tomography and coronary angiography. Circulation 2001;103:2230-2235.

Schwitter J, Wacker CM, van Rossum AC, et al: MR-IMPACT: Comparison of perfusion-cardiac magnetic resonance with single-photon emission computed tomography for the detection of coronary artery disease in a multicentre, multivendor, randomized trial. Eur Heart J 2008;29:480-489.

Shiode N, Kato M, Nakayama K, et al: Effect of adenosine triphosphate on human coronary circulation. Intern Med 1998;37:818-825.

Wolff SD, Schwitter J, Coulden R, et al: Myocardial first-pass perfusion magnetic resonance imaging: A multicenter dose-ranging study. Circulation 2004;110:732-737.

Chapter 18

Wall Motion Stress Magnetic Resonance

William O. Ntim, Rahul Aggarwal, Chirapa Puntawangkoon, and W. Gregory Hundley

KEY POINTS

- CMR can detect myocardial ischemia using exercise and pharmacologic stressors with accuracy comparable to nuclear and echocardiography.

- Accuracy of CMR wall motion stress testing for ischemia may be limited in patients with left ventricular hypertrophy, resting wall motion abnormalities, and severely reduced resting left ventricular systolic function. Addition of stress and rest perfusion protocols to wall motion assessment may improve the accuracy in these clinical situations.

- The prognostic value of CMR pharmacologic wall motion stress testing is well established.

- Further studies are needed to validate the prognostic implications of exercise wall motion CMR stress testing.

- Additional studies are needed to elucidate the diagnostic and prognostic values of combined wall motion–perfusion CMR stress testing.

- Myocardial scar and/or infarct assessment by late-gadolinium enhancement imaging from combined wall motion–perfusion CMR stress testing may provide additional prognostic implications.

- CMR wall motion stress testing is a suitable alternative for ischemia and viability assessments in patients with contraindications to gadolinium-based CMR perfusion stress testing as in moderate to severe kidney disease.

Cardiovascular magnetic resonance (CMR) has emerged as a viable alternate method of evaluating for myocardial ischemia, by the detection of stress-induced systolic wall motion abnormalities (Figure 18-1). Standardized myocardial nomenclature is used for segment and vascular territory identification (Figures 18-2 to 18-4).

CMR stressors used for wall motion stress tests include exercise, and pharmacologic agents (i.e., dobutamine and vasodilators such as adenosine and dipyridamole). Dobutamine ± atropine is the most common stressor used for assessment of inducible wall motion abnormalities (Figure 18-5). Performance of wall motion stress CMR requires standardized protocol, real-time display of wall motion, and safety protocols (Figures 18-6 to 18-9). Intraprocedural ECG tracing is mainly used for rhythm monitoring and not ischemic ST changes because of distortion of segments by CMR (Figure 18-10).

This chapter presents case studies of clinically available CMR methodologies using wall motion for the detection of myocardial ischemia.

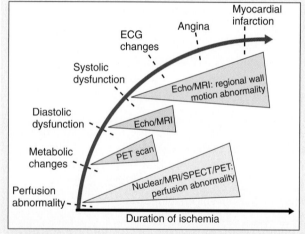

■ **Figure 18-1** The ischemic cascade represents the sequence of pathophysiologic events after ischemia.

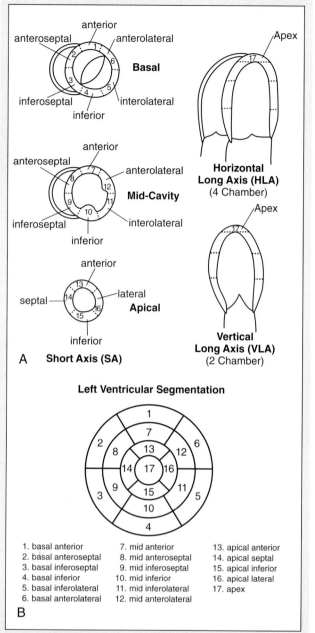

■ **Figure 18-2 A,** Diagram of vertical long-axis (VLA, approximating the two-chamber view), horizontal long-axis (HLA, approximating the four-chamber view), and short-axis (SA) planes showing the name, location, and anatomic landmarks for selection of the basal (tips of the mitral valve leaflets), mid-cavity (papillary muscles), and apical (beyond papillary muscles but before cavity ends) short-axis slices for the recommended 17-segment system. **B,** Display, on a circumferential polar plot, of the 17 myocardial segments and the recommended nomenclature for tomographic imaging of the heart. (*A is from Cerqueira MD, Weissman NJ, Dilsizian V, et al: Standardized myocardial segmentation and nomenclature for tomographic imaging of the heart. A statement for healthcare professionals from the Cardiac Imaging Committee of the Council on Clinical Cardiology of the American Heart Association. Circulation 2002;105:539-542.*)

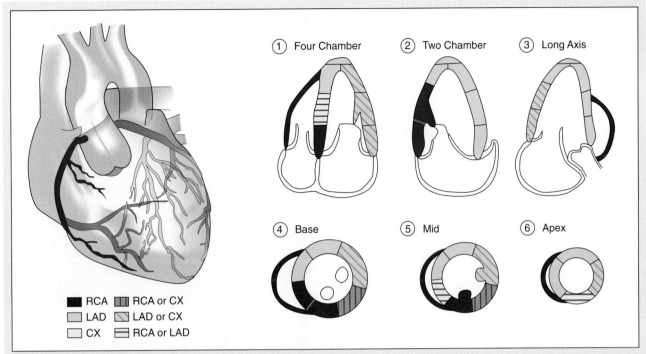

■ **Figure 18-3** Typical distributions of the right coronary artery (RCA), the left anterior descending (LAD), and the circumflex (CX) coronary arteries. The arterial distribution varies among patients. Some segments have variable coronary perfusion. *(From Recommendations for chamber quantification: A report from the American Society of Echocardiography's Guidelines and Standards Committee and the Chamber Quantification Writing Group, developed in conjunction with the European Association of Echocardiography, a branch of the European Society of Cardiology: J Am Soc Echocardiogr 2005;18:1440-1463.)*

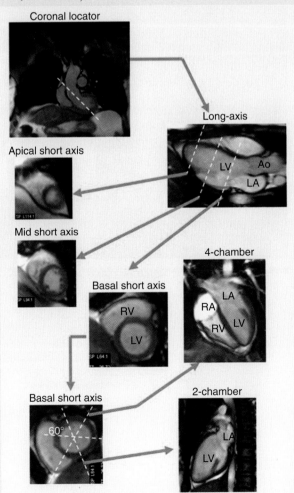

■ **Figure 18-4** Method for obtained standard views, obtaining three short-axis (basal, mid, and apical) and three apical long-axis views (long-axis, four-chamber, and two-chamber views). In all images the myocardium is gray and the blood pool is white. The *white dotted lines* indicate the slice positions for obtaining the subsequent views demarcated by the *gray arrows*. Ao, aorta; LA, left atrium; LV, left ventricle; RA, right atrium; RV, right ventricle.

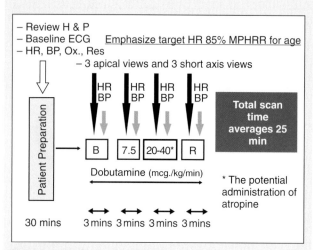

- Review H & P
- Baseline ECG   Emphasize target HR 85% MPHRR for age
- HR, BP, Ox., Res
                    – 3 apical views and 3 short axis views

Patient Preparation →

| B | 7.5 | 20-40* | R |

Dobutamine (mcg./kg/min)

Total scan time averages 25 min

* The potential administration of atropine

30 mins   3 mins 3 mins 3 mins 3 mins

■ **Figure 18-5** Protocol for DCMR.

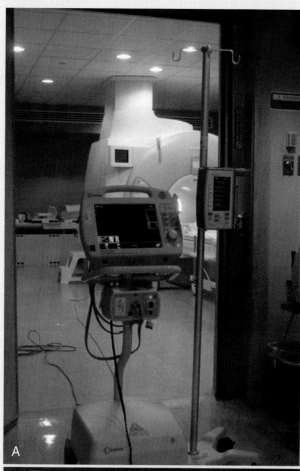

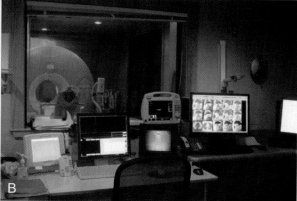

■ **Figure 18-7** Patient monitoring and image acquisition areas.

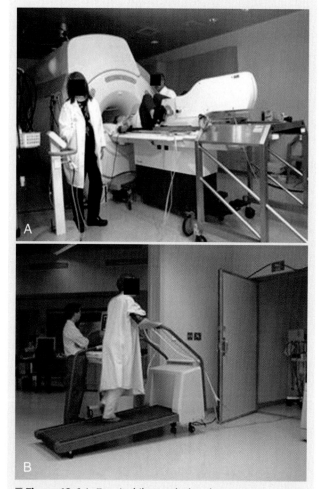

■ **Figure 18-6 A,** Exercise bike attached to the scanner.
B, Treadmill positioned outside the scan room.

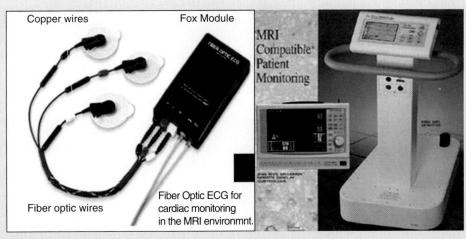

Figure 18-8 Patient monitoring devices.

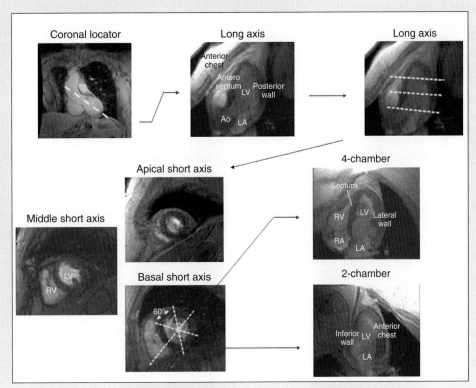

Figure 18-9 Various views obtained in wall motion stress CMR.

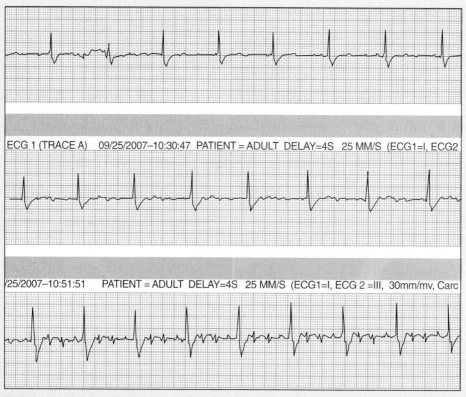

ECG 1 (TRACE A)   09/25/2007–10:30:47 PATIENT = ADULT DELAY=4S 25 MM/S (ECG1=I, ECG2

/25/2007–10:51:51   PATIENT = ADULT DELAY=4S 25 MM/S (ECG1=I, ECG 2 =III, 30mm/mv, Carc

■ **Figure 18-10** Magnetohydrodynamic effects. **A,** Telemetry outside of magnet. **B,** Telemetry during CMR scan. **C,** During pharmacologic stress test.

Case 1   Ischemia Evaluation by Dobutamine Stress Cardiac Magnetic Resonance

A 63-year-old woman with end-stage renal disease (ESRD) secondary to diabetic nephropathy and on maintenance hemodialysis presented for preoperative evaluation for renal transplantation. She underwent dobutamine stress cardiac magnetic resonance (DSCMR) for further preoperative cardiovascular risk stratification.

DSCMR revealed evidence of inducible ischemia in the apical inferior and inferolateral walls (Figure 18-11). A cardiac catheterization demonstrated significant three-vessel disease (Figure 18-12), necessitating a successful three-vessel CABG. She subsequently underwent a successful kidney transplant with an uneventful postoperative clinical course.

Comments

Wall motion stress test by CMR is considered an appropriate test for risk-stratifying patients with chest pain syndromes with intermediate pretest probability of coronary artery disease. Recent ACC/AHA guidelines on preoperative care before noncardiac surgery have also recommended stress test risk stratification among patients with at least three clinical risk factors (ischemic heart disease, compensated or prior heart failure, cerebrovascular disease, diabetes mellitus, renal insufficiency), poor functional capacity (less than 4 METs), and those undergoing vascular surgery.

DSCMR provides diagnostic accuracy and prognostic significance comparable with established tools such as nuclear imaging and echocardiography (Figure 18-13). DSCMR is also suitable in patients with contraindications to vasodilators such as adenosine and dipyridamole or in situations such as ESRD, in which administration of CMR contrast for perfusion is contraindicated.

DSCMR has sensitivity and specificity of 83% to 96% and 80% to 87%, respectively, for identifying significant epicardial coronary artery stenoses (≥50% luminal stenoses). The interpretation scheme for wall motion stress CMR is similar to stress echocardiography (Figure 18-14).

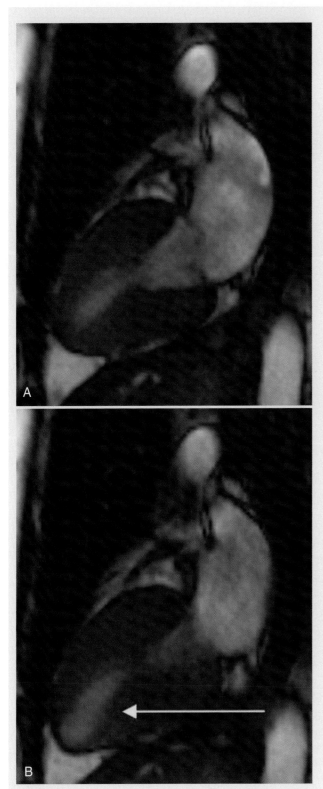

■ **Figure 18-11 A,** Resting parasternal angle demonstrates normal left ventricular contraction with no wall motion abnormalities. **B,** Peak dobutamine end-systolic cine view demonstrating hypokinesis of the inferoapical region.

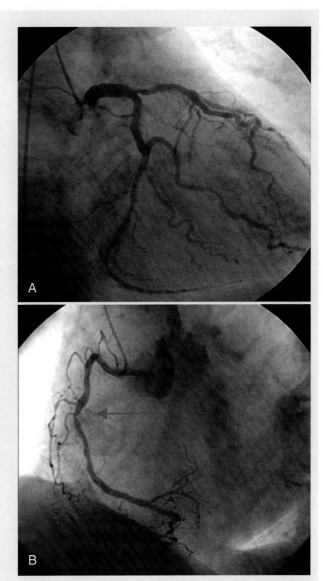

■ **Figure 18-12 A,** RAO caudal view demonstrating a 70% proximal LAD, 80% OM2, and 60% distal circumflex lesions. **B,** The red arrow demonstrates an 80% mid-RCA lesion.

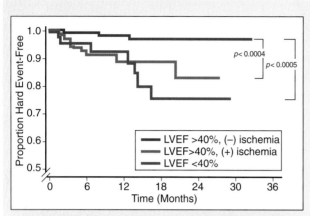

■ **Figure 18-13** Cardiac prognosis with dobutamine stress CMR. *(From Hundley WG, Morgan TM, Neagle CM, et al: Magnetic resonance imaging determination of cardiac prognosis. Circulation 2002;106:2328-2333, with permission.)*

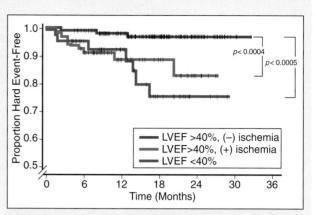

■ **Figure 18-15** Cardiac prognosis with dobutamine stress CMR. *(From Hundley WG, Morgan TM, Neagle CM, et al: Magnetic resonance imaging determination of cardiac prognosis. Circulation 2002;106:2328-2333, with permission.)*

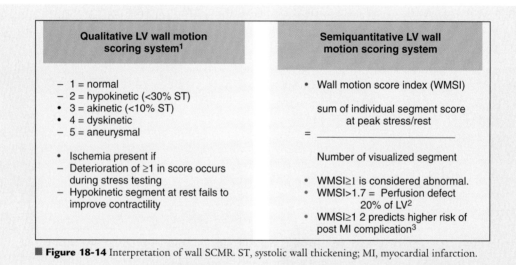

■ **Figure 18-14** Interpretation of wall SCMR. ST, systolic wall thickening; MI, myocardial infarction.

The utility of DSCMR in assessing cardiac prognosis is established. In a cohort 279 patients followed for 20 months, Hundley et al. (2002) reported that among those with LVEF ≥ 40% and no evidence of inducible ischemia, event-free survival was significantly better those with inducible ischemia (Figure 18-15). Jahnke et al. (2007) noted that among 513 patients with known or suspected coronary artery disease, inducible ischemia by DSCMR provided incremental prognostic information over clinical risk factors and resting wall motion abnormalities with a fivefold increase in major adverse cardiac events (MACE) (Figure 18-16).

Perioperative cardiac events result in significant mortality and morbidity. Rerkpattanapipat et al. (2002) studied the preoperative utility of DSCMR in 102 patients with suboptimal echocardiograms and intermediate clinical risk predictors before noncardiac surgery. Death, myocardial infarction, and heart failure were among MACEs assessed. Twenty-nine and seventy-three patients underwent vascular and nonvascular surgery, respectively. In a multivariate analysis including intermediate clinical risk factors for cardiac events, inducible ischemia during DSCMR was a significant predictor of cardiac events ($p = 0.04$). In contrast patients who achieved a heart rate response of 80% of the maximum predicted heart rate response for age during age, during stress, and no inducible ischemia had no MACE (Figure 18-17). Thus DSCMR is a suitable alternate for ischemia evaluation and prognostication among patients with intermediate pretest probability for coronary artery disease.

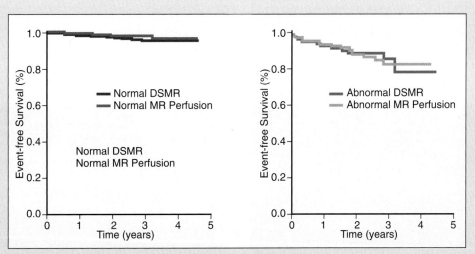

■ **Figure 18-16** Kaplan-Meier curves for comparison of normal and abnormal DSCMR and MRP. *(From Jahnke C, Nagel E, Gebker R, et al: Prognostic value of cardiac magnetic resonance stress tests: Adenosine stress perfusion and dobutamine stress wall motion imaging. Circulation 2007;115:1769-1776, with permission).*

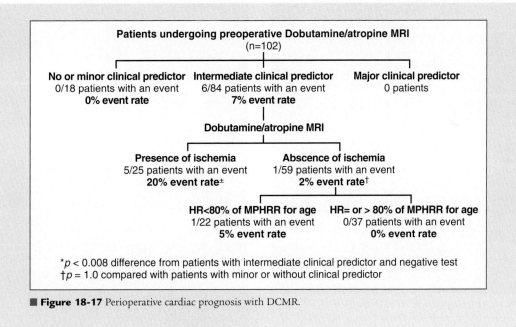

■ **Figure 18-17** Perioperative cardiac prognosis with DCMR.

Case 2 **Stress Wall Motion in a Patient with Left Ventricular Hypertrophy: The Role of Combined Wall Motion and Perfusion**

A 55-year-old white man with a history of coronary artery disease, status post two-vessel coronary artery bypass grafts, hypertension, hyperlipidemia, and obesity presented as an outpatient with increasing episodes of chest pressure not related to exertion. He also noted a progression of dyspnea on exertion as a possible angina equivalent. He underwent a dobutamine stress CMR. However, because of resting concentric LV hypertrophy, perfusion imaging was added. Stress and rest CINE did not demonstrate wall motion abnormalities. Contrast-enhanced first-pass perfusion revealed perfusion abnormalities in the anterior and inferior walls (Figure 18-18), which correlated with coronary artery disease (CAD) in the SVG to right coronary artery graft and left anterior descending artery (LAD) (Figure 18-19). Based on stress-induced perfusion abnormality, patient underwent successful PCI of SVG to RCA. Coronary angiography also revealed diffuse LAD disease, which was treated medically.

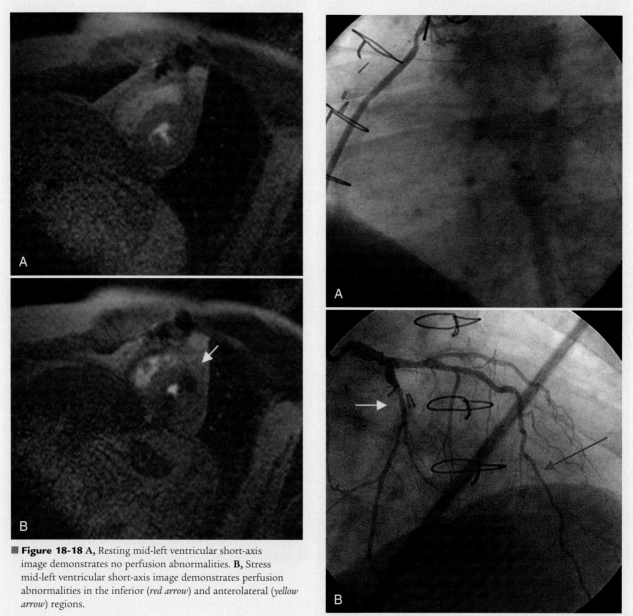

■ **Figure 18-18 A,** Resting mid-left ventricular short-axis image demonstrates no perfusion abnormalities. **B,** Stress mid-left ventricular short-axis image demonstrates perfusion abnormalities in the inferior (*red arrow*) and anterolateral (*yellow arrow*) regions.

■ **Figure 18-19 A,** LAO view of the SVG to distal RCA graft demonstrates a 70% lesion in the proximal body of the graft (*red arrow*). This lesion was successfully stented with a drug-eluting stent. **B,** RAO cranial view of the left coronary system demonstrates a 60% lesion in the mid-circumflex (*yellow arrow*) and diffuse disease in the mid-and distal LAD (*red arrow*). The SVG to the first OM (*not shown*) was patent.

Comments

The sensitivity, accuracy, and prognostic value of stress wall motion may be reduced in the presence of left ventricular hypertrophy (LVH). This has been attributed to the small left ventricular (LV) cavity, as well as abnormalities in LV geometry, wall stress, and coronary flow reserve among patients with LVH.

In a follow-up study of 174 subjects with normal LV function and no inducible ischemia who had undergone DSCMR, Walsh et al. (2007) noted that increased LV wall thickness (greater than 12 mm) predicted major adverse cardiac event (MACE) ($p = 0.0017$) (Figure 18-20). Myocardial stress perfusion imaging (MSP) provides independent information predicting death in patients with LVH. MSP is recommended in patients with LVH undergoing radionuclide stress testing. However, there is little information about the utility of combined wall motion and perfusion stress CMR in the setting of LVH. This case illustrates the possible utility of DSCMR with combined wall motion and perfusion for ischemia evaluation in patients with LVH.

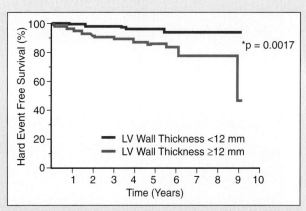

■ **Figure 18-20** Cardiac prognosis in patients with LVH. *(From Walsh TF, Morgan TM, Ntim W, Hundley WG: Poor cardiac prognosis in patients without inducible left ventricular wall motion abnormalities but with increased left ventricular wall thickness during IV dobutamine stress testing. J Am Coll Cardiol 2007;49:104A, with permission.)*

Case 3   Dobutamine Stress Cardiac Magnetic Resonance for Viability Assessment

A 58-year-old white man with a history of hypertension, hyperlipidemia, diabetes mellitus, coronary artery disease status post MI, and s/p percutaneous intervention to LAD and congestive heart failure presented with chest pain, shortness of breath, and no biochemical evidence of evolving MI. Transthoracic echocardiogram demonstrated severely reduced LV function with ejection fraction of 30%. He underwent cardiac catheterization demonstrating obstructive three-vessel disease (Figure 18-21). CMR performed to assess viability revealed evidence of nonviability in the LAD territory (Figure 18-22).

In another case, a 71-year-old white man with history of hypercholesterolemia and coronary artery disease (CAD) presented to the cardiology clinic with a 3-month history of angina and shortness of breath with severely reduced LV function. Cardiac catheterization showed significant two-vessel CAD (Figure 18-23). Dobutamine stress CMR with a viability protocol demonstrated significant myocardial viability (Figure 18-24). The patient subsequently received a two-vessel bypass with a LIMA to an LAD and a radial graft to the PDA.

Comments

In patients with ischemic cardiomyopathy, chronic LV dysfunction may result from infarct or myocardial hibernation. Evaluation of myocardial viability has become an integral part of the clinical and therapeutic management of patients with CAD and depressed LV function. This is important in the selection of patients for possible myocardial revascularization. Excellent agreement has been demonstrated between CMR, fludeoxyglucose positron

emission tomography (FDG-PET), and echocardiography for viability assessment in patients with chronic ischemic LV dysfunction.

Quantification of transmural extent of infarct by contrast-enhanced CMR techniques has been shown to predict likelihood of recovery of LV function after revascularization. However, infarcts with transmurality of 1% to 74% have demonstrated only an intermediate likelihood of recovery. In addition severe kidney disease or

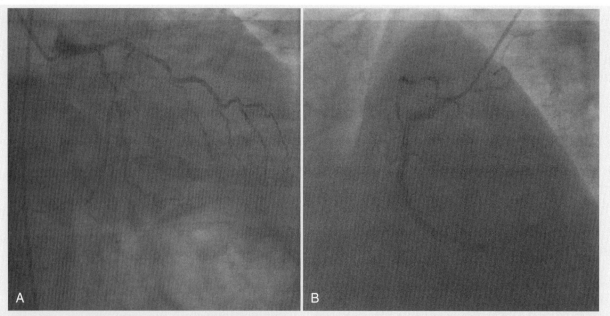

■ **Figure 18-21 A,** RAO caudal view demonstrates an occluded proximal LAD, an 80% proximal circumflex, 80% first marginal, and 90% proximal and mid-ramus lesions. **B,** RCA angiogram demonstrates 75% proximal and 80% distal lesions. An 80% lesion was noted in the PDA.

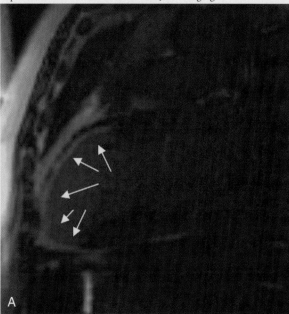

■ **Figure 18-22 A,** Delayed enhancement three-chamber view demonstrates a large transmural infarction involving the anteroseptal and apical walls consistent with LAD territory (*yellow arrows*). **B,** Delayed enhancement short-axis view demonstrates a large transmural infarction involving the anteroseptal wall (*yellow arrows*).

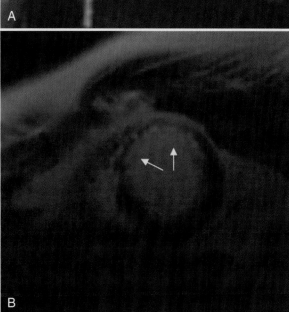

■ **Figure 18-23** Cardiac catheterization shows significant CAD.

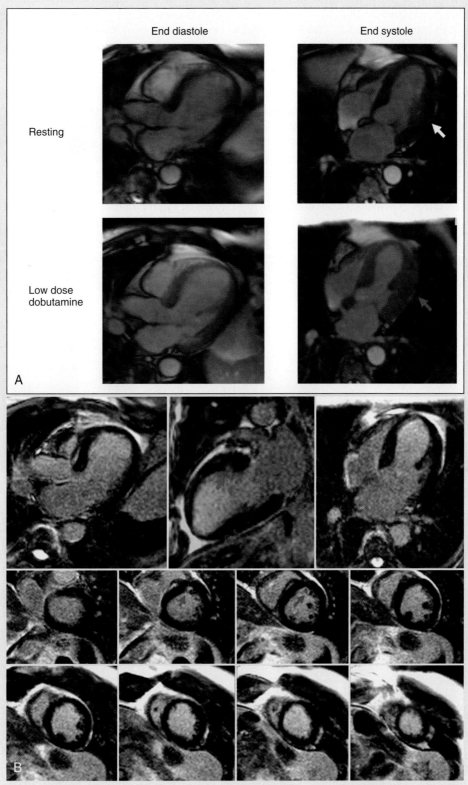

■ **Figure 18-24 A,** Dobutamine stress CMR result. The *white arrow* in right upper image shows the hypokinetic segment at the mid-inferolateral wall at rest; and the *red arrow* in the right lower image shows improved contraction of the mid-inferolateral wall during received low-dose dobutamine. **B,** Delayed hyperenhancement images showed small subendocardial scar at basal to mid-anterior wall scar (*red arrows*).

ESRD may preclude the use of CMR contrast because of the risk of nephrogenic systemic fibrosis.

Wall motion viability stress testing may provide improved diagnostic accuracy in viability assessment and serve as a suitable alternative in situations in which CMR contrast administration is contraindicated. Baer et al. (1995) reported that end-diastolic LV wall thickness less than 5.5 mm is an excellent marker of scar, and thus predicted lack of recovery of function with sensitivity and specificity of 92% and 56%, respectively.

In a prospective study of 29 patients with ischemic cardiomyopathy, Wellnhofer et al. (2004) reported superiority of low-dose DSCMR over delayed enhancement (DE) in predicting improvement in contractility after revascularization in non-transmural scars (1% to 74% transmurality). There was no significant difference between the two modalities for segments with no or extensive infarcts (Figure 18-25).

Low-dose DSCMR studies in patients with chronic LV ischemic dysfunction undergoing revascularization have predicted improvement in function with sensitivity 50% to 86%, specificity 70% to 100%. With advances in CMR technology, quantitative analysis of wall motion using tissue tagging may reduce the duration of the test with comparable results and improved sensitivity (Figure 18-26). A suggested viability algorithm incorporating wall motion and delayed enhancement imaging is outlined in Figure 18-27.

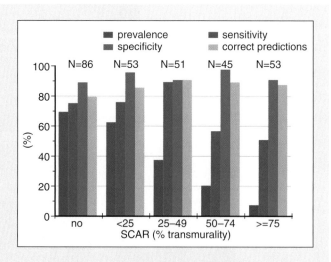

■ **Figure 18-25** Transmurality of scar and prediction of recovery of function by DSCMR. *(From Wellnhofer E, Olariu A, et al: Magnetic resonance low-dose dobutamine test is superior to scar quantification for the prediction of functional recovery. Circulation 2004;109:2172-2174, with permission.)*

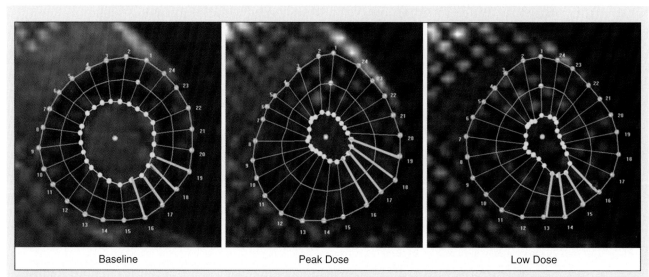

Baseline   Peak Dose   Low Dose

■ **Figure 18-26** Tagging images at end systolic phase of mid-LV level showed biphasic response to DSCMR at inferolateral region of mid-LV.

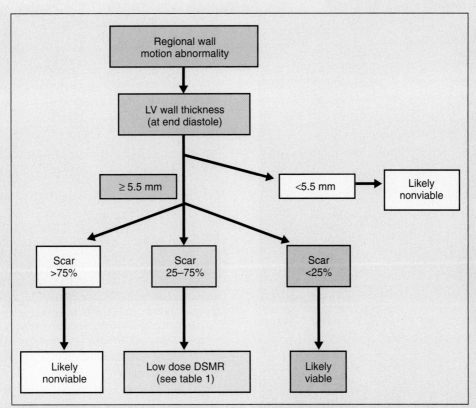

■ **Figure 18-27** Suggested algorithm for CMR viability assessment. DSMR, dobutamine stress CMR; scar percent, percentage of scar transmurality.

Case 4   **Exercise Stress Cardiac Magnetic Resonance**

A 61-year-old man with a history of smoking, hyperlipidemia, and a family history of premature coronary artery disease presented with substernal chest pain not associated with exertion. The patient underwent an exercise stress CMR, achieving 76% of his predicted heart rate at 10.5 METs. CINE CMR at peak stress demonstrated wall motion abnormalities in the apical and mid-lateral walls (Figure 18-28). The cardiac catheterization revealed an 80% lesion in the mid-LAD and an occluded OM2 with left-to-left collaterals (Figure 18-29). The mid-LAD was successfully stented. The OM2 could not be crossed with a wire and was subsequently treated medically.

Comments

ECG exercise stress testing (EEST) has provided a wealth of data on diagnostic accuracy and prognostic implications. However imaging in addition to EEST is recommended in clinical situations such as resting ECG abnormalities, female gender, intermediate to high pretest probability of CAD, and postcoronary revascularization to improve diagnostic accuracy. Echocardiography and radionuclide scintigraphy have been the main imaging modalities used in conjunction with ECG. CMR, with its heightened spatial and temporal resolution, has the potential of improving image quality when used with EEST. However, there is little information about the exercise CMR stress testing.

Rerkpattanapipat et al. (2003) proved the utility of upright treadmill exercise CMR using qualitative wall motion analysis in 27 patients. The sensitivity and specificity for detection of significant coronary stenosis (greater than 50%) were 79% and 85%, respectively. Although the prognostic value of EEST is known, the long-term outcomes of patients undergoing exercise CMR based on wall motion findings is unknown.

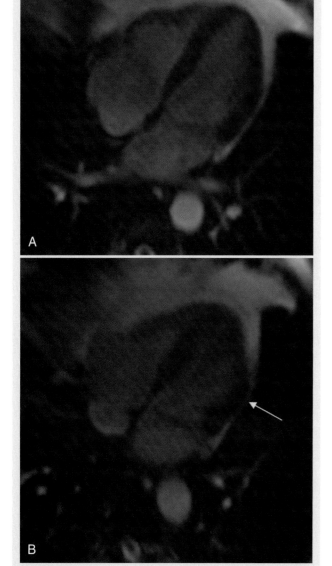

■ **Figure 18-28 A,** Apical four-chamber view with peak systolic realtime rest images demonstrating no wall motion abnormalities. **B,** Apical four-chamber view with real-time peak stress images demonstrating hypokinesis of the mid-lateral wall (*yellow arrow*) at peak systole.

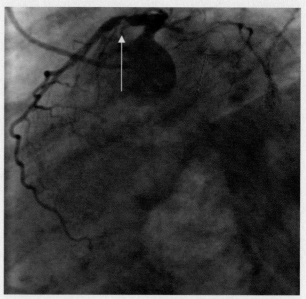

■ **Figure 18-29** LAO caudal view demonstrates an 80% mid-LAD lesion (*yellow arrow*) and an occluded second obtuse marginal branch (*red arrow*). Left-to-left collateral vessels are visualized.

CONCLUSIONS

1. CMR wall motion stress testing is an accurate method for identification of myocardial ischemia and viability. It also possesses excellent prognostic value.
2. Preliminary study with exercise stress CMR suggest potential for diagnostic accuracy similar to established tools such echocardiography and radionuclide imaging. Further studies are needed to elucidate its prognostic significance.

SUGGESTED READING

Cerqueira MD, Weissman WJ, Dilsizian V, et al: Standardized myocardial segmentation and nomenclature for tomographic imaging of the heart. Circulation 2002;105:539-542.

Darty S, Thomas MS, Neagle CM, et al: Nursing responsibilities during cardiovascular magnetic resonance imaging. Am J Nursing 2002;102(12):34-38.

Hendel RC, Patel MR, Kramer CM, et al: ACCF/ACR/SCCT/SCMR/ASNC/NASCI/SCAI/SIR Appropriateness criteria for cardiovascular computed tomography and cardiovascular magnetic resonance. J Am Coll Cardiol 2006;48:1475-1497.

Lang RM, Bierig M, Devereux RB, et al: Recommendations for chamber quantification: A report from the American Society of Echocardiography's Guidelines and Standards Committee and the Chamber Quantification Writing Group, developed in conjunction with the European Association of Echocardiography, a branch of the European Society of Cardiology: J Am Soc Echocardiogr 2005;18:1440-1463.

Mandapaka S, Hundley WG: Dobutamine cardiovascular magnetic resonance: A review. J Magn Reson Imaging 2006;24:499-512.

Paetsch I, Jahnke C, Wahl A, et al. Comparison of dobutamine stress magnetic resonance, adenosine stress magnetic resonance, and adenosine stress magnetic resonance perfusion. Circulation 2004;110:835-842.

Recent advances in parallel imaging have enhanced the performance of real-time white-blood imaging, with quantified LV function comparable with breath-hold segmented CMR. Real-time CINE imaging offers the ability to obtain non-ECG gated or non–breath-hold images at the peak exercise, although with lower spatial and temporal resolution. This imaging sequence may facilitate image acquisition at the peak exercise.

Dobutamine Stress Cardiac Magnetic Resonance

Browner WS, Li J, Mangano DT: In-hospital and long-term mortality in male veterans following non-cardiac surgery: the study of Perioperative Ischemia Research Group. JAMA 1992;268:228-232.

Fleisher LA, Beckman JA, Brown KA, et al: ACC/AHA 2007 Guidelines on perioperative cardiovascular evaluation and care for noncardiac surgery. J Am Coll Cardiol 2007;50:1707-1732.

Hendel RC, Patel MR, Kramer CM, et al: ACCF/ACR/SCCT/SCMR/ASNC/NASCI/SCAI/SIR Appropriateness criteria for cardiovascular computed tomography and cardiovascular magnetic resonance. J Am Coll Cardiol 2006;48:1475-1497.

Hundley WG, Morgan TM, Neagle CM, et al: Magnetic resonance imaging determination of cardiac prognosis. Circulation 2002;106:2328-2333.

Jahnke C, Nagel E, Gebker R, et al: Prognostic value of cardiac magnetic resonance stress tests. Adenosine stress perfusion and dobutamine stress wall motion imaging. Circulation 2007;115:1769-1776.

Rerkpattanapipat P, Morgan TM, Neagle CM, et al: Assessment of preoperative cardiac risk with magnetic resonance imaging. Am J Cardiol 2002;90(4):416-419.

Dobutamine Stress Imaging

Bangalore S, Yao S, Chaudhry F: Usefulness of stress echocardiography for risk stratification and prognosis of patients with left ventricular hypertrophy. Am J Cardiol 2007;100:536-543.

Elhendy A, Schinkel AFL, Domburg RT, et al: Prognostic implications of stress Tc-99m in patients with left ventricular hypertrophy. J Nucl Cardiol 2007;14:550-554.

Frohich ED: Pathophysiological considerations in left ventricular hypertrophy. J Clin Hypertens 1987;3:54-65.

Klocke FJ, Baird MG, Lorell BH, et al: ACC/AHA/ASNC guidelines for the clinical use of cardiac radionuclide imaging-executive summary: A report of the American College of Cardiology/American Heart Association Task Force on Practice Guidelines. J Am Coll Cardiol 2003;42:1318-1333.

Smart SC, Knickelbine T, Malik F, Sagar KB: Dobutamine-atropine stress echocardiography for the detection of coronary artery disease in patients with left ventricular hypertrophy. Importance of chamber size and systolic wall stress. Circulation 2000;101:258-263.

Walsh TF, Morgan TM, Ntim W, Hundley WG: Poor cardiac prognosis in patients without inducible left ventricular wall motion abnormalities but with increased left ventricular wall thickness during IV dobutamine stress testing. J Am Coll Cardiol 2007;49:104A.

Dobutamine Stress Cardiac Magnetic Resonance for Viability Assessment

Baer FM, Voth E, Schneider CA, et al: Comparison of low-dose dobutamine-gradient echo magnetic resonance imaging and positron emission tomography with [18F] fluorodeoxyglucose in patients with chronic coronary artery disease. A functional and morphological approach to the detection of residual myocardial viability. Circulation 1995;91:1006-1015.

Bax JJ, van der Wall EE, de Roos A, Poldermans D: Comparison with non-nuclear techniques. In: Zaret BL, Beller GA (eds). Clinical nuclear cardiology: State of the art and future directions, 3rd ed. St Louis, Mosby, 2005, 535-555.

Kim RJ, Wu E, Rafael A, et al: The use of contrast-enhanced magnetic resonance imaging to identify reversible myocardial dysfunction. N Engl J Med 2000;343:1445-1453.

Lin S, Brown JJ: MR contrast agents: Physical and pharmacologic basics. J Magn Reson Imag 2007;25:884-899.

Mandapaka S, Hundley WG: Dobutamine cardiovascular magnetic resonance: A review. J Magn Reson Imag 2006;24:499-512.

Saito I, Watanabe S, Masuda Y: Detection of viable myocardium by dobutamine stress tagging with three-dimensional analysis by automatic trace method. Jpn Circ J 2000;64:487-494.

Wellnhofer E, Olariu A, Klein C, et al: Magnetic resonance low-dose dobutamine test is superior to scar quantification for the prediction of functional recovery. Circulation 2004;109:2172-2174.

Exercise Stress Cardiac Magnetic Resonance

Epstein FH: MRI of left ventricular function. J Nucl Cardiol 2007;14:729-744.

Gibbons RD, Balady GJ, Bricker T, et al: ACC/AHA 2002 Guideline update for exercise testing. Circulation 2002;106:1883-1892.

Kaju S, Yang PC, Kerr AB, et al: Rapid evaluation of left ventricular volume and mass without breath-holding using real-time interactive cardiac magnetic resonance imaging system. J Am Coll Cardiol 2001;38:527-533.

Rerkpattanapipat P, Darty SN, Hundley WG, et al: Feasibility to detect severe coronary artery stenoses with upright treadmill exercise magnetic resonance imaging. Am J Cardiol 2003;92:603-606.

Chapter 19

Delayed-Enhancement Magnetic Resonance

Chetan Shenoy, Annamalai Senthilkumar, and Raymond J. Kim

KEY POINTS

- Delayed-enhancement cardiac magnetic resonance (DE-CMR) can identify reversible myocardial dysfunction before coronary revascularization, predict improvement in contractile function in patients with reperfused acute myocardial infarction, and predict response to β-blocker therapy in patients with heart failure.

- DE-CMR involves T1-weighted imaging of the heart after administration of gadolinium contrast media using a segmented inversion-recovery gradient echo sequence where infarcted or scarred myocardium accumulates gadolinium and appears as "hyperenhanced" or bright.

- DE-CMR allows the identification of the presence, location, and extent of acute and chronic myocardial infarction with high accuracy relative to histopathology.

- The pattern of hyperenhancement is useful in differentiating ischemic from nonischemic cardiomyopathy. Frequently the specific etiology responsible for nonischemic cardiomyopathy also may be ascertained.

- DE-CMR improves the specificity and accuracy of stress perfusion CMR for the detection of coronary artery disease.

- Emerging applications for DE-CMR include the detection of intracardiac thrombus and the assessment of patients with intraventricular dyssynchrony for potential cardiac resynchronization therapy.

- Myocardial scarring detected by DE-CMR has been associated with adverse prognosis in patients both with ischemic and nonischemic heart disease.

Magnetic resonance imaging of the heart after administration of gadolinium contrast media has been described in the literature for over 20 years. This approach was predicated on the concept that injured tissue accumulates gadolinium and appears as "hyperenhanced" or bright on T1-weighted images acquired at least 10 minutes after injection of gadolinium. A major limitation of the initial approach was poor contrast between normal and injured myocardium. More recently a segmented inversion-recovery gradient echo sequence has been developed that significantly improves in vivo detection of hyperenhanced regions. This technique, known as delayed-enhancement cardiac magnetic resonance (DE-CMR), can identify the presence, location, and extent of both acute and chronic myocardial infarction with high spatial resolution. This technique has been extensively validated with comparisons to histopathology.

Accurate assessment of viable myocardium is important in patients with contractile dysfunction. In these patients if substantial viable myocardium is found, left ventricular function can improve following coronary revascularization and the functional improvement may be accompanied by survival benefits. Identification of nonviable myocardium is also important, because infarcted or scarred tissue may provide a substrate for ventricular tachyarrhythmias and sudden cardiac death. Thus the evaluation of both viable and nonviable myocardium provides important guidance for clinical decision making.

In this chapter we will first illustrate the physiologic basis for DE-CMR, and describe the protocol and typical imaging parameters. Then well-established applications of DE-CMR in patients with ischemic and nonischemic heart disease will be discussed, as well as some newer emerging applications. Finally recent reports demonstrating the prognostic significance of DE-CMR findings will be briefly reviewed.

TABLE 19-1 Typical DE-CMR Scanning Parameters

PARAMETER	TYPICAL VALUES
Gadolinium dose	0.10-0.20 mmol/kg
Field of view	300-380 mm
In-plane voxel size	1.2-1.8 × 1.2-1.8 mm
Slice thickness	6 mm
Flip angle	20-30 degrees
Segments	13-31
Inversion time (IT)	Variable
Bandwidth	90-250 Hz/pixel
Echo time (TE)	3-4 msec
Repetition time (TR)	8-9 msec
Gating factor	2
K-space ordering	Linear
Fat saturation	No
Asymmetric echo	Yes
Gradient moment refocusing	Yes

The dose of gadolinium given is usually 0.10 to 0.20 mmol/kg. Higher doses result in better SNR, but the bright LV blood pool may obscure subendocardial infarcts. The field-of-view (FOV) in both read and phase-encode directions is minimized to improve spatial resolution without resulting in wrap-around artifact in the area of interest. For patients with heart rates less than 90 beats per minute, we typically acquire 23 lines of k-space data during the mid-diastolic portion of the cardiac cycle. For a repetition time of 8 msec, the data acquisition window is 184 msec in duration (8 × 23 = 184). Because the middiastolic period of relative cardiac standstill is reduced in patients with faster heart rates, we decrease the number of segments (k-space lines) acquired per cardiac cycle in order to reduce the length of the imaging window. This eliminates blurring from cardiac motion during the k-space collection. In order to allow for adequate longitudinal relaxation between successive 180-degree inversion pulses, inversion pulses are applied every other heartbeat (gating factor of 2). In our experience an in-plane resolution of 1.2 to 1.8 mm by 1.2 to 1.8 mm with a slice thickness of 6 mm provides an adequate signal-to-noise balance while avoiding significant partial volume effects. As stated previously, the flip angle is kept shallow to retain the effects of the inversion prepulse, but it can be relatively greater (30 degrees) if larger doses of gadolinium are given (0.2 mmol/kg) and the IT of myocardium is correspondingly shorter.

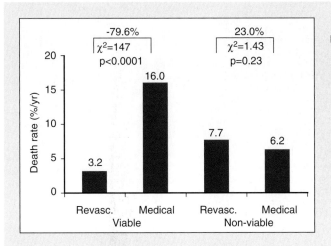

■ **Figure 19-1** The importance of myocardial viability assessment. This figure shows data pooled from 24 studies examining late survival with revascularization versus medical therapy after myocardial viability testing in patients with severe coronary artery disease and left ventricular dysfunction. This metaanalysis in 3088 patients demonstrated that in patients with viability, revascularization was associated with a 79.6% reduction in annual mortality (16% versus 3.2%, *p* less than 0.0001) compared with medical therapy. Patients without viability had intermediate mortality, trending to higher rates with revascularization versus medical therapy (7.7% versus 6.2%, *p* = NS). Mean left ventricular ejection fraction at baseline was 32 ± 8%, and patients were followed for 25 ± 10 months. (*From Allman et al: J Am Coll Cardiol 2002;39:1151-1158, with permission.*)

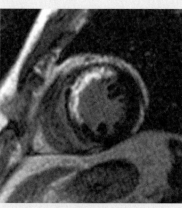

DE-CMR protocol

TIME

- Insert peripheral IV
- Place patient in scanner
- Obtain scout images
- Obtain cine images
- Inject gadolinium (0.1–0.2 mmol/kg)
- Wait 10 minutes
- Obtain delayed enhancement images

■ **Figure 19-2** Overall DE-CMR protocol. Imaging starts with scouting and typically a complete set of short- and long-axis cine images are acquired before contrast media is administered. Gadolinium is usually given at a dose of 0.1 to 0.2 mmol/kg of body weight. Ideally, delayed enhancement images are obtained at least 10 minutes after contrast administration in order to better separate bright myocardium from bright left ventricular blood pool. Cine and delayed enhancement images are taken at the same anatomic levels to enable direct comparison.

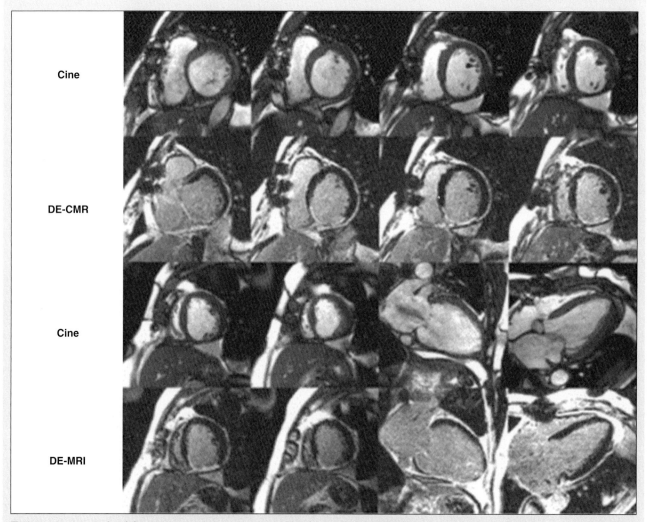

Cine

DE-CMR

Cine

DE-MRI

■ **Figure 19-3** Typical viability scan. Interpretation is improved by alternating cine with delayed enhancement images to allow side-by-side comparison of dysfunctional regions (cine) with areas of infarction (delayed enhancement). In this patient example the diastolic still frames from the cine movies show regional thinning of the inferior and inferoseptal walls, which corresponds to the area of transmural infarction on the delayed enhancement images.

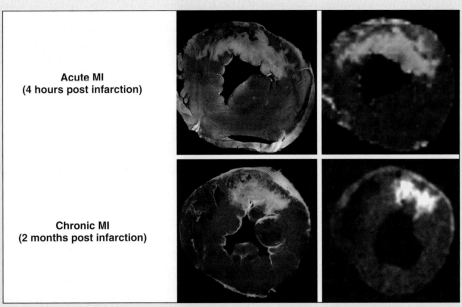

■ **Figure 19-4** Comparison with histopathology. Multiple studies of both acute and chronic myocardial infarction have compared DE-CMR with histopathology and observed that the size and shape of hyperenhanced regions by DE-CMR closely match those of irreversible injury defined by histopathology. Short-axis histopathology sections of the heart are shown on the left, with corresponding delayed enhancement images on the right. The pale yellow/white regions on histopathology represent myocardial infarction, which closely match the bright areas on DE-CMR. *(From Fieno et al: J Am Coll Cardiol 2000;36:1985-1991, with permission.)*

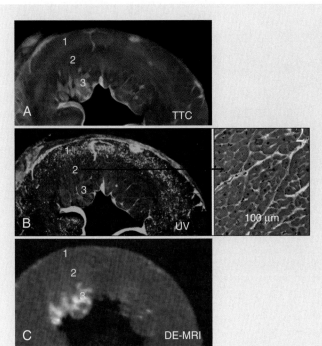

■ **Figure 19-5** DE-CMR delineates irreversible from reversible injury. Three pathophysiologically distinct regions are depicted. Region "1" represents normal noninfarcted myocardium. Region "2" represents myocardium that has suffered temporary hypoperfusion and reversible injury—the "at risk but not infarcted" region. Viability of this region was confirmed by light microscopy. Region "3" represents infarcted myocardium. Panel **A** shows a portion of the left ventricular anterior wall following triphenyl tetrazolium chloride (TTC) staining for histopathology identification of viable myocardium. Panel **B** shows the same myocardial section under ultraviolet light. Note that both regions "2" and "3" lack fluorescent microparticles depicting hypoperfusion. Panel **C** shows ex vivo delayed enhancement imaging of the section. Importantly, region "2" does not hyperenhance by DE-CMR. This example demonstrates that areas suffering reversible injury do not hyperenhance by DE-CMR. *(From Fieno et al: J Am Coll Cardiol 2000;36:1985-1991, with permission.)*

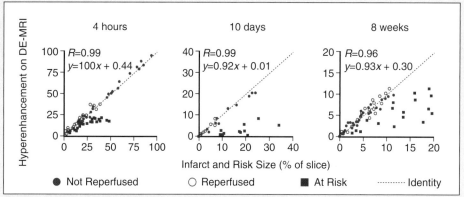

■ **Figure 19-6** There is a close match between the extent of hyperenhancement by DE-CMR and infarct size (*blue circles*) in the acute (4 hours), subacute (10 days), and chronic (8 weeks) time points, independent of reperfusion status. Conversely, the area at risk (*red squares*) is nearly always larger than the area of hyperenhancement. In this study the infarct size was determined by triphenyl tetrazolium chloride (TTC) staining and the myocardium at risk of infarction was identified by injecting fluorescent microparticles into the left atrium after reoccluding the coronary artery before sacrificing the animal for histopathology. These data are consistent with the principle that hyperenhancement only occurs in regions of irreversible injury. (*Adapted from Fieno et al: J Am Coll Cardiol 2000;36:1985-1991, with permission.*)

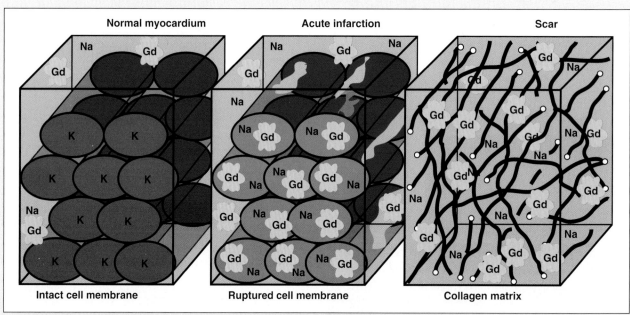

■ **Figure 19-7** The physiologic basis of hyperenhancement in DE-CMR. In normal myocardium, two points should be noted. First, myocytes are densely packed, and total tissue volume is predominantly intracellular ($\approx$ 80% of the water space). Second, gadolinium contrast media does not cross cellular membranes, and thus is limited to the extracellular (intravascular and interstitial) space. The result is that the volume of distribution of gadolinium contrast in normal myocardium is quite small ($\approx$ 20% of water space), and one can consider viable myocytes as actively excluding contrast media. In acutely infarcted regions the myocyte membranes are ruptured, allowing gadolinium to passively diffuse into the intracellular space. The result is an increased concentration of gadolinium at the tissue level and therefore hyperenhancement occurs. Myocardial scar is characterized by a dense collagenous matrix; however, at a cellular level the interstitial space between collagen fibers may be significantly greater than the interstitial space between the living myocytes that is characteristic of normal myocardium. Thus the concentration of gadolinium in scar is greater than in normal myocardium because of the expanded volume of distribution and the regions of scar appear hyperenhanced by DE-CMR.

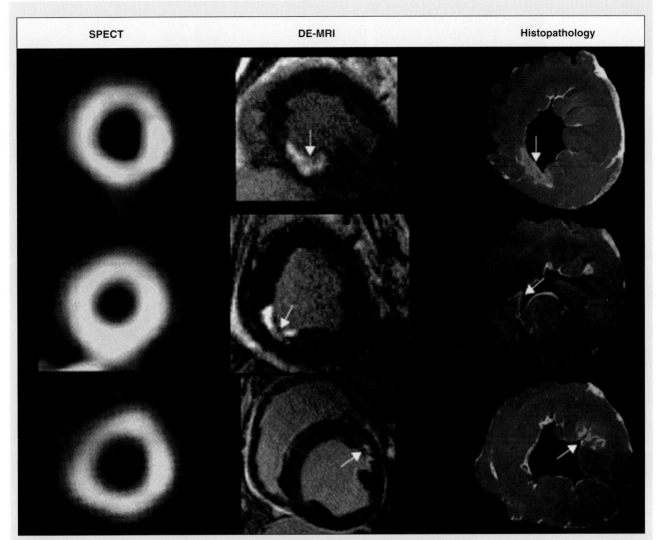

| SPECT | DE-MRI | Histopathology |

■ **Figure 19-8** Comparison of single photon emission computed tomography (SPECT) and DE-CMR with histology in three canines with subendocardial infarcts (*arrows*). Note that the infarcts are not evident on SPECT. It is often reported that the mechanism by which subendocardial infarcts are routinely missed by SPECT is limited spatial resolution. However, the primary mechanism may relate to the inability of SPECT to directly visualize both viable and infarcted myocardium. Measuring only the amount of viability is problematic because there is a large intrinsic variation in the amount of viability in normal regions. Hence, although tracer activity "on average" may be modestly reduced in the setting of subendocardial infarction, for any specific patient or region, the level of reduction may be smaller than the normal regional variation, rendering the subendocardial infarction "invisible." With DE-CMR, both viable (unenhanced) and infarcted (enhanced) myocardium are visualized simultaneously. Note on the DE-CMR images that hyperenhanced regions correspond to infarcted regions by histopathology. Note also, on both DE-CMR and histopathology, that even the regions completely free of infarction have variable wall thickness, representing variable absolute amounts of viability. *(Adapted from Wagner et al: Lancet 2003;361:374-379, with permission.)*

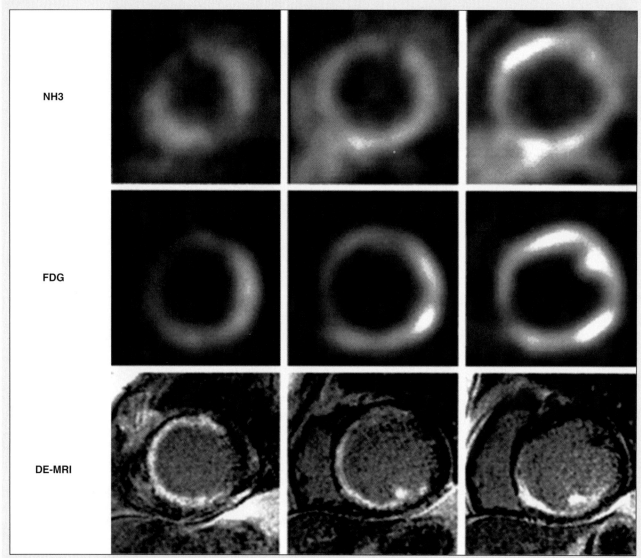

NH3

FDG

DE-MRI

■ **Figure 19-9** Comparison with positron emission tomography (PET) imaging. The top panels show three short-axis views of a PET viability study with assessment of rest perfusion (NH3) and glucose metabolism (FDG). The bottom panel shows DE-CMR images in the corresponding slices. Note that in segments with matched reduced perfusion and metabolism, there is hyperenhancement on DE-CMR. However, the border between normal and defect areas is less distinct on PET compared with DE-CMR. Although the investigators concluded that CMR hyperenhancement as a marker of myocardial scar closely agrees with PET data, the study also showed that more than half of segments showing a subendocardial infarct by DE-CMR were classified as normal by PET. *(From Klein et al: Circulation 2002;105:162-167, with permission.)*

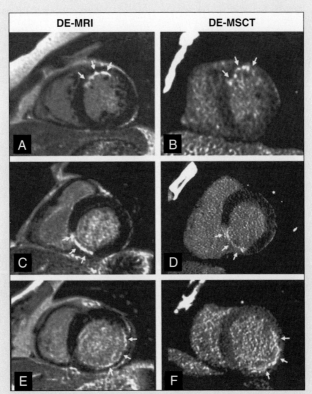

Figure 19-10 Comparison with CT imaging. Recently the delayed-enhancement concept has been extended to multislice spiral computed tomography (MSCT). The interpretation of delayed enhancement patterns on MSCT (DE-MSCT) appear quite similar to that for DE-CMR, and is likely based on the same underlying mechanism because the iodinated contrast media used for MSCT has nearly identical pharmacokinetics as that of "extracellular" gadolinium contrast. Short-axis DE-CMR and DE-MSCT images from three different patients with acute myocardial infarction attributable to the left anterior descending (**A, B**) and right coronary artery (**C, D**), and left circumflex artery (**E, F**) occlusion after successful revascularization are shown. There is an excellent agreement between the two, albeit with reduced contrast-to-noise ratio and image quality for MSCT. *(From Mahnken et al: J Am Coll Cardiol 2005;45:2042-2047, with permission.)*

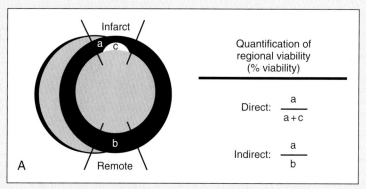

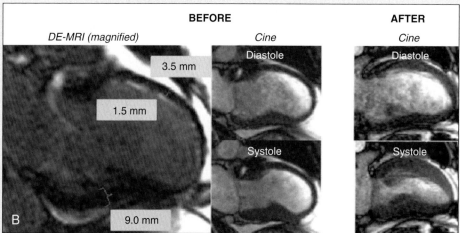

■ **Figure 19-11** It is important to recognize that the use of different techniques of viability assessment often lead to differences in the way in which viability is quantified although the nomenclature used may be the same. For instance, when only viable myocardium can be visualized, the percentage of viability in any given segment is assessed indirectly and generally refers to the amount of viability in the segment normalized to the segment with the maximum amount of viability ("remote" zone in the figure in panel **A**) or to data from a gender-specific database of controls. Conversely, when both viable (*black in the cartoon*) and nonviable (*white in the cartoon*) myocardium can be visualized, the percentage of viability can be assessed directly and expressed as the amount of viability in the segment normalized to the amount of viability plus infarction in the same segment. These differences in the way in which viability is measured can alter clinical interpretation, as illustrated in the patient example in panel **B** showing long-axis DE-CMR images of a patient before and 2 months after revascularization. Although the akinetic anterior wall is "thinned" (diastolic wall thickness 5 mm; remote zone 9 mm), DE-CMR demonstrates that there is only subendocardial infarction (1.5 mm thick). Direct assessment of viability would show that the anterior wall is predominately viable (3.5/5 mm = 70% viable), whereas the indirect method would show that the anterior wall is predominately nonviable (3.5/9 mm = 39% viable). Cine views after revascularization demonstrate that the direct method is more accurate because there is recovery of wall motion.

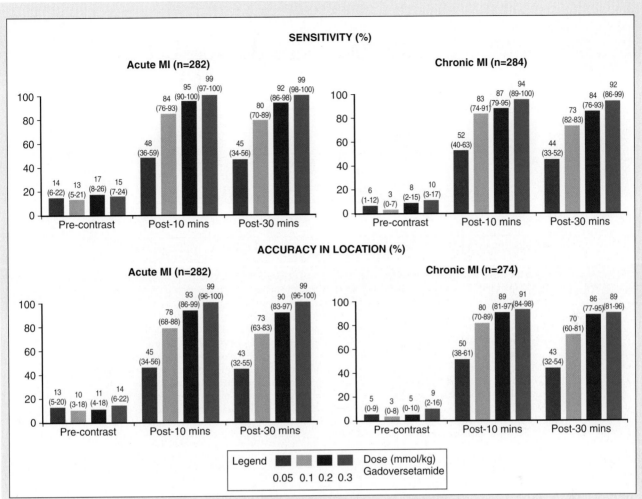

■ **Figure 19-12** The performance of DE-CMR for the detection of MI was studied in an international, multicenter, double-blinded, randomized trial. Patients with their first MI were enrolled in an acute (≤ 16 days after MI; n = 282) or chronic (17 days to 6 months; n = 284) arm and then randomized to 1 of 4 doses of gadolinium contrast: 0.05, 0.1, 0.2, or 0.3 mmol/kg. Standard delayed-enhancement CMR was performed before contrast (control) and 10 and 30 minutes after gadolinium contrast. The infarct-related artery perfusion territory was scored from x-ray angiograms separately. The sensitivity of CMR for detecting MI increased with rising dose of gadolinium contrast (p less than 0.0001), reaching 99% (acute) and 94% (chronic) after contrast compared with 11% (pooled) before contrast. Likewise, the accuracy of CMR for identifying MI location (compared with infarct-related artery perfusion territory) increased with rising dose of gadolinium contrast (p less than 0.0001), reaching 99% (acute) and 91% (chronic) after contrast compared with 9% (pooled) before contrast. For gadolinium doses ≥0.2 mmol/kg, 10- and 30-minute images provided equal performance, and peak creatine kinase-MB levels correlated with CMR infarct size (p less than 0.0001). *(From Kim et al: Circulation 2008;117:629-637, with permission.)*

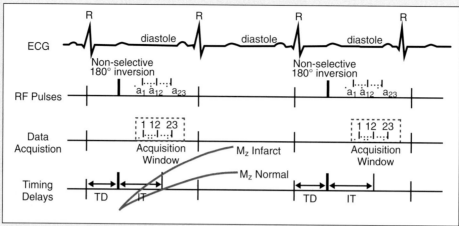

■ **Figure 19-13** This diagram illustrates the typical timing employed by DE-CMR—a segmented inversion-recovery fast gradient echo pulse sequence. Immediately after the onset of the R wave trigger, there is a delay or wait period (the trigger delay or TD) before a nonselective 180-degree radiofrequency inversion pulse is applied, which inverts the longitudinal magnetization from the +z-axis to the −z-axis. Following this inversion pulse, a second variable wait period (the inversion time or IT) occurs corresponding to the time between the inversion pulse and the center of the data acquisition window (for linearly ordered k-space acquisition). The data acquisition window is generally 140 to 200 msecs long, depending on the patient heart rate, and is placed during middiastole when the heart is relatively motionless. A group of k-space lines are acquired during this acquisition window, where the flip angle used for radio-frequency excitation for each k-space line is shallow (≈ 20 degrees) to retain regional differences in magnetization that result from the inversion pulse and IT delay. The number of k-space lines in the group is limited by the repetition time between each k-space line (≈ 8 ms) and the duration of middiastole. In the implementation shown here, 23 lines of k-space are acquired during each data acquisition window, which occurs every other heartbeat. Every other heartbeat imaging is employed to allow for recovery of magnetization. Typically a breath hold duration of 12 cardiac cycles is required to obtain all the k-space lines for the image matrix. ECG, electrocardiogram; RF, radiofrequency; TD, trigger delay; IT, inversion time delay; a, shallow flip angle excitation. *(Adapted from Simonetti et al: Radiology 2001;218:215-223, with permission.)*

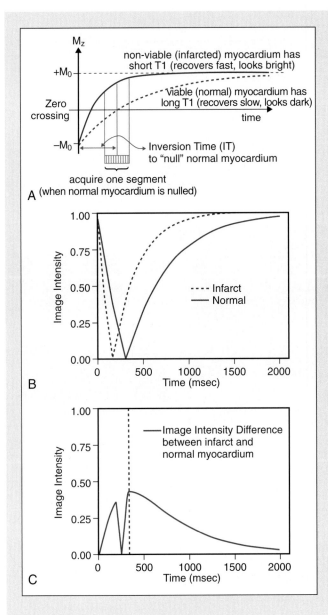

■ **Figure 19-14** "Nulling" the myocardium. One of the most important parameters that needs to be set correctly for DE-CMR is the time between the inversion pre-pulse and the center of data readout, known as the inversion time or IT. The IT is chosen so that the center of image readout (for linear k-space acquisition) occurs when the magnetization of normal myocardium reaches the zero crossing (i.e., normal myocardium is "nulled"). Panel **A** illustrates the inversion recovery curves of normal and infarcted myocardium. It is at this point (or immediately just after) that the image intensity difference between infarcted and normal myocardium is maximized as seen in panel **C** showing the difference in image intensities between infarcted and normal myocardium as a function of inversion time. If the IT is set too short, normal myocardium will be below the zero crossing and will have a negative magnetization vector at the time of k-space data acquisition. Because the image intensity corresponds to the magnitude of the magnetization vector, the image intensity of normal myocardium will increase as the IT becomes shorter and shorter, whereas the image intensity of infarcted myocardium will decrease until it reaches its own zero crossing. At this point infarcted myocardium will be nulled and normal myocardium will be hyperenhanced. On the opposite extreme, if the IT is set too long, the magnetization of normal myocardium will be above zero and will appear gray (not nulled). Although areas of infarction will have high image intensity, the relative contrast between infarcted and normal myocardium will be reduced. Panel **B** shows image intensities resulting from an inversion prepulse with various inversion delay times. In principle, the optimal IT at which normal myocardium is nulled must be determined by imaging iteratively with different inversion times. In practice, however, only one or two "test" images needs to be acquired, because with experience one can estimate the optimal IT based on the amount of contrast agent that is administered and the time after contrast agent administration. *(From Kim et al: J Cardiovasc Magn Reson 2003;5:505-514, with permission.)*

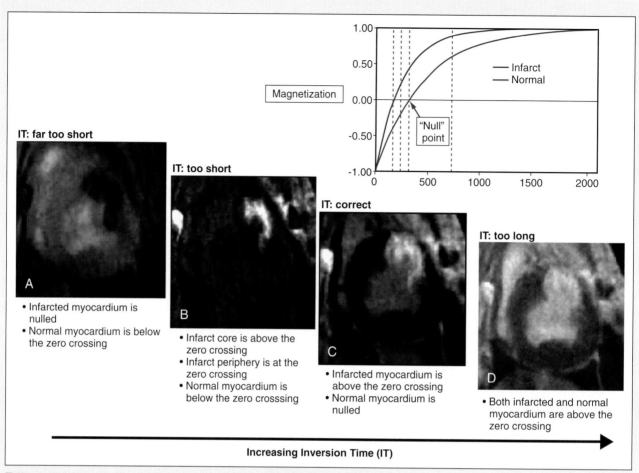

■ **Figure 19-15** Images of a subject with an anterior wall myocardial infarction in which the IT has been varied from too short to too long. Note that with the IT set far too short **(A),** the infarcted myocardium is nulled and appears dark instead of bright. With the IT set moderately too short **(B),** the anterior wall does have some regions that are hyperenhanced; however, the total extent of hyperenhancement is less than that seen when the IT is set correctly **(C).** This is due to the periphery of the infarcted region passing through a zero-crossing, thereby affecting its apparent size. If the IT is set too long **(D),** although the relative contrast between infarcted and normal myocardium is reduced as previously stated, the total extent of hyperenhancement does not change. Thus it is better to err on the side of setting the IT too long rather than too short. *(From Kim et al: J Cardiovasc Magn Reson 2003;5:505-514, with permission.)*

■ **Figure 19-16** Single-shot DE-CMR technique. DE-CMR can also be performed using an ultrafast technique that can acquire subsecond, "snapshot" images during free breathing. ECG gating is also not required. This technique could be considered the preferred approach in patients who are more acutely ill or unable to hold their breath. However, compared with standard imaging, sensitivity for detecting MI is mildly reduced, and the transmural extent of infarction may be underestimated. The overall diagnostic performance of the two techniques is displayed in the figure. Compared to a sensitivity of 98% and specificity of 100% for the diagnosis of MI by the standard DE-CMR technique, the single-shot technique had a sensitivity of 87% and specificity of 96%. *(From Sievers et al: Circulation 2007;115:236-244, with permission.)*

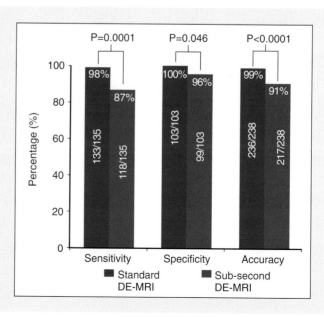

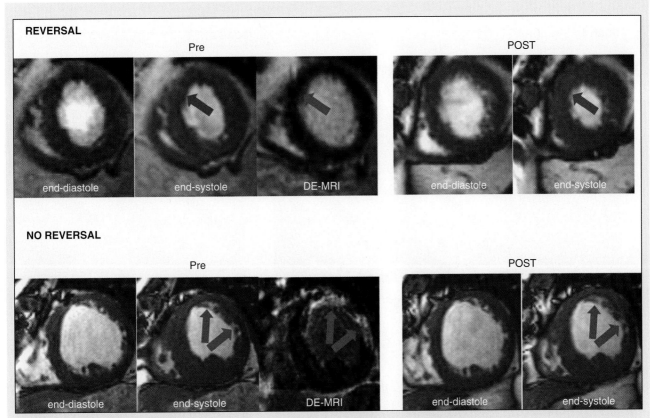

■ **Figure 19-17** The interpretation of DE-CMR for assessing the likelihood of contractile improvement following coronary revascularization. Representative cine images and DE-CMR images in a patient with reversible left ventricular dysfunction (top row) and in another patient with irreversible left ventricular dysfunction (bottom row) are shown. The patient with reversible dysfunction had severe hypokinesia of the anteroseptal wall (*arrows*), and this area was not hyperenhanced before revascularization. The contractility of the wall improved after revascularization. The patient with irreversible dysfunction had akinesia of the anterolateral wall (*arrows*), and this area was hyperenhanced before revascularization. The contractility of the wall did not improve after revascularization. (*From Kim et al: N Engl J Med 2000;343:1445-1453, with permission.*)

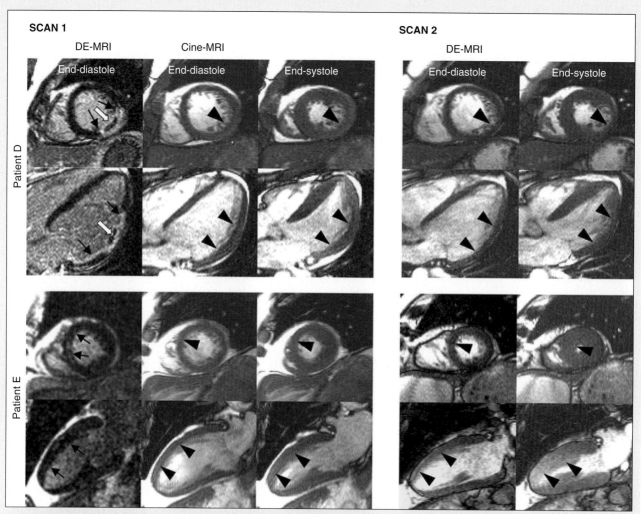

■ **Figure 19-18** The transmural extent of infarction defined by DE-CMR predicts improvement in contractile function in patients with acute reperfused myocardial infarction. This was a study of 24 patients following their first myocardial infarction. All patients underwent successful reperfusion. Patients underwent both an acute and a chronic scan; scan 1 was within 7 days of their myocardial infarction and scan 2 at 8 to 12 weeks. Improvement in segmental contractile function on scan 2 was inversely related to the transmural extent of infarction on scan 1 ($p = 0.001$). Improvement in global contractile function, as assessed by ejection fraction and mean wall thickening score, was not predicted by peak creatine kinase-MB ($p = 0.66$) or by total infarct size, as defined by CMR ($p = 0.70$). The best predictor of global improvement was the extent of dysfunctional myocardium that was not infarcted or had infarction comprising less than 25% of left ventricular wall thickness (p less than 0.005 for ejection fraction, p less than 0.001 for mean wall thickening score). Patient D in the figure had transmural extent of infarction of greater than 75% of LV wall thickness within the dysfunctional region on scan 1 (*arrows*) and had minimal improvement in contractile function in this region on scan 2. Note the subendocardial hypoenhanced region surrounded by hyperenhancement in this patient, indicating "no-reflow" at the infarct core (*white arrow*). Patient E, conversely, had transmural extent of infarction of less than 25% of LV wall thickness within the dysfunctional region on scan 1 (*arrows*) and had significant improvement in contractile function on scan 2. (*From Choi et al: Circulation 2001;104:1101-1107, with permission.*)

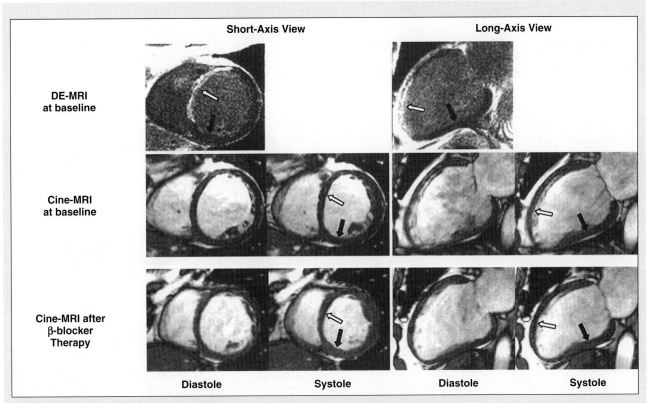

■ **Figure 19-19** DE-CMR can predict the response in LV function and remodeling from ß-blocker therapy for heart failure patients. This was a study of 45 patients with chronic heart failure before and after 6 months of ß-blockade. The study included patients with either ischemic or nonischemic cardiomyopathy. DE-CMR demonstrated scarring in 30 of 45 patients (67%). Scarring was found in 100% of patients with ischemic cardiomyopathy (28 of 28) but in only 12% with nonischemic cardiomyopathy (2 of 17). In the 35 patients who were maintained on ß-blockers and had a second study, there was an inverse relation between the extent of scarring at baseline and the likelihood of contractile improvement 6 months later (p less than 0.001). For instance, contractility improved in 56% (674 of 1207) of regions with no scarring but in only 3% with greater than 75% scarring (8 of 232). Multivariate analysis showed that the amount of dysfunctional but viable myocardium by DE-CMR was an independent predictor of the change in ejection fraction ($p = 0.01$), mean wall motion score ($p = 0.0007$), LV end-diastolic volume index ($p = 0.007$), and LV end-systolic volume index ($p = 0.0001$). In the above patient example showing representative images before and 6 months after ß-blocker therapy, hyperenhanced myocardium (*white arrows*) does not improve after ß-blocker therapy, whereas non-hyperenhanced regions (*black arrows*) do improve. *(From Bello et al: Circulation 2003;108:1945-1953, with permission.)*

■ **Figure 19-20** Characteristic hyperenhancement patterns of scarring and/or necrosis can help differentiate between ischemic and nonischemic etiologies of cardiomyopathy. The typical pattern of hyperenhancement in ischemic heart disease can be explained by the pathophysiology of ischemia. Little or no cellular necrosis is found until about 15 minutes after coronary occlusion. After 15 minutes, a "wavefront" of necrosis begins in the subendocardial layer and extends toward the epicardium over the next few hours. During this period, the necrotic region within the ischemic zone grows until it becomes a transmural infarction. Hence myocardial cell death resulting from epicardial coronary artery disease should involve the subendocardium. Conversely, scarring or necrosis that is limited to the mid-wall or epicardial layer and spares the subendocardium is not consistent with myocardial infarction and a nonischemic etiology should be considered. In some types of nonischemic cardiomyopathy, the subendocardium may be involved; however, the distribution often is global (i.e., throughout the entire LV). Even with diffuse, three-vessel coronary artery disease, a global subendocardial infarction would be distinctly uncommon; therefore a nonischemic etiology should also be considered in the setting of global subendocardial hyperenhancement. The figure illustrates common hyperenhancement patterns that may be encountered in clinical practice along with a partial list of their differential diagnoses *(From Mahrholdt et al: Eur Heart J 2005;26:1461-1474, with permission.)*

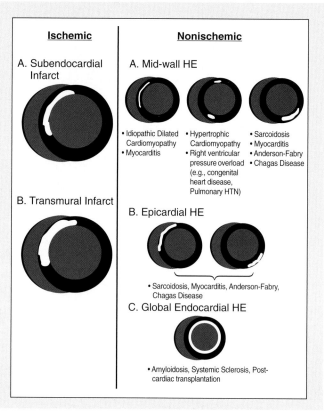

■ **Figure 19-21** Typical patient examples of scarring in nonischemic cardiomyopathy are shown. Patient A has hypertrophic cardiomyopathy (HCM). Note hyperenhancement in the hypertrophied septum, predominantly involving the middle third of the ventricular wall in a patchy, multifocal distribution. Additionally, note that the junctions of the right ventricular free wall and the interventricular septum are involved. This is a common finding in HCM patients. Patient B has idiopathic dilated cardiomyopathy (IDCM). A distinctive linear striae of hyperenhancement is seen in the midwall of the basal septum. This finding is seen in up to 30% of IDCM patients. Patient C has myocarditis with two separate regions of hyperenhancement. The lateral wall has epicardial involvement and the interventricular septum has midwall involvement. Not all myocarditis patients have both patterns. A third pattern, consisting of multiple midwall regions of patchy involvement throughout the LV, is also common in myocarditis. Patient D has cardiac amyloidosis. The hyperenhancement is global but predominantly affects the subendocardium. *(Adapted from White et al: Cardiol Clin 2007;25:71-95, with permission.)*

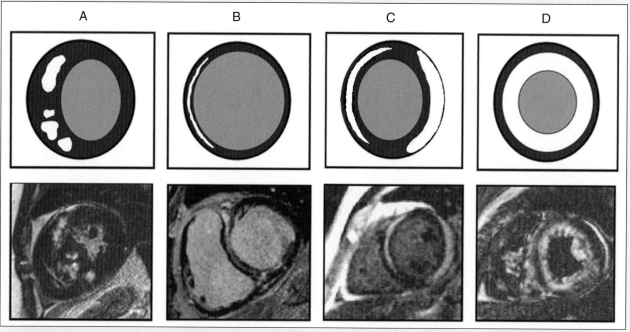

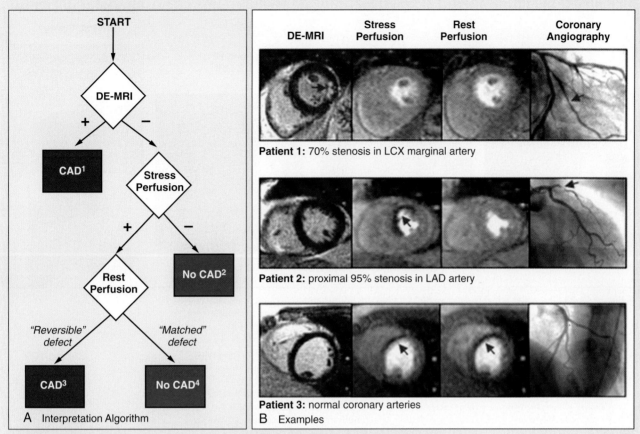

■ **Figure 19-22** DE-CMR improves the specificity and accuracy of stress perfusion CMR for the detection of coronary artery disease (CAD) when performed as a combined exam and interpreted with an algorithm as shown. Panel **A** shows the schema of the algorithm, which is based on visual interpretation. Panel **B** demonstrates DE-CMR, stress, and perfusion CMR images and the coronary angiography in three patient examples. There are four possible pathways depending on the results of the individual CMR tests. (1) Positive DE-CMR study. Hyperenhanced myocardium consistent with a prior myocardial infarction (MI) is detected. This does not include isolated midwall or epicardial hyperenhancement, which can occur in nonischemic disorders as mentioned above. (2) Standard negative stress study. No evidence of prior MI or inducible perfusion defects. (3) Standard positive stress study. No evidence of prior MI, but perfusion defects are present with adenosine that are absent or reduced at rest. (4) Artifactual perfusion defect. Matched stress and rest perfusion defects without evidence of prior MI on DE-CMR. Panel **B** shows patient examples using the algorithm. The top row shows a patient with positive DE-CMR study demonstrating an infarct in the inferolateral wall (*red arrow*), although perfusion CMR is negative. The interpretation algorithm (step 1) classified this patient as positive for CAD. Coronary angiography verified disease in a circumflex marginal artery. Cine CMR demonstrated normal contractility. The middle row shows a patient with a negative DE-CMR study but with a prominent reversible defect in the anteroseptal wall on perfusion CMR (*red arrow*). The interpretation algorithm (step 3) classified this patient as positive for CAD. Coronary angiography demonstrated a proximal 95% left anterior descending coronary artery stenosis. The bottom row shows a patient with a matched stress-rest perfusion defect (*blue arrows*) but without evidence of prior MI on DE-CMR. The interpretation algorithm (step 4) classified the perfusion defects as artifactual. Coronary angiography demonstrated normal coronary arteries. (*From Klem et al: J Am Coll Cardiol 2006;47:1630-1638, with permission.*)

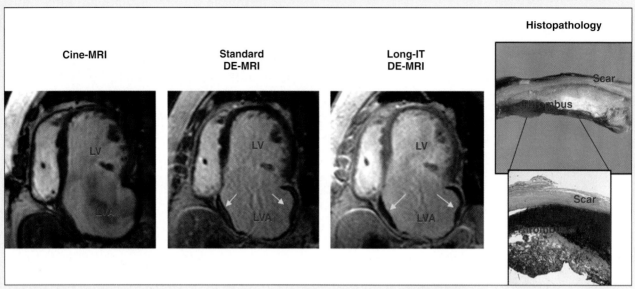

■ **Figure 19-23** DE-CMR is a highly sensitive tool for detecting LV thrombus. Because of its avascularity, thrombus has essentially no gadolinium uptake, and this fact can be used to discern thrombus from myocardium. The figure shows short-axis images from a patient with a large mural thrombus adherent to a left ventricular inferior wall aneurysm (LVA). The thrombus was detected by DE-CMR but missed by cine-CMR. Thrombus was verified by pathology (gross examination [overlay] and histopathology [inset, Masson trichrome stain]). Note that thrombus may have an "etched" appearance with a black border and a central grey zone on standard IT (inversion-time) DE-CMR, whereas it appears homogeneously black on long-IT imaging. Long-IT imaging involves use of a modified DE-CMR sequence in which the inversion time is increased from that needed to null viable myocardium (approximately 350 msec) to a fixed time of 600 msec, which nulls avascular tissue such as thrombus. With this "long inversion time" (long-IT) sequence, regions with contrast uptake such as viable myocardium increase in image intensity (i.e., appear grey rather than black), thrombus appears homogeneously black, and there is improved thrombus delineation. *(From Weinsaft et al: J Am Coll Cardiol 2008.)*

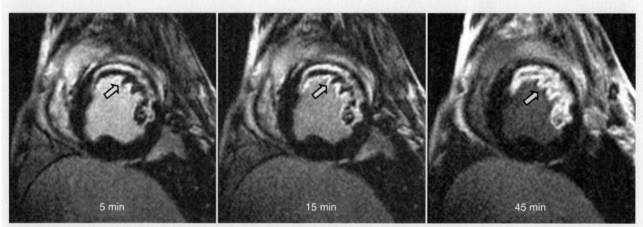

■ **Figure 19-24** DE-CMR detects areas of acute myocardial infarction with microvascular obstruction, called "no-reflow" zones. These areas appear as a filling defect with no contrast uptake, similar to thrombus. However, the differentiating features are (a) surrounding structures—no-reflow zones should be completely encompassed in 3D space by hyperenhanced myocardium or LV cavity; this is not an absolute finding for thrombus; (b) appearance—no-reflow occurs within the myocardium; thrombus can occur in the LV cavity and features such as protruding structures and abrupt transitions suggest thrombus; and (c) stability of size on consecutive DE-CMR acquisitions—no-reflow size shrinks from gadolinium contrast fill-in at the periphery as seen in the above example (*yellow arrows*), whereas thrombus size is stable. The figure shows DE-CMR of a short axis view of the heart showing areas of microvascular obstruction in the anterior and anterolateral walls, which fill in with gadolinium contrast with the passage of time as seen on the images obtained at 15 and 45 minutes.

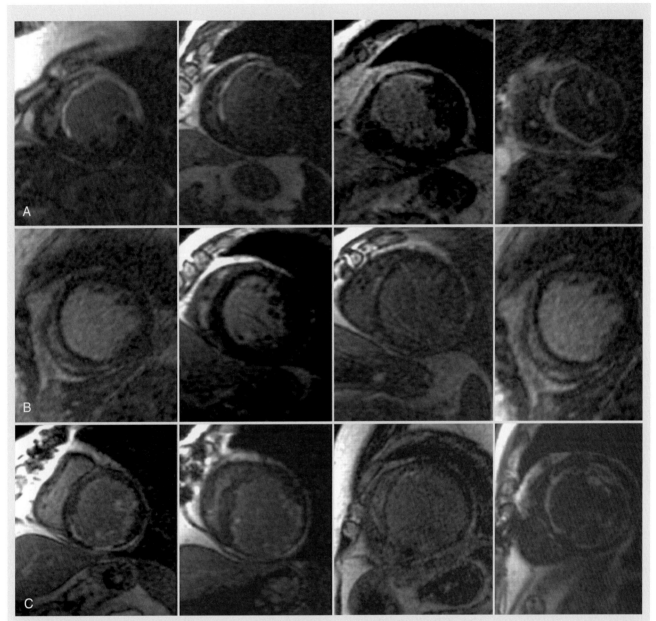

■ **Figure 19-25** DE-CMR predicts clinical response to cardiac resynchronization therapy (CRT) in patients with intraventricular dyssynchrony. This was a study of 23 patients (mean age 64.9 ± 11.7 years), of whom 13 (57%) met response criteria. Percent total scar was significantly higher in the nonresponse versus response group (median and interquartile range of 24.7% [18.1 to 48.7] versus 1.0% [0.0 to 8.7], *p* = 0.0022) and predicted nonresponse by receiver-operating characteristic analysis (area = 0.94). At a cutoff value of 15%, percent total scar provided a sensitivity and specificity of 85% and 90%, respectively, for clinical response to CRT. Similarly, septal scar 40% provided a 100% sensitivity and specificity for response. Regression analysis showed linear correlations between percent total scar and change in each of the individual response criteria. In the figure, panel **A** shows DE-CMR images of nonresponders, who have large amounts of total scar and scarring of the septal and anteroseptal walls. Panels **B** and **C** show examples of clinical responders, who have a percent total scar of ≤ 15% or a percent septal scar ≤ 40%, respectively. *(From White et al: J Am Coll Cardiol 2006;48:1953-1960, with permission.)*

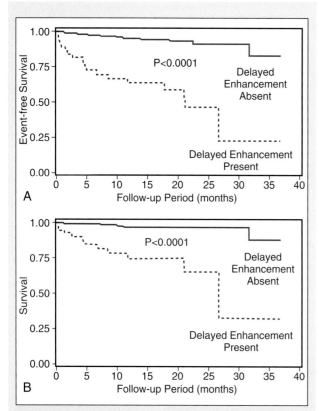

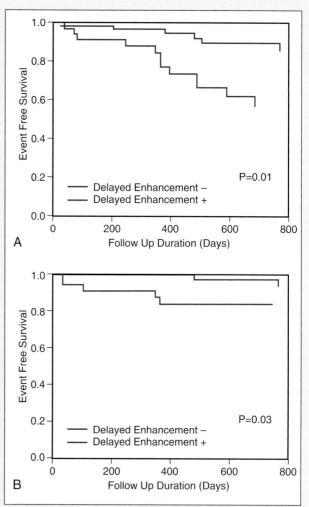

■ **Figure 19-26** In patients without a known prior MI and presenting with clinical suspicion of CAD, the presence and extent of myocardial scar as detected by DE-CMR is a strong predictor of major adverse cardiovascular events and cardiac death. Kwong et al. *(Circulation 2006;113:2733-2743, with permission)* studied 195 patients without a known prior MI and assessed the prognostic value of delayed enhancement. During a median follow-up of 16 months, 31 patients (18%) experienced major adverse cardiac events (MACE), including 17 deaths. Delayed enhancement demonstrated the strongest unadjusted associations with MACE and cardiac mortality (hazard ratios of 8.29 and 10.9, respectively; both *p* less than 0.0001). By multivariable analyses, delayed enhancement was independently associated with MACE beyond the clinical model (*p* less than 0.0001). Panel **A** shows the Kaplan-Meier curves for MACE. Panel **B** shows the Kaplan-Meier curves for cardiac mortality. Thus delayed enhancement may improve risk stratification of patients who present with a clinical suspicion of CAD but without a history of MI.

■ **Figure 19-27** In patients with nonischemic dilated cardiomyopathy, midwall fibrosis determined by DE-CMR may be helpful in predicting clinical outcome. Assomull et al. *(J Am Coll Cardiol 2006;48:1977-1985, with permission)* studied 101 patients with dilated cardiomyopathy for 658 ± 355 days for events. Midwall fibrosis was present in 35% of patients and was associated with a higher rate of the primary end point—a composite of all-cause death and hospitalization for a cardiovascular event (hazard ratio 3.4, *p* = 0.01). Multivariate analysis showed midwall fibrosis as the sole significant predictor of death or hospitalization. Perhaps because of limited sample size, there was no significant difference in all-cause mortality between the two groups. Midwall fibrosis was also associated with the secondary outcome measure—a composite of sudden cardiac death (SCD) and sustained ventricular tachycardia (VT) (hazard ratio 5.2, *p* = 0.03). Midwall fibrosis remained predictive of SCD/VT after correction for baseline differences in left ventricular ejection fraction between the two groups. Panel **A** shows the Kaplan-Meier curves for the combined end point of all-cause mortality or hospitalization resulting from cardiovascular causes. Panel **B** shows the Kaplan-Meier curves for the combined end point of sudden cardiac death or ventricular tachycardia. These data suggest that DE-CMR may improve risk stratification of patients with nonischemic dilated cardiomyopathy.

SUGGESTED READING

Allman KC, Shaw LJ, Hachamovitch R, Udelson JE: Myocardial viability testing and impact of revascularization on prognosis in patients with coronary artery disease and left ventricular dysfunction: a meta-analysis. J Am Coll Cardiol 2002;39:1151-1158.

Assomull RG, Prasad SK, Lyne J, et al: Cardiovascular magnetic resonance, fibrosis, and prognosis in dilated cardiomyopathy. J Am Coll Cardiol 2006;48:1977-1985.

Bello D, Shah DJ, Farah GM, et al: Gadolinium cardiovascular magnetic resonance predicts reversible myocardial dysfunction and remodeling in patients with heart failure undergoing beta-blocker therapy. Circulation 2003;108:1945-1953.

Kim RJ, Albert TS, Wible JH, et al: Performance of delayed-enhancement magnetic resonance imaging with gadoversetamide contrast for the detection and assessment of myocardial infarction: an international, multicenter, double-blinded, randomized trial. Circulation 2008;117:629-637.

Kim RJ, Fieno DS, Parrish TB, et al: Relationship of MRI delayed contrast enhancement to irreversible injury, infarct age, and contractile function. Circulation 1999;100:1992-2002.

Kim RJ, Shah DJ, Judd RM: How we perform delayed enhancement imaging. J Cardiovasc Magn Reson 2003;5:505-514.

Kim RJ, Shah DJ: Fundamental concepts in myocardial viability assessment revisited: When knowing how much is "alive" is not enough. Heart 2004;90:137-140.

Kim RJ, Wu E, Rafael A, et al: The use of contrast-enhanced magnetic resonance imaging to identify reversible myocardial dysfunction. N Engl J Med 2000;343:1445-1453.

Klein C, Nekolla SG, Bengel FM, et al: Assessment of myocardial viability with contrast-enhanced magnetic resonance imaging: Comparison with positron emission tomography. Circulation 2002;105:162-167.

Klem I, Heitner JF, Shah DJ, et al: Improved detection of coronary artery disease by stress perfusion cardiovascular magnetic resonance with the use of delayed enhancement infarction imaging. J Am Coll Cardiol 2006;47:1630-1638.

Kwong RY, Chan AK, Brown KA, et al: Impact of unrecognized myocardial scar detected by cardiac magnetic resonance imaging on event-free survival in patients presenting with signs or symptoms of coronary artery disease. Circulation 2006;113:2733-2743.

Mahnken AH, Koos R, Katoh M, et al: Assessment of myocardial viability in reperfused acute myocardial infarction using 16-slice computed tomography in comparison to magnetic resonance imaging. J Am Coll Cardiol 2005;45:2042-2047.

Mahrholdt H, Wagner A, Judd RM, et al: Delayed enhancement cardiovascular magnetic resonance assessment of non-ischaemic cardiomyopathies. Eur Heart J 2005;26:1461-1474.

Sievers B, Elliott MD, Hurwitz LM, et al: Rapid detection of myocardial infarction by subsecond, free-breathing delayed contrast-enhancement cardiovascular magnetic resonance. Circulation 2007;115:236-244.

Simonetti OP, Kim RJ, Fieno DS, et al: An improved MR imaging technique for the visualization of myocardial infarction. Radiology 2001;218:215-223.

Srichai MB, Junor C, Rodriguez LL, et al: Clinical, imaging, and pathological characteristics of left ventricular thrombus: A comparison of contrast-enhanced magnetic resonance imaging, transthoracic echocardiography, and transesophageal echocardiography with surgical or pathological validation. Am Heart J. 2006;152:75-84.

Wagner A, Mahrholdt H, Holly TA, et al: Contrast-enhanced MRI and routine single photon emission computed tomography (SPECT) perfusion imaging for detection of subendocardial myocardial infarcts: An imaging study. Lancet 2003;361:374-379.

White JA, Yee R, Yuan X, et al: Delayed enhancement magnetic resonance imaging predicts response to cardiac resynchronization therapy in patients with intraventricular dyssynchrony. J Am Coll Cardiol 2006;48:1953-1960.

Chapter 20

Peripheral Magnetic Resonance Angiography

Rajiv Agarwal and Scott D. Flamm

KEY POINTS

- Peripheral arterial disease (PAD) is prevalent, particularly in the elderly.

- X-ray angiography has definite risks and limitations, including exposure to radiation and administration of iodinated contrast.

- Magnetic resonance angiography (MRA) has emerged as a popular alternative in the diagnostic work-up of patients with PAD.

- The most common techniques employed for MRA include time of flight (TOF-MRA), phase contrast (PC-MRA), and contrast-enhanced (CE-MRA) angiography.

- TOF-MRA is most commonly used to image the carotid and intracranial circulation.

- CE-MRA is less sensitive to artifacts and can be performed rapidly.

- The sensitivity and specificity of CE-MRA in PAD is greater than 90%.

- Disadvantages of CE-MRA in PAD include timing of gadolinium administration, need for IV access, and concerns regarding gadolinium-induced nephrogenic systemic fibrosis.

Peripheral arterial disease (PAD) is prevalent, particularly in the elderly population. Typical symptoms include claudication and nonhealing ulcers or wounds. Multiple imaging modalities are now available for diagnostic evaluation of the peripheral vasculature. Traditional x-ray angiography has been considered the "gold-standard" technique to define vascular anatomy. However, x-ray angiography has definite risks and limitations, including exposure to radiation and administration of iodinated contrast that may result in allergic reactions and contrast nephropathy. Contrast nephropathy is particularly important in this patient population as many patients with PAD also have renal insufficiency. Therefore noninvasive alternatives, such as magnetic resonance angiography (MRA), have emerged as popular alternatives in the diagnostic work-up of patients with PAD.

Magnetic resonance angiography (MRA) can be accomplished with a variety of techniques. The most common techniques employed include time of flight (TOF-MRA), phase contrast (PC-MRA), and contrast-enhanced (CE-MRA) angiography. Each technique has its distinct advantages, disadvantages, and preferred indications.

TOF-MRA manipulates longitudinal magnetization of stationary spins, thus providing contrast within the vasculature. TOF-MRA is most commonly used to image the carotid and intra-cranial circulation. PC-MRA uses velocity changes, and hence phase shifts to provide contrast within the vasculature. CE-MRA typically utilizes a gadolinium chelate, a T1 shortening agent that, in conjunction with a T1 weighted sequence (typically a conventional or fast gradient echo sequence), leads to high signal intensity of the arteries compared with the surrounding tissue. The two main distinguishing factors in favor of CE-MRA compared with the other two techniques are: CE-MRA is not affected by artifacts caused by in-plane saturation and turbulence, and reduction in examination time (entire study can be completed in less than 15 minutes). Multiple studies have consistently shown the sensitivity and specificity of CE-MRA are greater than 90%. Hence CE-MRA is widely used to evaluate peripheral arterial disease. The disadvantages include problems with timing of gadolinium administration relative to image acquisition, and the need for intravenous access. Recently there also has been concern about gadolinium-induced nephrogenic systemic fibrosis in patients with renal insufficiency.

Case 1   Normal Peripheral MR Angiogram

A 49-year-old patient presented with a 5-day history of bilateral calf pain with exertion and at rest. On examination there was severe tenderness on palpation of bilateral lower extremities. Peripheral pulses (femoral, popliteal, anterior tibial, and dorsalis pedis) were normal in amplitude and contour. Laboratory data revealed significantly elevated serum creatine kinase level, white blood cell count, and erythrocyte sedimentation rate. The referring physician was concerned about the integrity of the lower extremity vasculature and ordered a CMR/MRA (Figure 20-1).

Case 2   Superficial Femoral Artery Occlusion

A 65-year-old patient presented with a 2-month history of claudication and a nonhealing wound in his right foot. On examination, the ankle-brachial index was 0.56 on the right side and 0.96 on the left side (normal ankle-brachial index = 0.95-1.2). On the right side, the femoral pulse was normal; however, the popliteal, dorsalis pedis, and posterior tibial pulses were not palpable. A weak signal was obtained by Doppler ultrasound technique. The referring physician was concerned about peripheral vascular disease involving the right superficial femoral artery and ordered a CMR/MRA (Figure 20-2). Because of abnormal findings on the MR angiogram, a traditional x-ray angiogram was performed for therapeutic intervention.

■ **Figure 20-1 A,** Normal abdominal aorta and iliac branch
vessels. Contrast enhanced magnetic resonance angiogram of
patient with bilateral calf pain demonstrating a normal aorta and
branch vessels. Note the smooth walls of the aorta, indicating no
significant atherosclerosis. Pictured are distal abdominal aorta
(A), common iliac arteries (C), external iliac arteries (E), and
internal iliac arteries (I). **B,** Normal femoral artery and branch
vessels. Contrast enhanced magnetic resonance angiogram
demonstrating a normal lumen of the femoral arteries. Again,
note the smooth walls of the vasculature, indicating no significant
atherosclerosis. Pictured are common femoral artery (C), profunda
femoris (P), and superficial femoral artery (S). **C,** Popliteal artery
and infrapopliteal outflow branch vessels. Contrast enhanced
magnetic resonance angiogram demonstrating normal lumen
of the popliteal artery (P) and infrapopliteal trifurcation, which
includes the anterior tibial (A), peroneal (R), and posterior tibial
(T) arteries. Note the smooth walls of the vasculature on the right
side, indicating no significant atherosclerosis. However, there
is partial signal dropout of the left popliteal region. This was
confirmed as artifact based on the raw images.

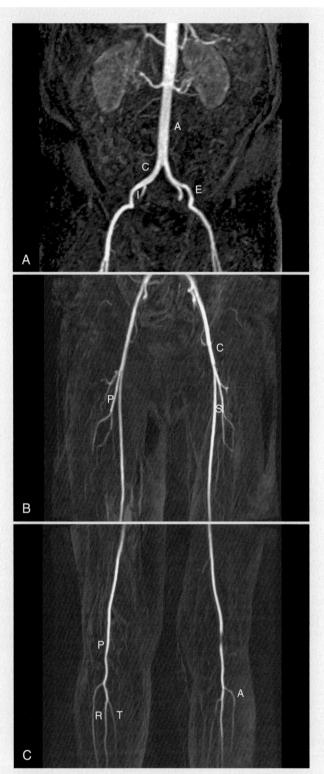

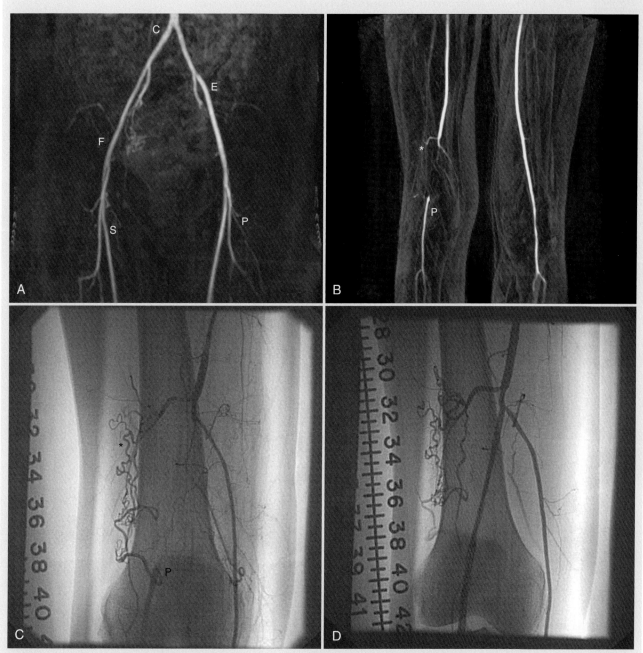

■ **Figure 20-2 A,** Normal iliac, common femoral, and proximal superficial femoral arteries. Contrast-enhanced magnetic resonance angiogram demonstrating normal lumen of the bilateral common (C), external (E), and internal iliac arteries. The common femoral (F), profunda femoris (P), and proximal superficial femoral (S) arteries are all patent. The walls of the visualized vessels are smooth, indicating no significant atherosclerosis. **B,** Occluded distal right superficial femoral artery with reconstitution via collaterals. Contrast-enhanced magnetic resonance angiogram demonstrating complete occlusion of the distal right superficial femoral artery with collateral formation (*), and subsequent reconstitution of the popliteal (P) artery. The left superficial femoral and popliteal arteries are patent and contain only luminal irregularities. **C,** Occluded distal right superficial femoral artery with reconstitution via collaterals. Corresponding contrast-enhanced x-ray angiogram demonstrating complete occlusion of the distal right superficial femoral artery with collateral formation (*), and subsequent reconstitution of the popliteal (P) artery. Note the extensive tortuosity of the collateral vessels before reconstitution. **D,** Postpercutaneous transluminal angioplasty of the occluded segment. Contrast-enhanced x-ray angiogram obtained immediately after angioplasty of the occluded segment, now demonstrating recanalization of the distal superficial femoral artery. The collateral vessels are still present and will likely diminish or occlude as blood will travel toward the path of least resistance.

Case 3 Patent Proximal Superficial Femoral Artery to Posterior Tibial Artery Graft

A 77-year-old patient presented 3 years ago with severe claudication in the right calf region with limited exertion. The patient was found to have severe diffuse atherosclerosis involving the entire right superficial femoral and popliteal arteries. Additionally, disease was noted in the proximal infrapopliteal branch vessels. Therefore surgical approach was deemed the best option and the patient underwent bypass grafting from the proximal superficial femoral artery to the right posterior tibial artery. Recently the patient presented with intermittent right calf pain at rest that improves with exertion. The referring physician was concerned about patency of the bypass graft and ordered a CMR/MRA (Figure 20-3).

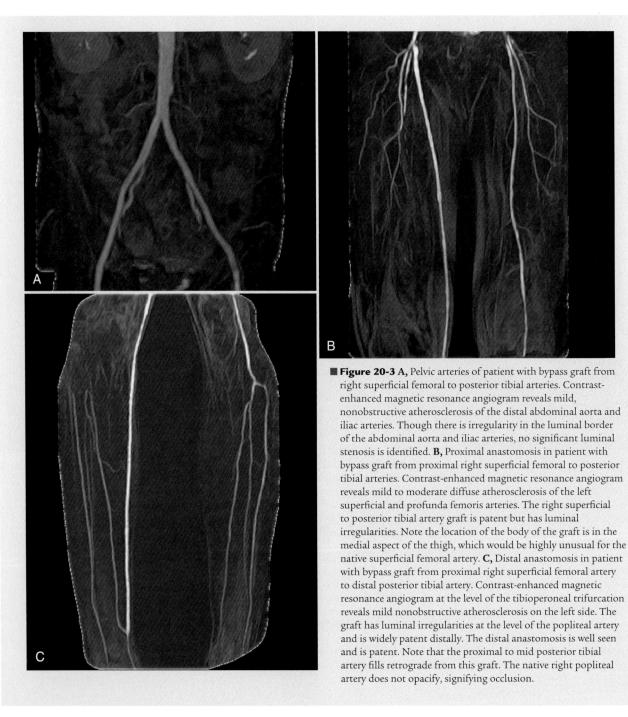

■ **Figure 20-3 A,** Pelvic arteries of patient with bypass graft from right superficial femoral to posterior tibial arteries. Contrast-enhanced magnetic resonance angiogram reveals mild, nonobstructive atherosclerosis of the distal abdominal aorta and iliac arteries. Though there is irregularity in the luminal border of the abdominal aorta and iliac arteries, no significant luminal stenosis is identified. **B,** Proximal anastomosis in patient with bypass graft from proximal right superficial to posterior tibial arteries. Contrast-enhanced magnetic resonance angiogram reveals mild to moderate diffuse atherosclerosis of the left superficial and profunda femoris arteries. The right superficial to posterior tibial artery graft is patent but has luminal irregularities. Note the location of the body of the graft is in the medial aspect of the thigh, which would be highly unusual for the native superficial femoral artery. **C,** Distal anastomosis in patient with bypass graft from proximal right superficial femoral artery to distal posterior tibial artery. Contrast-enhanced magnetic resonance angiogram at the level of the tibioperoneal trifurcation reveals mild nonobstructive atherosclerosis on the left side. The graft has luminal irregularities at the level of the popliteal artery and is widely patent distally. The distal anastomosis is well seen and is patent. Note that the proximal to mid posterior tibial artery fills retrograde from this graft. The native right popliteal artery does not opacify, signifying occlusion.

Case 4   **Severe Diffuse Peripheral Vascular Disease**

A 65-year-old patient with history of coronary artery bypass surgery and ischemic cardiomyopathy presented with nonhealing ulcers on both feet. On examination there was evidence for bilateral dry gangrene involving the lateral malleoli. The distal pulses in the feet were not palpable. The ankle-brachial index was less than 0.55 bilaterally. The referring physician ordered a CMR/MRA to evaluate for peripheral vascular disease (Figure 20-4).

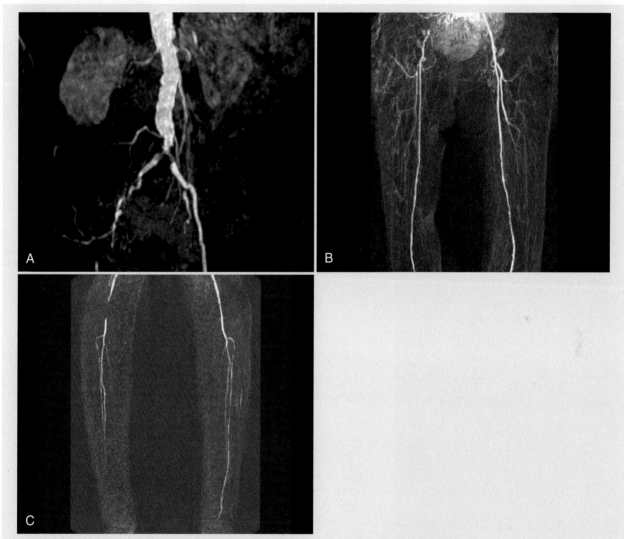

■ **Figure 20-4 A,** Severe diffuse aortoiliac disease. Contrast-enhanced magnetic resonance angiogram reveals marked irregularities of the distal mid to distal abdominal aorta. Note that the abdominal aorta tapers and measures 1.2 cm in diameter at the bifurcation into the common iliac arteries. There are severe stenoses involving bilateral proximal common iliac arteries. Additionally, the right external iliac artery has severe diffuse atherosclerosis and is occluded distally. **B,** Severe diffuse peripheral vascular disease. Contrast-enhanced magnetic resonance angiogram reveals reconstitution of the right common femoral artery, likely secondary to deep collateral vessels. Bilateral superficial femoral and proximal popliteal arteries have luminal irregularities but are free from significant luminal stenosis.
C, Severe diffuse peripheral vascular disease involving the outflow vessels. Contrast-enhanced magnetic resonance angiogram reveals 2.5 cm long occlusion of the right popliteal artery with subsequent reconstitution. Bilateral posterior tibial arteries are only seen proximally and then are not visualized, consistent with severe stenotic disease. Also, there is severe diffuse atherosclerosis involving bilateral anterior tibial and peroneal arteries.

Case 5   **Artifacts and Miscellaneous**

Figure 20-5 presents instances of bilateral iliac artery stents, right common and left external iliac artery stents, and diffuse atherosclerosis involving the right anterior tibial artery.

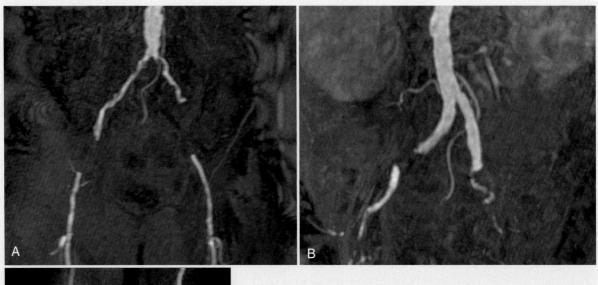

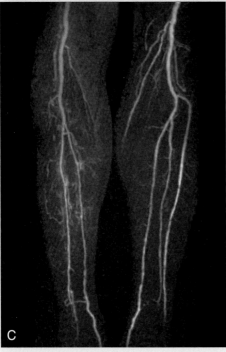

■ **Figure 20-5 A,** Bilateral iliac artery stents. Contrast-enhanced magnetic resonance angiogram reveals bilateral signal dropout at the level of the external iliac arteries. Note that there is abrupt cessation (without tapering) and reconstitution of flow without any observed collateral circulation. These findings are consistent with this patient's history of stent implantation in bilateral external iliac arteries. X-ray angiography confirmed full patency of stents bilaterally. **B,** Right common and left external iliac artery stents. Contrast-enhanced magnetic resonance angiogram reveals bilateral signal dropout at the level of the right common and left external iliac arteries. Note again that there is abrupt cessation and reconstitution of flow without apparent collateral circulation. These findings are consistent with this patient's history of stent implantation. X-ray angiography confirmed full patency of both stents. **C,** Diffuse atherosclerosis involving the right anterior tibial artery. Contrast-enhanced magnetic resonance angiogram reveals only luminal irregularities of the left popliteal and infra-popliteal vessels. Three-vessel runoff is present on the left side. However, the right anterior tibial artery has severe diffuse atherosclerosis and appears occluded proximally. Collateral vessels are noted in the mid anterior tibial artery region. Two-vessel runoff is present in the right leg.

SUGGESTED READING

Ersoy H, Zhang H, Prince MR: Peripheral MR angiography. J Cardiovasc Magn Reson 2006;8(3):517-528.

Gozzi M, Amorico MG, Colopi S, et al: Peripheral arterial occlusive disease: Role of MR angiography. Radiol Med (Torino) 2006;111(2):225-237.

Leiner T, Ho KY, Nelemans PJ, et al: Three-dimensional contrast-enhanced moving-bed infusion-tracking (MoBi-track) peripheral MR angiography with flexible choice of imaging parameters for each field of view. J Magn Reson Imaging 2000;11:368-377.

Nelemans PJ, Leiner T, de Vet HCW, et al: Peripheral arterial disease: Meta-analysis of the diagnostic performance of MR angiography. Radiology 2000;217:105-114.

Prince MR, Yucel EK, Kaufman JA, et al: Dynamic gadolinium-enhanced three-dimensional abdominal MR arteriography. J Magn Reson Imaging 1993;3:877-881.

Zhang H, Maki JH, Prince MR. 3D contrast-enhanced MR angiography. J Magn Reson Imaging 2007;26(3):816.

Chapter 21

Diseases of the Aorta

Mark A. Lawson

KEY POINTS

- Be familiar with the anatomy of the normal aorta and branch vessels

- Appreciate that the comprehensive evaluation of the aorta includes examination of the heart for other comorbid conditions

- Identify and describe major pathologic findings of diseases of the aorta on CMR/MRA studies

- Understand the challenges of contrast-enhanced magnetic resonance angiography

Cardiovascular magnetic resonance (CMR) is recognized as a useful tool for the noninvasive evaluation of the aorta by providing clinicians with high quality diagnostic images, in any imaging plane, without interference from surrounding soft tissue or bone, using only a peripheral IV catheter and administration of CMR contrast agents characterized by a favorable safety profile. Recent technological advances in magnet design allow for short acquisition times, high signal-to-noise and contrast-to-noise ratios, and improved spatial and temporal resolution. With images resembling conventional x-ray angiography, contrast-enhanced MRA (CE-MRA) is the preferred currently available MRA technique used today. This technique does not rely on the flow characteristic of blood but rather on T1-shortening effects of a circulating CMR contrast agent, making it less prone to flow-related artifacts. Successful CE-MRA requires the coordination of an intravenously administered CMR contrast agent bolus with image acquisition during the arterial phase of the first-pass transit of the CMR contrast agent. With a short acquisition time, the scan can be completed before venous enhancement occurs. For vascular applications, CE-MRA can depict often complex and entwined vascular anatomy because of the free choice of imaging planes by the scan operator and the acquisition of 3D data sets that overcome many limitations of projection techniques. CE-MRA contains little information about the morphology of the aortic wall, and should be complemented by T1- or T2-weighted precontrast and, in some cases, postcontrast images.

One of the strengths of CMR is the ability to obtain dynamic information regarding blood flow and heart function. A cardiac cine CMR study (whether complete or abbreviated) should be performed before CE-MRA to examine left ventricular cavity size, mass, and global and segmental function as clues of other comorbid conditions. Cine CMR is also invaluable for determining aortic valve morphology (such as bicuspid or calcific valves) and, in cases of aortic dissection and aneurysm, the mechanism of aortic regurgitation (e.g., dilatation of the aortic root and annulus, tearing of the annulus or valve cusps, downward displacement of one cusp below the line of valve closure, loss of support of the cusp, and physical interference in the closure of the aortic valve by an intimal flap). Phase contrast methods through the aortic root can be used to calculate the regurgitant fraction or estimate aortic stenosis severity by measuring peak transaortic velocity.

Unlike CT angiography or conventional x-ray angiography, CMR is not associated with concerns related to ionizing radiation exposure (whether to the patient, operator, or staff), or to the unfavorable side effect profile of iodinated contrast (including nephrotoxicity, anaphylactoid allergic response, and adverse hemodynamic effects of lowering blood pressure, increasing left ventricular end diastolic pressure, and depressing myocardial contractility). X-ray angiography carries the risks associated with arterial puncture, vascular injury in patients with difficult vascular access, hemorrhage, and catheter-induced thromboembolic or atheroembolic ischemic complications. There is no aftercare of the patient following a CMR examination, and compared with conventional x-ray angiography, it is virtually painless.

NORMAL ANATOMY OF THE AORTA AND BRANCH VESSELS

In order to cover large vascular territories, CE-MRA can be performed using several overlapping contiguous CE-MRA acquisitions, so-called multistation MRA. In Figure 21-1, the initial station is centered on the neck and the first scan is initiated with arrival of gadolinium in the aortic arch. Each subsequent MRA station is acquired in rapid succession moving caudally to capture the arterial transit of gadolinium down the aorta. A stepping table is essential to perform this "bolus chase" and consists of the progressive movement of the imaging field of view to coincide with gadolinium run-off. The main challenge of multistation MRA is to image quickly to avoid enhancement in the venous vessels, which overlap arterial vessels. The ascending aorta takes its origin from the left ventricle. At its beginning, the aortic root comprises the aortic annulus and the sinuses of Valsalva (three localized dilatations or sinuses), and from the right and left sinuses arise the right and left coronary arteries. The sinuses lie above and behind the aortic semilunar valve leaflets. The sinuses join the tubular ascending aorta at the sinotubular junction, and from there the aorta is directed upward and forward. The ascending aorta is mobile for the most part and is enclosed by the pericardium up to the level of the sternal angle (angle of Louis). The aortic arch is the continuation of the ascending aorta and emerges from the pericardium traveling first upward, then backward and to the left, before turning downward just to the left side of the fourth thoracic vertebra. Aortae that cross over the left pulmonary artery and pass left of the trachea are termed left-sided, and right-sided when crossing over the right pulmonary artery and to the right of the trachea. For the most part, adult patients will have normal ventriculoarterial concordance and left-sided aortae. In all forms of aortic disease, it is important to identify the origins of the branch vessels. Branch ostia may originate from the body of the aneurysm or from the false lumen in cases of dissection. It is important to identify the branch vessel origins in these cases because a complete surgical repair will be determined in part by this information. Branches of the aortic arch are the innominate artery (or brachiocephalic trunk), left common carotid artery, and the left subclavian artery. This pattern is found in about 65% to 70% of people. Attached to the underside of the arch opposite the origin of the left subclavian artery and directed toward the root of the left pulmonary artery is the *ligamentum arteriosum*, which is a band of connective tissue about 3 to 5 mm in diameter and represents

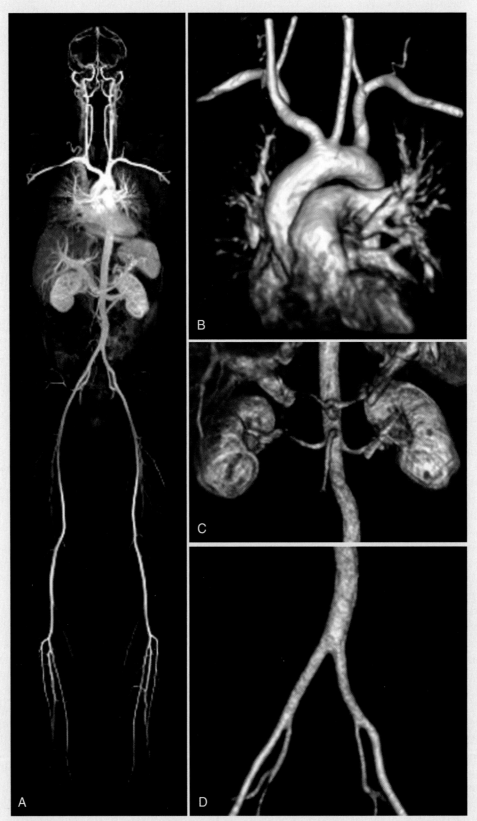

■ **Figure 21-1** Normal anatomy of the aorta and branch vessels.

the remains of the fetal *ductus arteriosus*. Here a focal narrowing of the lumen of the aorta may be found called the aortic isthmus. The aorta is fixed to the thorax at this point. The descending aorta then travels caudally to the left of the spine until it penetrates the diaphragm at the aortic hiatus near the level of the twelfth thoracic vertebra. Below the level of the diaphragm, the aorta becomes the abdominal aorta and ends by dividing into the two common iliac arteries at the bifurcation. Three ventral unpaired branches of larger size supply the gastrointestinal tract: the celiac trunk, the superior mesenteric artery, and the inferior mesenteric artery. The celiac trunk arises from the front of the aorta just below the aortic hiatus. The classic anatomic branches of the celiac trunk (occurring in about 50% to 60% of patients) are the splenic, left gastric, and common hepatic arteries. The superior mesenteric artery (SMA) is the second of the unpaired branches of the aorta, originating caudal to the celiac trunk, and supplies branches to the pancreas, all of the small bowel (except the proximal duodenum), and the right and mid colon. The renal arteries arise one on each side of the aorta at the upper level of the second lumbar vertebra about 1 cm below the SMA. They pass transversely to the hilum of each kidney where they divide typically into three branches that then break into numerous secondary branches. Multiple renal arteries are present in 30% of the population, usually arising as accessory renal arteries from the aorta. Left accessory renal arteries are encountered more often than right sided ones. As a rule, aortic origins of accessory renal arteries occur caudal to the main renal artery. The abdominal aorta bifurcates into the right and left common iliac arteries at the level of the umbilicus, typically near the level of the fourth lumbar vertebra. Atherosclerosis commonly first involves the arteries of the lower extremities at or near the aortic bifurcation. Normal aortic dimensions are listed in Table 21-1.

A common anatomic variation of the arch vessels is the so-called "bovine" arch where the innominate and left common carotid arteries share a common origin (Figure 21-2). In this example the left common carotid artery originates off the innominate artery, the second arch vessel is the left vertebral artery, and the third arch vessel is the left subclavian artery. This branching pattern is found in about 25% to 27% of people, and interest-ingly, in most apes. Less common are four separate ostia for each of the arch vessels (2.5%) and the "avian" arch characterized by only two branches, or bi-innominate anatomy (1.2%).

AORTIC ANEURYSM

A 50-year-old man with hypertension treated with an ACE inhibitor and diuretic presented with mild chest pain across the mid chest. ECG demonstrated sinus bradycardia with voltage criteria for left ventricular hypertrophy, inferior T-wave inversion, and J-point and ST-segment elevation in leads V3-V4. Bright blood CMR images were taken (Figure 21-3).

Aneurysms are areas of focal or diffuse dilatation of the aorta that develop at sites of medial weakness. The aneurysmal sack is composed of fibrous tissue. Aneurysms can be fusiform (uniform, symmetric, circumferential shape) or saccular (eccentric, focal, outpouching shape). The most common etiologies of aneurysmal development are atherosclerosis and hypertension. The atherosclerotic process is thought to erode the aortic wall and destroy the medial elastic elements that leads to weakening of the wall and dilatation; whereas hypertension imposes increase mechanical wall stress. Ascending thoracic aortic aneurysms can occur from Marfan's syndrome (or other connective tissue diseases), longstanding aortic stenosis, and rarely, traumatic or mycotic etiologies.

For contrast-enhanced MRA (CE-MRA) to be successful, a high concentration of contrast agent (a chelate of gadoliunium) should be maintained in the aorta during the entire image acquisition time. Contrast volume, delivery rate, delay time from injection to image acquisition, and saline flush are important for good image quality. To make blood appear bright compared with the background tissues, it is necessary to inject a sufficient dosage (or volume) of gadolinium at a sufficient rate.

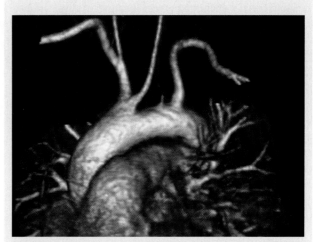

■ **Figure 21-2** Normal anatomic variation of the arch vessels.

TABLE 21-1 Normal Aortic Dimensions

	MEN	WOMEN
Aortic annulus	26 ± 3 mm	23 ± 2 mm
Aortic root	31 ± 5 mm	28 ± 3 mm
Ascending aorta	34 ± 6 mm	28 ± 4 mm
Descending aorta	25 ± 4 mm	20 ± 4 mm

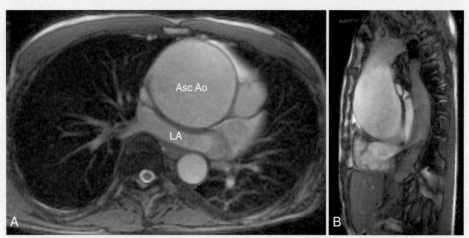

■ **Figure 21-3** Bright blood CMR images through the chest in a patient with an ascending thoracic aortic aneurysm. **A,** Compression of adjacent structures such as vertebrae, tracheobronchial tree, esophagus, duodenum, pulmonary vessels, and vena cavae can occur and erosion of the aneurysm into these structures has been reported. In this example, axial bright blood CMR images demonstrate a large fusiform aneurysm of the ascending thoracic aorta (Asc Ao) that compresses the left atrium (LA). **B,** The risk for rupture of thoracic aortic aneurysms is directly related to the aortic diameter with a 5-year risk of rupture of 16 % for aneurysms between 40 to 60 mm and 31% in those greater than 60 mm in diameter. Therefore the size should be measured in its maximal cross-sectional dimensions perpendicular to the long axis of the aorta as well as the cranial-caudal extent of the aneurysm. Ascending thoracic aortae measuring greater than 40 mm in diameter are aneurysmal (aortae measuring between 35 to 40 mm are sometimes described as ectatic) and greater than 30 mm for descending thoracic and abdominal aortae. In this example the maximal cross-sectional dimension is 78 mm and extends 150 mm in the cranial-caudal dimension. Prophylactic surgical repair would be indicated for ascending thoracic aortic aneurysms exceeding 50 mm in diameter.

The arterial phase of the gadolinium bolus injection is the optimal time to acquire MRA data to take advantage of the higher arterial SNR and to eliminate overlapping venous enhancement. An extremely fast MRA acquisition is essential to capture the gadolinium bolus during the brief moment that the agent is present in the aorta but not yet in the venous system. Circulation times are variable from patient to patient because of differences in cardiac output, blood flow profiles, and plasma volume. Coordination of image acquisition and the arrival of the gadolinium bolus in the aorta are crucial to achieve good image quality. Imaging prematurely can result in incomplete vascular depiction. Imaging too late can result in insufficient signal within the aorta (caused by washout of the gadolinium and diffusion into the tissue) and enhancement of the veins and soft tissues, which can obscure the aorta. Different strategies have been developed to optimize the proper timing of synchronizing arterial enhancement with image acquisition in order to avoid enhancement of any unwanted structures. A real time method of timing the bolus arrival is MR fluoroscopy (Figure 21-4).

An aortic aneurysm can be described in regards to its site or location along with its morphology or shape (fusiform versus saccular). It may be helpful to reference the location to another anatomical landmark. Aortic dilatation may extend into branch vessels (Figure 21-5).

One of the strengths of CMR is the ability to obtain dynamic information regarding the blood flow and heart function. A complete CMR/MRA evaluation for aortic disease includes scans to evaluate not only the aorta and aortic lumen but also the heart. Aortic insufficiency is common with ascending aortic aneurysms (Figures 21-6 and 21-7).

Depending on the patient's age and risk factors for coronary artery disease, many cardiothoracic surgeons recommend coronary artery angiography before aneurysm repair. Conventional x-ray coronary angiography may be challenging because of distorted aortic anatomy and a limited selection of available angiographic catheters of sufficient length and angulation to engage the coronary arteries. Whereas current coronary MRA techniques do not evaluate the entire coronary tree, coronary MRA is sufficient to illustrate the origins of the coronary arteries and help the proceduralist avoid technical pitfalls while performing conventional x-ray coronary angiography (Figures 21-8 and 21-9).

Ascending thoracic aortic aneurysms are typically larger at the time of diagnosis compared with descending aneurysms, although ascending aneurysm tend to expand

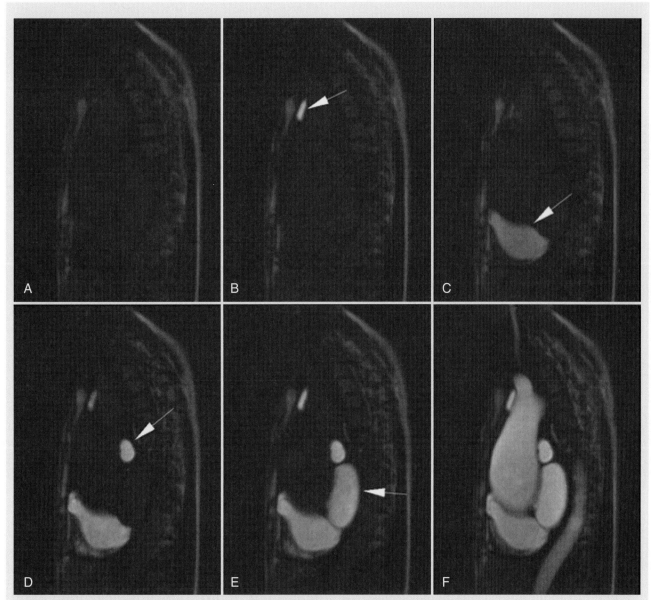

■ **Figure 21-4** Bolus tracking techniques used in acquiring CE-MRA. In this case MR fluoroscopy demonstrates the appearance of the central circulation (**A**) before arrival of the contrast, then the sequential appearance of contrast (*arrow*) into the (**B**) superior vena cava, (**C**) right atrium, (**D**) pulmonary artery, (**E**) left atrium, and (**F**) finally into the aorta. At this point, the operator can manually trigger the start of the CE-MRA image acquisition once enhancement from the arrival of gadolinium into the aorta is visualized.

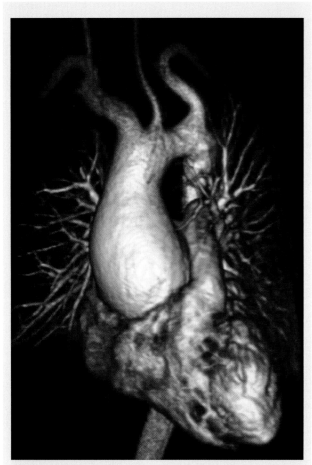

Figure 21-5 Three-dimensional volume-rendered CE-MRA of an ascending thoracic aortic aneurysm. A large fusiform aneurysm of the ascending aorta involves much of the ascending thoracic aorta. The innominate (first arch branch artery) and left subclavian (third arch branch artery) arteries are dilated as well.

chest pain, diaphoresis, or syncope. On arrival, her heart rate was 87 bpm; blood pressure was 124/72 mm Hg in the right arm and 175/50 mm Hg in the left arm. She had 2+ radial and femoral pulses and a 2/6 systolic murmur. Her ECG demonstrated sinus rhythm, left anterior fascicular block, and late R-wave transition and nonspecific T-wave changes across the anterior precordial leads. Dark-blood and bright-blood CMR images were obtained (Figure 21-11).

Classic aortic dissection is the longitudinal cleavage of the aortic media by a dissecting column of blood forming a true and false lumen. The false lumen communicates with the true lumen through an intimal tear or laceration usually located near its proximal end. It is typically single and transverse, but exceptions are frequent with secondary and reentry tears occurring distally. CMR imaging of aortic dissections is shown in Figures 21-12 to 21-14. Chronic systemic hypertension (believed to accentuate the degenerative process of aging to promote weakness of the aortic wall) is the most common factor predisposing the aorta to dissection and is present in 62% to 78% of patients with aortic dissection. Aortic diseases, such as aortic dilatation, aneurysms, annuloaortic ectasia, chromosomal aberrations, coarctation, arch hypoplasia, arteritis, bicuspid aortic valve, and hereditary connective tissue diseases are other predisposing factors for the development of dissection. Atherosclerosis does not appear to pose a high risk for classic spontaneous aortic dissection, but the development of two variants (intramural hematoma and aortic ulcer) is strongly associated with the presence and severity of atherosclerosis.

The DeBakey and Stanford classification systems describe the origin and extent of thoracic aortic dissections. Stanford Type A dissections involve the ascending thoracic aorta. The DeBakey system further characterizes these into Type I (tears originating in the ascending aorta and extending distally into the descending aorta) and Type II (tears and extent limited to just to the ascending aorta). Stanford Type B and DeBakey Type III dissections account for 25% of aortic dissection with the intimal tear beginning just beyond the origin of the left subclavian artery and extending distally. Only 10% of dissections involve the aortic arch where entry just beyond the left subclavian artery extends retrograde (or proximally). Complications occur randomly and the outcome is frequently fatal. Death from dissection can occur from rupture of the outer wall of the false lumen. Other complications of Type I dissections include hemopericardium and tamponade or from dissection planes that undermine the aortic valve leading to acute severe aortic insufficiency. Complications of Type III dissections include hemorrhagic left pleural effusion.

more slowly (Figure 21-10). Kommerell's diverticulum is a consequence of regression in the fourth left aortic arch (between the left carotid and left subclavian arteries) and is prominent because the fetal *ductus arteriosus*, near the origin of the aberrant left subclavian artery, carries a large volume of blood. The left subclavian artery arises from a diverticulum at the junction of the right-sided aortic arch and the descending aorta and passes obliquely upward, behind the esophagus, toward the left arm. At first glance, Kommerell's diverticulum in Figure 21-10C has a similar appearance to the proximal descending thoracic aneurysm in Figure 21-10B except that the aberrant left subclavian artery originates from the diverticulum.

AORTIC DISSECTION

A 58-year-old woman with hypertension and a myxomatous mitral valve presented following acute onset of severe upper and lower back pain. She denied anterior

AORTIC ATHEROSCLEROSIS

A 64-year-old previously healthy man presented following 2 weeks of progressive dyspnea on exertion, orthop-

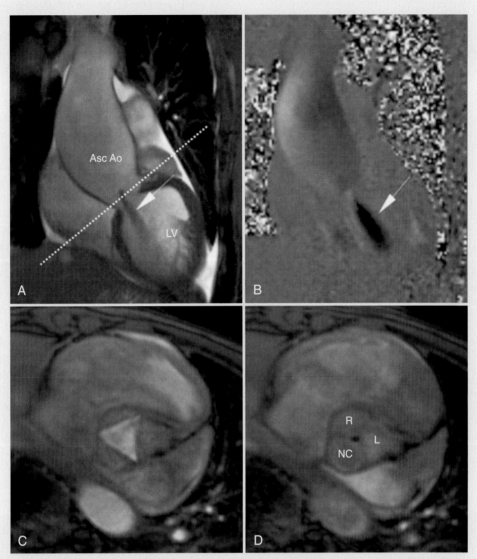

■ **Figure 21-6** The comprehensive CMR/MRA examination: aortic valve structure. **A,** A central jet of aortic insufficiency is denoted by the diastolic signal void (*arrow*) within the left ventricle on bright blood cine CMR. **B,** Phase contrast methods create contrast between stationary and moving hydrogen spins as a result of velocity-induced phase shifts of moving spins acquired along a magnetic gradient. Stationary tissue will experience no net phase shift by the combination of positively and negatively applied gradients. Flowing blood accumulates a phase shift that is directly proportional to the velocity and direction of blood flow. The central jet of aortic insufficiency (*arrow*) is again demonstrated during diastole on phase contrast cine CMR. **C,** By imaging parallel with the aortic annulus (*dashed line*) and perpendicular to the long axis of the aorta, a cross-sectional view of the aortic valve can be obtain. A tricuspid aortic valve opens normally during systole in the example case. **D,** The right (R), left (L), and noncoronary (NC) cusps fail to coapt completely during diastole resulting in the central jet of aortic insufficiency.

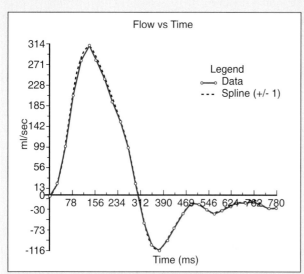

Figure 21-7 The comprehensive CMR/MRA examination: aortic insufficiency severity. Phase contrast cine CMR techniques calculate blood flow volume and depict in graphic form blood flow profiles across the aortic valve during the cardiac cycle. The technique is analogous to Doppler evaluation of blood flow waveforms. A single imaging plane parallel to the aortic annulus is selected to calculate the cross-sectional blood flow through the aortic valve. Blood flow volume can be calculated by circumscribing a region of interest around the aortic valve (volume = velocity × area). In this example, the forward stroke volume (area under the curve above the x-axis on the graph) is 100 ml, whereas the regurgitant volume (area under the curve below the x-axis) is 14 ml. This yields a regurgitant fraction of 14% for this patient.

nea with paroxysmal nocturnal dyspnea, and edema. He is a painter and has smoked one pack per day for the past 40 years. On review of systems, he describes claudication when walking or climbing the ladder when painting. He was found to be hypertensive with a blood pressure of 153/70 mm Hg (Figure 21-15).

Atherosclerotic lesions may be quite heterogeneous even within the same patient and all subtypes of atherosclerotic lesions likely coexist together but in unpredictable proportions. The proportional distribution of different plaque types is inherently variable within individual patients because of the continuous, evolutionary nature of atheroma formation. Scattered stenoses from atherosclerotic lesions may be evident in many older patients. Leriche originally described complete obliteration of the aortic bifurcation, but Leriche syndrome is commonly used to describe obstruction at any level of the infrarenal aorta. It typically results from plaque rupture and subsequent mural thrombus leading to gradual progressive lumenal narrowing. On rare occasions, it can be caused by infrarenal coarctation, aortitis, in situ thrombosis, or embolism. The process is often chronic allowing time for the development of periaortic collateral circulation. Collateral vessels are sufficient to prevent gangrene and amputation for ischemia is seldom required. MRA is an ideal image modality for this condition because gadolinium contrast remains visible in very low concentrations secondary to the vast difference in T1 between tissue and contrast-enhanced blood.

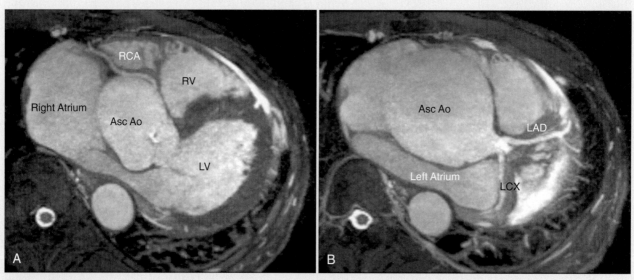

Figure 21-8 The comprehensive CMR/MRA examination: coronary angiography. **A,** The right coronary artery (RCA) originates from the right aortic sinus perhaps more left lateral than typically observed and courses toward the right atrioventricular groove. **B,** The left coronary artery originates in its typical location from the left aortic sinus and quickly bifurcates into the left anterior descending (LAD) coronary artery that courses in the interventricular groove and left circumflex (LCx) coronary artery that courses in the left atrioventricular groove.

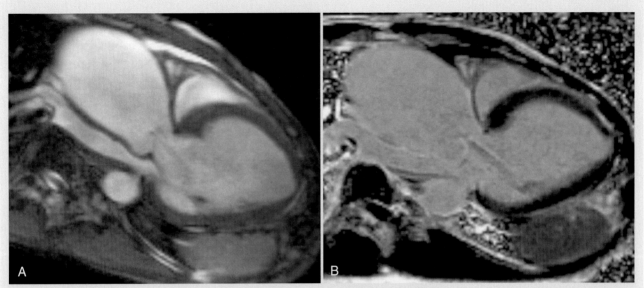

■ **Figure 21-9** The comprehensive CMR/MRA examination: left ventricular size, function, and myocardial delayed enhancement. Beyond an evaluation for the presence of aortic insufficiency, bright blood CMR depicts the left ventricle for clues of other comorbid conditions including ventricular cavity size, mass, and global and segmental function. Left ventricular hypertrophy may be an indication of uncontrolled hypertension. Segmental wall motion abnormalities may provide a clue for previously undiagnosed coronary artery disease. Left ventricular enlargement may indicate concurrent hypertensive, valvular, or ischemic heart disease. **A,** In this example patient, an end-diastolic image of the left ventricle in the LVOT orientation demonstrates left ventricular dilatation (left ventricular end-diastolic dimension 64 mm, end-diastolic volume 286 ml) and eccentric hypertrophy (left ventricular mass 230 grams). Left ventricular systolic function was moderately depressed (LVEF 34%) with moderate global hypokinesis. **B,** Because the patient received gadolinium contrast for CE-MRA, myocardial delayed enhancement images complete the comprehensive CMR/MRA examination by demonstrating no prior myocardial infarction or occult myocardial fibrosis.

A prominent feature of advanced atherosclerosis is superficial ulcerations limited just to the intima. Aortic ulcer typically occurs in elderly patients, often men, who have histories of hypertension, hyperlipidemia, and severe aortic atherosclerosis. It is characterized by ulceration of an atherosclerotic plaque that penetrates through the intima of the aortic wall and is thought to occur as the result of intimal fracture of atherosclerotic plaque. Penetrating aortic ulcer (PAU) is used to describe an ulcer that erodes through the media. Progressive penetration deep into the aortic wall may result in hematoma and a weakening of the aortic wall, which in turn may result in aortic enlargement and aneurysm formation and even be a precursor to dissection. On CMR, aortic ulcer is seen as an outpouching or "crater" extending beyond the contour of the aortic lumen, typically located in the descending aorta, and is invariably surrounded by extensive atherosclerosis (Figure 21-16).

INFLAMMATORY DISEASE OF THE AORTA

A 34-year-old woman presented with gradual worsening of left arm and jaw claudication, intermittent blurred vision, and headaches. Her left radial pulse was not palpable. Laboratory investigation revealed an ESR 62 mm/hr, CRP 28 mg/L, ANA greater than 1:160 (speckled pattern), RF less than 10 IU/ml, negative ANCA, HDL cholesterol 68 mg/dl, and LDL cholesterol 92 mg/dl.

Inflammatory processes show increased aortic wall thickness and enhancement of the aortic wall and surrounding periaortic soft tissues on T1- and T2-weighted sequences (Figure 21-17). These CMR characteristics when associated with elevated serum markers of inflammation without definite adjacent atheromata suggest aortitis. Takayasu arteritis is a primary arteritis of unknown etiology that commonly affects the aorta and its major branches (Figure 21-18). It is more commonly seen in the Orient but has a worldwide distribution. This is a condition of marked intimal proliferation, degeneration of elastin, cellular infiltrate, and fibrosis leading to fibrotic scarring and obliterative lumenal changes of the aorta. The adventitia thickens and *vasa vasorum* becomes obliterated. The etiology of this disease is unknown, but rheumatic fever, rheumatoid arthritis, prior streptococcal or tuberculous infection, and collagen-vascular disease have been postulated.

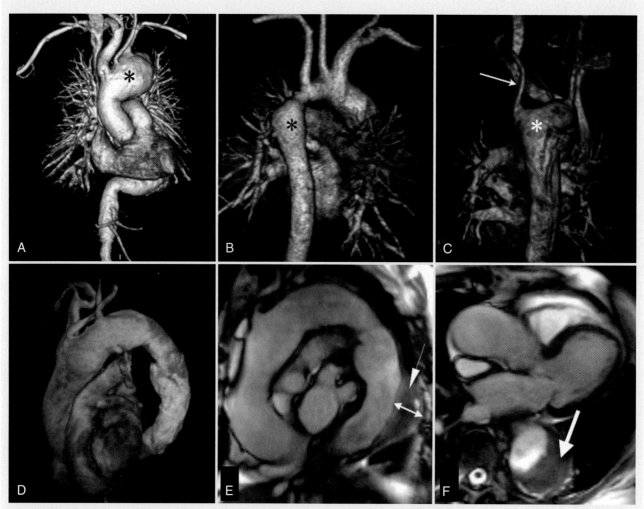

■ **Figure 21-10** Other examples of aortic aneurysms. **A,** Coronal CE-MRA of an aneurysm of the aortic arch that spares the ascending aorta. **B,** RPO CE-MRA of a patient with a small focal fusiform aneurysm of the proximal descending thoracic aorta. **C,** RPO CE-MRA of a patient with Kommerell's diverticulum. **D,** LAO CE-MRA of a patient with descending thoracic aortic aneurysm lined with mural thrombus. Laminated thrombus often lines the aneurysm. Gadolinium opacification of the lumen alone does not completely delineate the size and extent of the aneurysm. **E, F,** On bright blood CMR, thrombus (*arrow*) appears hypointense compared with the flowing blood in the aortic lumen that appears bright. The cross-sectional diameter of the aneurysm is much greater than would be apparent on CE-MRA alone. (*RPO,* right posterior oblique. *LAO,* left anterior oblique.)

COARCTATION OF THE AORTA

An active 18-year-old man presented for evaluation of hypertension and intermittent nose bleeds. Blood pressure measured 162/82 mm Hg in the right arm and 162/81 mm Hg in the left. Although radial pulses were normal, the femoral pulses were absent. A systolic femoral blood pressure of 78 mm Hg could only be obtained using a Doppler probe.

Coarctation of the aorta is classically described as a congenital narrowing of the proximal descending aorta adjacent to the site of the *ligamentum arteriosum* that is of sufficient severity to develop a pressure gradient across the coarctation. Coarctation of the aorta is thought to occur either from (1) muscular tissue of the ductus arteriosus incorporating into the aorta that contracts as the ductus closes, (2) abnormal involution of the left dorsal aorta, (3) failure of the aortic isthmus to enlarge with the rest of the aorta, or (4) underdevelopment of the aortic arch. Although the arch may have a steep angulated configuration (often accompanied by arch hypoplasia), coarctation occurring proximally in the aortic arch between the left common carotid and left subclavian arteries is uncommon. Coarctation can be described using measurements of the aorta, the spatial relationship between the aortic narrowing and the origin of the major arch

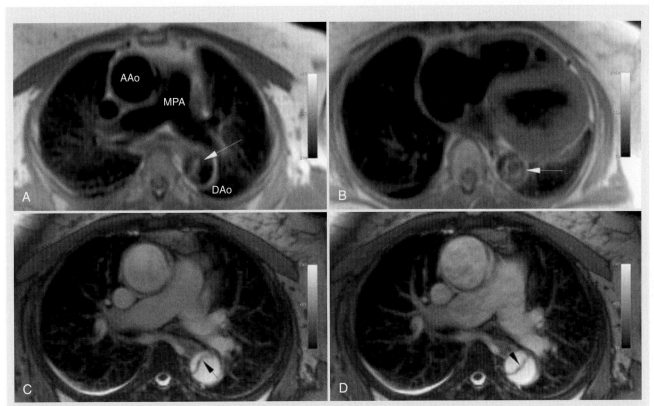

■ **Figure 21-11** Dark blood and bright blood images of an aortic dissection. **A,** On typical black blood pulse sequences, the blood appears black because of the washout of blood before the refocusing pulse and sampling of the echo. In this example case, aortic dissection is suspected on black blood images because of the presence of intraaortic signal. On black blood imaging, intraaortic signal may be high caused by mural thrombus, slow flow, or a combination of the two. In the example case, at the level of the pulmonary bifurcation, altered flow along the medial aspect of the aorta (*arrow*) is present in the true lumen in part because of partial compression of the true lumen by the false lumen (**C**). **B,** A lower axial slice at the level of the coronary sinus demonstrates slower flow this time along the lateral aspect of the descending thoracic aorta (*arrow*) in the false lumen. Also, note the presence of left ventricular hypertrophy that may be an indication of uncontrolled hypertension. **C-D,** The *sine qua non* of aortic dissection is the documentation of an intimal flap and systolic expansion of the true lumen. The location and extent of the tear should be determined accompanied by measurements of the true and false lumen dimensions in the various parts of the affected aorta. In the example case, the dissection flap (*arrow*) during diastole (**C**) is in a neutral position between the true and false lumens. The intimal flap is usually not circumferential but typically occupies about half the aortic circumference and it encroaches upon the true lumen. During systole (**D**), the dissection flap (*arrow*) expands toward the false lumen. Extravasation of blood into the pericardial, pleural, or mediastinal space often signals an emergency because of the high likelihood of the rupture into these spaces. In the example case, a small right-sided pleural effusion is present.

vessels, and visualization of collateral vessels bypassing the coarctation (Figures 21-19 to 21-21).

Percent lumenal stenosis of the coarctation does not always predict hemodynamic importance because a 50% reduction in cross-sectional area of a localized coarctation may be equally notable as a longer tubular coarctation of lesser narrowing (Figure 21-22). Because coarctations can vary in severity, they are considered hemodynamically significant when (1) a pressure gradient of more than 20 mm Hg across the coarctation is present, or (2) collateral flow development is present. Flow volumes in the normal descending aorta should decrease from the arch to the diaphragm. A complete CMR examination of coarctation should include 2D phase contrast imaging just distal to the coarctation and at the level of the diaphragm. If the aortic flow measured at the level of the diaphragm is more than that immediately distal to the coarctation, then collateral flow (mostly through intercostals arteries) is present.

As is characteristic to other forms of congenital heart disease, there are often other coexisting cardiac anomalies. Bicuspid aortic valve is encountered in 50% to 85% of patients with coarctation (Figure 21-23).

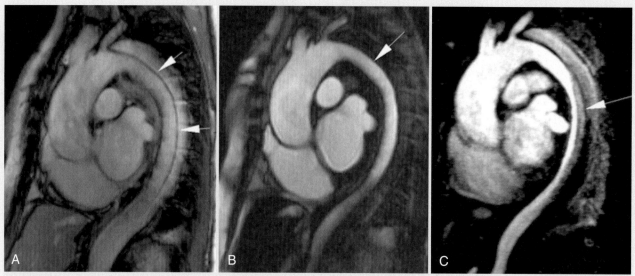

■ **Figure 21-12** Cine and multiphase contrast-enhanced MRA of a patient with aortic dissection viewed in the LAO orientation. **A,** The primary tear exposes the media to aortic luminal pressure and resulting shear forces that propagate the medial cleavage down the aorta. In the example case, LAO bright blood cine CMR demonstrates an intimal flap (*arrows*) extending down the descending aorta. **B,** During MR fluoroscopy, gadolinium initially fills the true aortic lumen. **C,** Contrast blush noted in the false lumen later during the arterial phase of the first-pass of gadolinium.

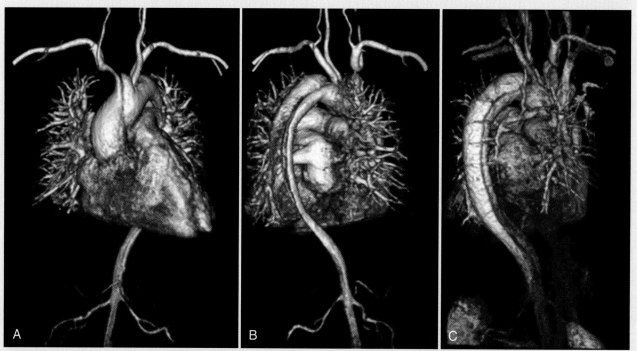

■ **Figure 21-13** Three-dimensional volume rendered CE-MRA of aortic dissection. **A,** Coronal view demonstrating dissection beginning in the aortic arch. **B,** RPO view demonstrating a narrow true lumen coursing caudally down the aorta. Note the lack of initial enhancement of the kidneys suggesting organ hypoperfusion. **C,** Following acquisition of the initial arterial phase CE-MRA, routine repeating of a second and even a third MRA acquisition (so-called "equilibrium phases") is useful. Equilibrium phase CE-MRA is recommended because flow within a patent false channel may be slow and not adequately filled with gadolinium during the arterial phase acquisition. In the example case, contrast eventually appears in the false lumen on the second CE-MRA acquisition.

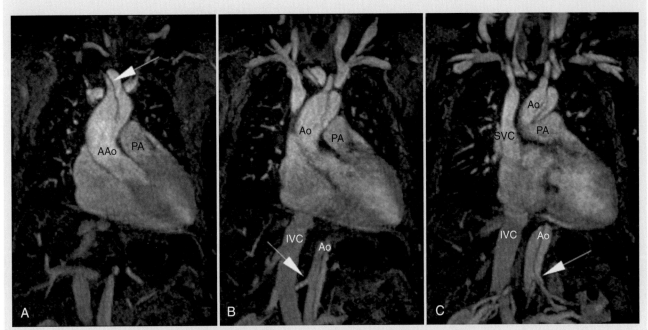

■ **Figure 21-14** Branch involvement in aortic dissection. Involvement of branch vessels is also of concern in cases of aortic dissection. The frequency of branch vessel obstruction after dissection is as high as 27%. Branch vessels may become obstructed from (1) the intimal flap extending into the branch artery, separating the branch vessel into two lumens, one which is supplied by the true lumen and the other by the false lumen, (2) thrombosis of the false lumen or compression of the true lumen, (3) compression of the branch artery by external hematoma, (4) prolapsing dissected intimal flap across the origin of the branch artery, covering it like a curtain overlying the orifice, or (5) reduced flow in the true branch vessel lumen caused by collapse of the aortic true lumen. **A,** Dissection extending up innominate artery (*arrow*). The left common carotid and left subclavian arteries originate from the true lumen. **B,** The right renal artery (*arrow*) originates from the true lumen along the medial aspect of the abdominal aorta. **C,** Dissection extending down the left renal artery (*arrow*).

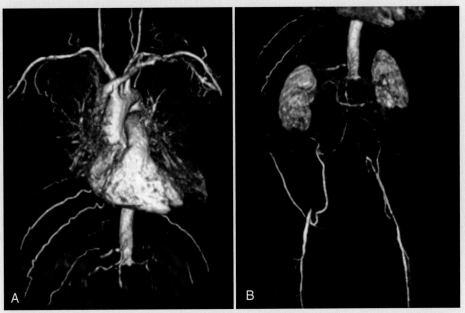

■ **Figure 21-15** Abdominal aortic occlusion. **A,** Coronal CE-MRA of the chest demonstrates right subclavian stenosis and prominent intercostal and upper lumbar arteries. **B,** Coronal CE-MRA of the abdomen demonstrates infrarenal aortic occlusion with reconstitution of the iliofemoral arteries via collateral filling.

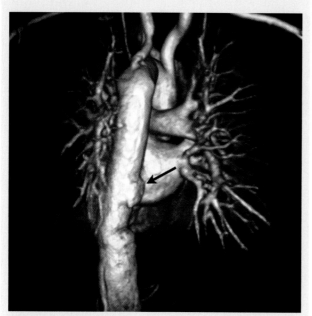

Figure 21-16 Aortic ulcer. In this case of a 51-year-old man with low HDL cholesterol and hypertension, an aortic ulcer (*arrow*) is noted on the posterior aspect of the descending thoracic aorta with adjacent atheromatous disease mildly obstructing the aortic lumen just caudal to the ulcer.

AORTIC THROMBUS

A 55-year-old woman treated for Crohn's disease over the past 22 years presented with an ischemic left fourth finger (Figure 21-24). Her left radial pulse was as strong as her right. A transesophageal echocardiogram demonstrated no valvular vegetation, patent foramen ovale, or left ventricular apical or left atrial appendage thrombus.

POSTOPERATIVE APPEARANCE OF THE AORTA

A detailed knowledge of the surgical technique and its anatomic consequences are required to accurately evaluate postoperative images (Figure 21-25). In some patients, variations seen after surgery may suggest complications, whereas in others they may be the result of routine postoperative findings. The two most widely used surgical techniques to repair the aorta involve placement of an interposition graft (with excision of the diseased segment) or an inclusion graft (with closure of the diseased aorta around the graft, creating a potential space between the graft and the aortic wall that may contain thrombus). The length of graft does not always match the extent of the aneurysm or dissection and residual dilatation or dissection of the remaining native aorta is often encountered.

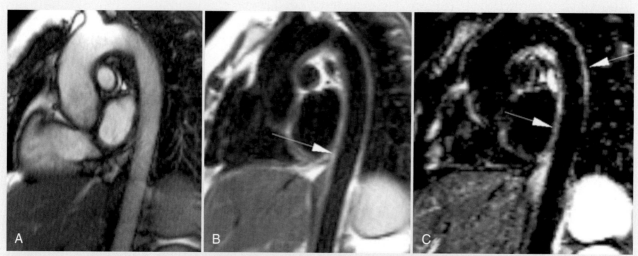

Figure 21-17 Bright blood, dark blood, and STIR CMR of the aorta viewed in the LAO orientation. **A,** Bright blood CMR excludes aortic dissection in this patient with differential upper extremity pulses although the aortic wall is not well visualized. **B,** Black blood CMR demonstrates thickened aortic wall (*arrow*). Thickening, edema, and contrast enhancement of the aortic wall are markers of early vascular inflammation that precedes arterial stenosis and ischemia. T2W-weighted images show high signal intensity in and around the aorta during the acute and active phase of Takayasu arteritis. **C,** STIR images demonstrate a bright aortic wall (*arrow*) indicative of periaortic inflammation and edema.

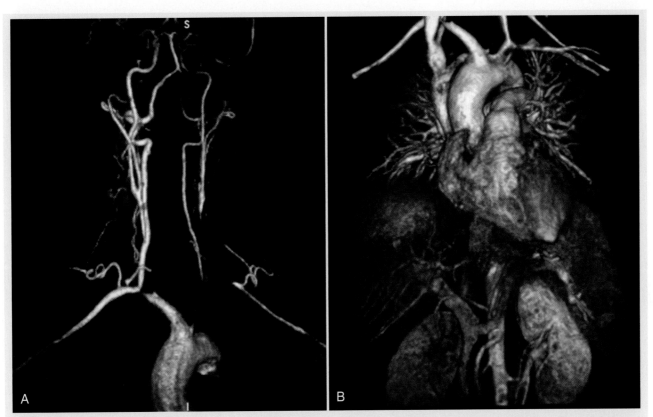

■ **Figure 21-18** CE-MRA of Takayasu's arteritis. CE-MRA contains little information about the morphology of the aortic wall, which was better visualized on T1- or T2-weighted images. CE-MRA strength is in delineating the location and severity of branch vessel disease. **A,** Coronal CE-MRA of the neck demonstrates Takayasu's arteritis predilection for affecting the arch vessels. There is severe stenosis of the right subclavian artery and occlusion of the proximal left common carotid and subclavian arteries. The left internal carotid and distal left subclavian artery reconstitute through collateral filling. Much of the cerebral circulation appears to come from a dominant right vertebral artery that originates distal to the high-grade right subclavian artery stenosis. **B,** Coronal CE-MRA of the abdomen demonstrates patent celiac, SMA, and bilateral renal arteries.

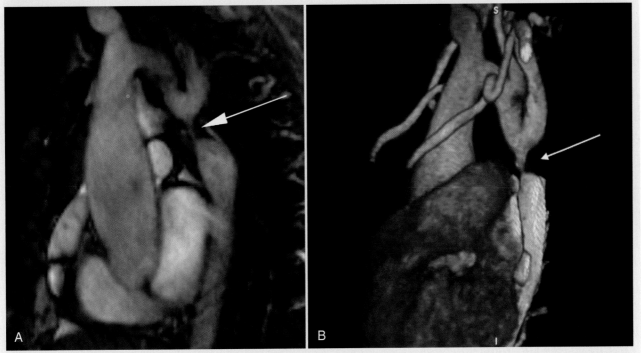

■ **Figure 21-19** Bright blood and CE-MRA of coarctation of the aorta viewed in the LAO orientation. **A,** The primary CMR feature of classic untreated coarctation is a localized shelf or projection of aortic media into the lumen of the aorta, which occurs along the posterior and leftward wall of the aorta just opposite the *ligamentum arteriosum*. In the example case, bright blood CMR demonstrates marked luminal narrowing of the proximal descending thoracic aorta (*arrow*) immediately distal to a downwardly displaced left subclavian artery. The coarctation measures only 5 mm wide and about 12 to 13 mm long. There is borderline dilatation of the ascending aorta (35 mm diameter) and arch hypoplasia. **B,** On CE-MRA, coarctation appears as an indentation or waisting (*arrow*) of the proximal descending thoracic aortic wall.

■ **Figure 21-20** Coronal chest CE-MRA of coarctation of the aorta. Collateral circulation develops between the aorta proximal and distal to the coarctation. Collateral circulation inflow pathways rely on the subclavian arterial branches: vertebral artery (to anterior spinal artery), internal mammary artery, lateral thoracic artery, costocervical trunk (to the supreme intercostal artery), and thyrocervical trunk (to the transverse cervical and transverse scapular arteries). These inflow channels anastomose with the intercostals arteries, which in turn reverse flow to drain into the descending aorta.

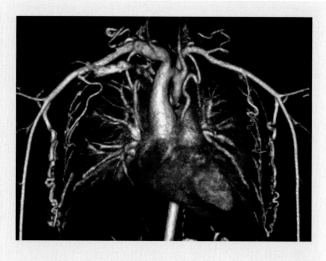

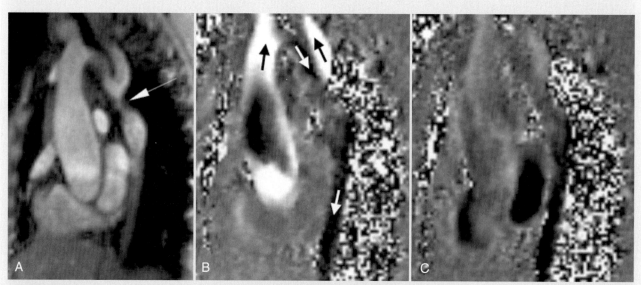

■ **Figure 21-21** Coarctation physiology and CMR. **A,** Bright blood magnitude image of the aorta demonstrating the tight coarctation (*arrow*). **B-C,** Corresponding velocity-encoded images of the aorta in (**B**) systole and (**C**) late diastole. Blood flowing superiorly is represented by white flowing blood and inferiorly flowing blood is depicted as black. Even in late diastole, persistent diastolic blood flow can still be demonstrated in the descending thoracic and abdominal aorta of the example case.

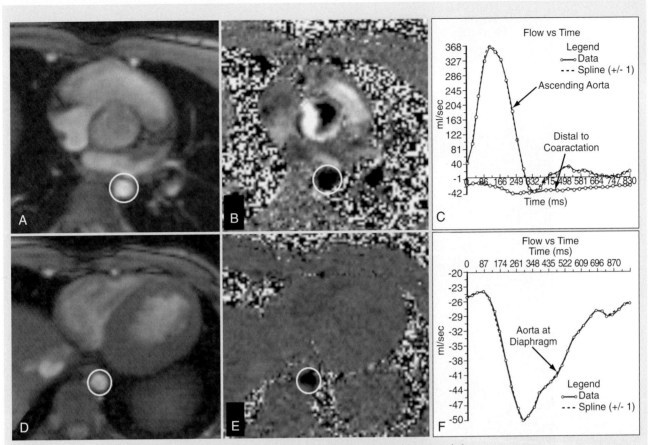

■ **Figure 21-22** Aortic flow graphs in coarctation. Cross-sectional magnitude (**A**) and velocity-encoded (**B**) images of the descending thoracic aorta (*circle*) just distal to the coarctation. **C**, Blood flow profile (y-axis) over the cardiac cycle (x-axis) demonstrating minimal flow through the coarctation. By integrating the area under the curves, the forward stoke volume through the ascending aorta is 70 ml per cardiac cycle and flow down the upper descending thoracic aorta is about 20 ml per cardiac cycle in the example case. Cross-sectional magnitude (**D**) and velocity-encoded (**E**) images of the descending thoracic aorta (*circle*) at the level of the diaphragm. **F**, Blood flow profile over the cardiac cycle demonstrating persistent diastolic flow in the aorta at the level of the diaphragm. Rather than decreasing blood flow volume in the aorta, the flow through the aorta at the level of the diaphragm is higher (about 32 ml per cardiac cycle), suggesting the presence of collateral flow.

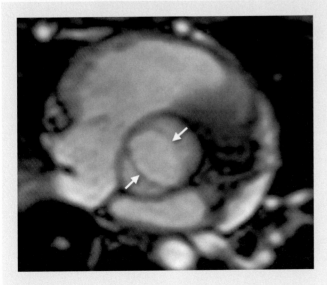

■ **Figure 21-23** Bicuspid aortic valve and coarctation. *Arrows* point to the anterior and posterior commissures of this patient's bicuspid valve imaged during mid systole.

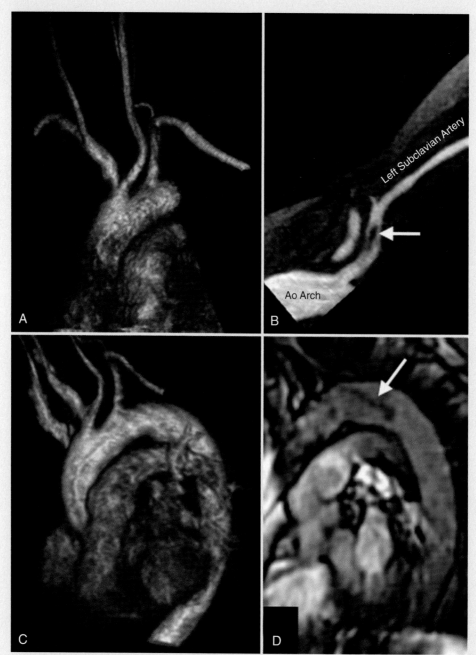

■ **Figure 21-24** Left subclavian artery thrombus. **A,** Aortic thrombus formation in a seemingly otherwise normal aorta is rare. Cases of mobile thrombus formation with peripheral embolization in the absence of aortic atheromata have been reported in patients with hypercoagulable states or inflammatory diseases (such as Crohn's disease). In the example case, intraluminal aortic disease may be missed on MRA data processed into the typical three-dimensional volume rendered images pictured earlier in this chapter. **B,** Curved planar reformatted image constructed from the MRA data set that lays out the course of left subclavian artery. An intraluminal filling defect (*arrow*) is present in the proximal left subclavian artery. **C,** LAO CE-MRA demonstrates an apparently normal aorta. **D,** A long, mobile aortic thrombus (*arrow*) is also present, originating from the proximal descending aorta just distal to the left subclavian artery.

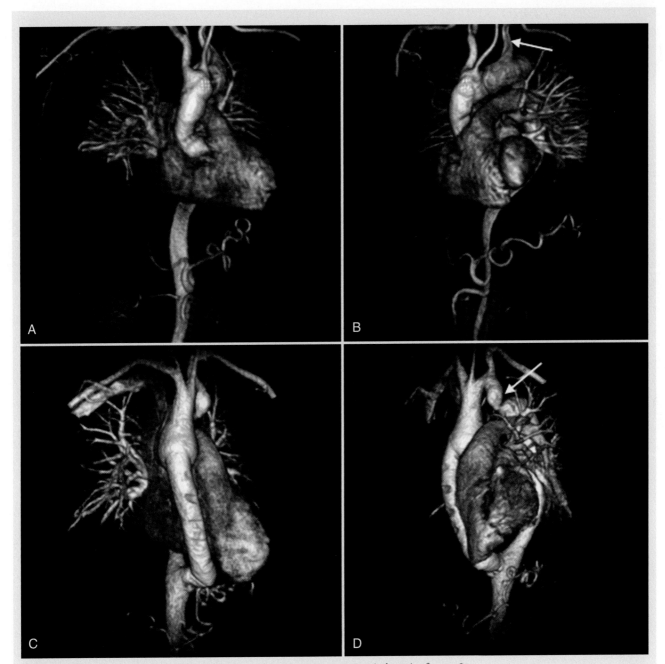

■ **Figure 21-25** Postoperative CE-MRA of two cases of aortic repairs. **A-B,** Surgical repair of a type I aortic dissection. The ascending aorta was repaired by insertion of a short segment of graft material between the sinuses and the proximal arch. The segment of graft is seen between two small areas of aortic constriction of the vessel wall at the site of proximal and distal anastomoses. In Type A dissection, a persistent intimal flap may be seen distal to the graft in up to 75% of cases. Residual dissection (*arrow*) extends up the left subclavian artery. The celiac trunk and SMA originate from the small true lumen. **C-D,** Surgical repair of aortic coarctation. For aortic coarctation, an interposition graft, Dacron patch, or bypass graft can be used. In this example case, the native coarctation (*arrow*) was not repaired. Rather, a graft was fashioned between the ascending aorta and mid descending aorta coursing anterior to the heart.

SUGGESTED READING

Araoz PA, et al: Magnetic resonance findings of collateral circulation are more accurate measures of hemodynamic significance than arm-leg blood pressure gradient after repair of coarctation. J Magn Reson Imaging 2003;17:177-183.

Bogaert J, et al: Follow-up of aortic dissection: contribution of MR angiography for evaluation of the abdominal aorta and its branches. Eur Radiol 1997;7:695-702.

Carr JC, Finn JP: MR imaging of the thoracic aorta. Magn Reson Imaging Clin N Am 2003;11:135-148.

Chan SK, et al: Scan reproducibility of magnetic resonance imaging assessment of aortic atherosclerosis burden. J Cardiovasc Magn Reson 2000;3:331-338.

Choe YH, et al: Takayasu arteritis: diagnosis with MR imaging and MR angiography in acute and chronic active stages. J Magn Reson Imaging 1999;10:751-757.

Didier D, et al: Coarctation of the aorta: pre and postoperative evaluation with MRI and MR angiography; correlation with echocardiography and surgery. Int J Cardiovasc Imaging 2006;22:457-475.

Ganaha F, et al: Prognosis of aortic intramural hematoma with and without penetrating atherosclerotic ulcer: A clinical and radiological analysis. Circulation 2002;106:342-348.

Grist TM. MRA of the abdominal aorta and lower extremities. J Magn Reson Imaging 2000;11:32-43.

Hayashi H, et al: Penetrating atherosclerotic ulcer of the aorta: imaging features and disease concept. Radiographics 2000;20:995-1005.

Ho VB, Corse WR: MR angiography of the abdominal aorta and peripheral vessels. Radiol Clin North Am 2003;41(1):115-144.

Schneider G, Price MR, Meaney JFM, HoVB (eds): Magnetic Resonance Angiography. Milan, Springer, 2005.

Neimatallah MA, Ho VB, Dong Q, et al: Gadolinium-enhanced 3D magnetic resonance angiography of the thoracic vessels. J Magn Reson Imaging 1999;10:758-770.

Nienaber CA, et al: The diagnosis of thoracic aortic dissection by non-invasive imaging procedures. N Engl J Med 1993;328:1-9.

Prince MR, Grist TM, Debatin JF (eds): 3D Contrast Angiography, 3rd Edition. Milan, Springer, 2003.

Prince MR, Narasimham DL, Jacoby WT, et al: Three dimensional gadolinium-enhanced MR angiography of the thoracic aorta. AJR Am J Roentgenol 1996;166:1387-1397.

Rajagopalan S, Prince M: Magnetic resonance angiographic techniques for the diagnosis of arterial disease. Cardiol Clin 2002;20(4):501-512.

Riederer SJ, et al: Three-dimensional contrast-enhanced MR angiography with real-time fluoroscopic triggering: Design specifications and technical reliability in 330 patient studies. Radiology 2000;215:584-593.

Tatli S, et al: MR imaging of aortic and peripheral vascular disease. Radiographics 2003;23:S59-S78.

Vogt FM, Goyen M, Debatin JF, et al: MR angiography of the chest. Radiol Clin North Am 2003;41(1):29-41.

Weber OM, Higgins CB: MR evaluation of cardiovascular physiology in congenital heart disease: Flow and function. J Cardiovasc Magn Reson 2006;8:607-617.

Chapter 22

Renal Arteries

Christopher J. François and Thomas M. Grist

KEY POINTS

- Contrast-enhanced renal MRA is an accurate, noninvasive technique for detecting renal artery stenosis.

- Phase contrast MRA techniques can be used to assess the hemodynamic significance of a stenosis.

- MRA plays an important role in the evaluation of vascular complications following renal transplant.

- Non–contrast-enhanced MRA techniques can be used to noninvasively evaluate the renal vasculature in patients who cannot receive MR contrast agents.

Renal Artery Stenosis

A 65-year-old woman was referred for renal magnetic resonance angiography (MRA) because of suspected renovascular hypertension (Figure 22-1 A-C). In another case, a 52-year-old with acute left flank pain and elevated serum creatinine was referred for contrast enhanced renal MRA (Figure 22-1 D-E). Further, we review the case of an 18-month-old boy presenting with fever and hypertension who was referred for contrast enhanced renal MRA. Work-up confirmed a diagnosis of Takayasu arteritis (Figure 22-1 F). The last case in this section is that of a 76-year-old woman who was referred for CE-MRA with a history of recurrent hypertension following endovascular treatment of left renal artery stenosis with stent (Figure 22-1 G-H).

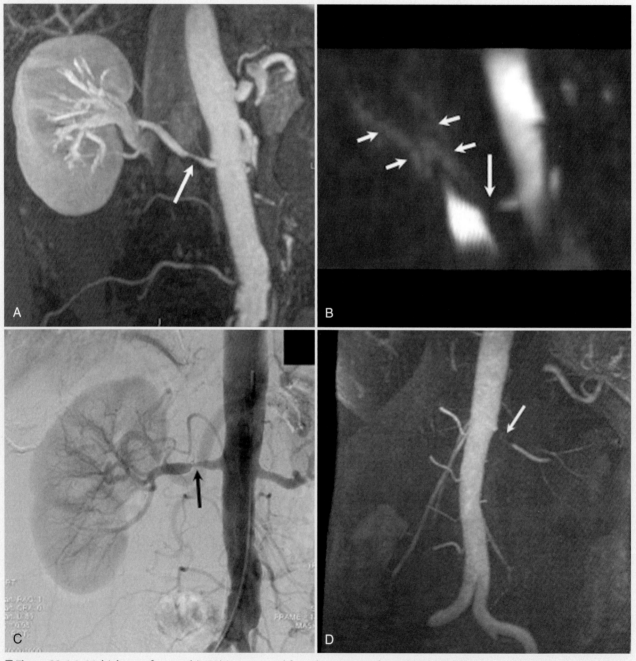

■ **Figure 22-1 A,** Multiplanar reformatted (MPR) image created from the contrast-enhanced (CE) MRA data set reveals a severe (greater than 70%) stenosis in the proximal right renal artery (*arrow*). **B,** MPR image created from the three-dimensional (3D) phase contrast (PC) MRA data set. The image demonstrates signal dropout at the stenosis (*long arrow*) because of aliasing from turbulent, high-velocity flow indicating a hemodynamically significant stenosis. Signal distal to the stenosis is also decreased (*short arrows*) because of decreased flow. **C,** Images from digital subtraction angiography in the same patient confirms a severe (greater than 70%) stenosis in the proximal right renal artery (*arrow*). Pressure measurements confirmed a hemodynamically significant stenosis, which was subsequently stented. **D,** Maximum intensity projection (MIP) image from CE-MRA reveals near occlusive stenosis in the proximal left renal artery (*arrow*).

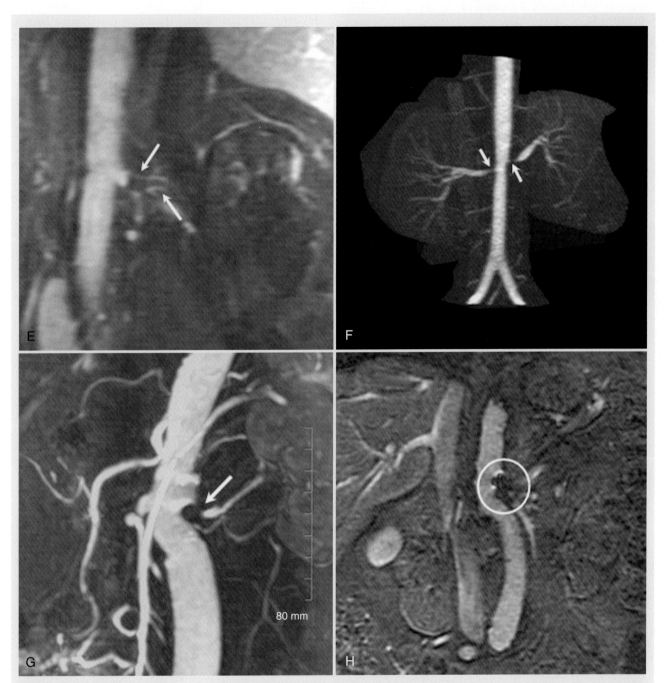

■ **Figure 22-1, cont'd E,** Image from a coronal postcontrast T1-weighted spoiled gradient echo sequence with fat saturation shows a central filling defect (*arrows*) in the left renal artery, extending into the first segmental arteries, consistent with a left renal artery embolus. **F,** MIP image from CE-MRA shows smoothly tapered severe stenosis in the proximal left renal artery and moderate stenosis in the proximal right renal artery (*arrows*). **G,** MIP image from CE-MRA shows an apparent severe stenosis in the proximal left renal artery (*arrows*). The left renal artery distal to this apparent stenosis is well opacified and normal in caliber. **H,** Coronal source image from CE-MRA shows left renal artery stent causing susceptibility artifact (*circle*). The high signal intensity at the margin of the stent is indicative of susceptibility artifact. Renal artery stents have a variable appearance on CMR, depending on their content. For example, nitinol stents have less susceptibility artifact than steel stents.

Comments

MRA is an accurate and safe technique for evaluating the main renal artery for renal artery stenosis. High sensitivities (85% to 100%) and specificities (86% to 100%) have been reported for the detection of hemodynamically significant renal artery stenosis compared with digital subtraction angiography (DSA). Because of the relatively small size of the renal arteries, grading of renal artery stenosis with MRA is typically done using qualitative (normal, mild, moderate, severe, occlusion) descriptors rather than quantitative measures. In addition, the accuracy of CE-MRA is greater for stenoses located in the proximal renal artery, where its diameter is largest, than stenoses located in the mid or distal renal artery branches. Because of the effects of respiratory motion, CE-MRA techniques are generally preferred over time-of-flight and PC techniques. Although CE-MRA accurately depicts the morphology of the renal vasculature, it does not provide physiologic or hemodynamic information. Hemodynamic information can be obtained with the use of PC-MRA techniques or by using dynamic, time-resolved CE-MRA techniques. In patients with renal artery stents, the images must be reviewed with caution because susceptibility artifact from the metal can mislead one into diagnosing a severe stenosis.

Case 2 Renal Artery Fibromuscular Dysplasia

A 32-year-old woman was referred for renal magnetic resonance angiography (MRA) because of suspected renovascular hypertension (Figure 22-2).

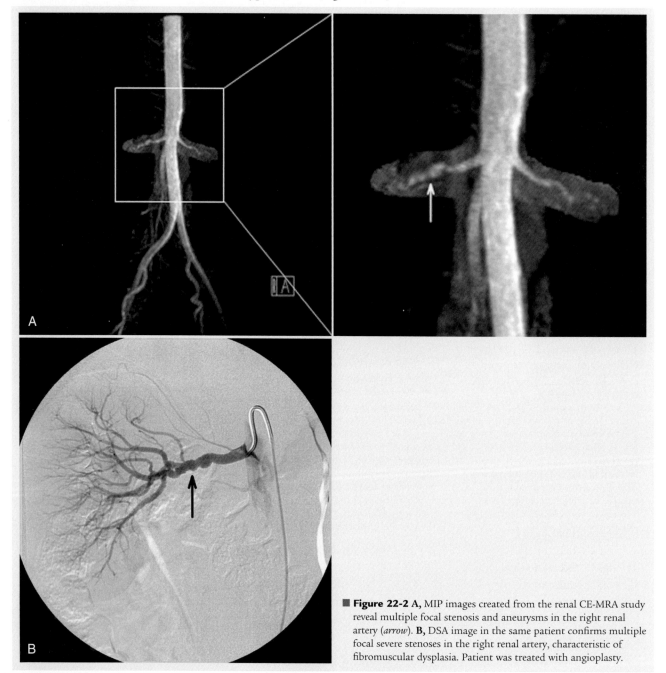

■ **Figure 22-2 A,** MIP images created from the renal CE-MRA study reveal multiple focal stenosis and aneurysms in the right renal artery (*arrow*). **B,** DSA image in the same patient confirms multiple focal severe stenoses in the right renal artery, characteristic of fibromuscular dysplasia. Patient was treated with angioplasty.

Comments

Renal fibromuscular dysplasia (FMD) is typically diagnosed with DSA. The most common form of renal FMD, medial fibromuscular disease, characteristically has a beaded or "string-of-pearls" appearance because of the multiple focal stenoses, without or with aneurysms. Perimedial, medial hyperplasia, and isolated intimal or adventitial forms of FMD are less common and usually present as smoothly tapered stenoses. A limitation of MRA in the diagnosis of renal FMD remains its lower spatial resolution compared with DSA and computer tomography angiography (CTA). However, recently developed three-dimensional (3D) CE-MRA techniques have resulted in improved spatial resolution and, therefore, improved sensitivity and specificity for diagnosing this disease.

Case 3   Renal Artery Aneurysms

A 47-year-old man with hypertension was referred for contrast-enhanced MRA (Figure 22-3 A-B). In another case, a 19-year-old woman with polyarteritis nodosa and hypertension was referred for contrast-enhanced renal MRA (Figure 22-3 C-D).

Comments

Renal artery aneurysms are most often a result of atherosclerotic disease. Other causes of renal artery aneurysms include FMD, polyarteritis nodosa, and neurofibromatosis. Although aneurysms of the main renal arteries and larger aneurysms of the segmental branches are easily detected with CE-MRA, the small aneurysms typically seen in patients with polyarteritis nodosa are less reliably detected with CE-MRA.

Case 4   Transplant Renal Arteries

A 42-year-old man with left iliac fossa renal transplant and hypertension was referred for CE-MRA to detect transplant artery stenosis (Figure 22-4 A). In other cases, a 52-year-old man with a history of right iliac fossa renal transplant and hypertension was referred for CE-MRA to detect transplant artery stenosis (Figure 22-4 B-C), and a 52-year-old woman with left iliac fossa renal transplant and bilateral lower extremity swelling was referred for CE-MRA to detect transplant artery stenosis (Figure 22-4 D).

Comments

Vascular complications following renal transplants—including transplant artery stenosis, arteriovenous fistulas (AVF), pseudoaneurysms, and graft thrombosis—are relatively common, with a reported prevalence of approximately 1% to 23%. The most common of these complications, transplant renal artery stenosis, may be either an early or late complication following transplant and has many different causes. Renal transplant AVF have been reported to occur in up to 18% of patients following percutaneous biopsies. Traditionally, the diagnosis of renovascular complications has been made with color Doppler ultrasound or conventional catheter angiography. MR angiography has emerged as a safer and more accurate noninvasive alternative. In patients with normal renal function, CE-MRA techniques are used to evaluate the transplant vasculature. Alternatively, non–contrast-enhanced (NCE-MRA) techniques can be used to evaluate the transplant vasculature.

Case 5   Non–Contrast-Enhanced (NCE) MRA

A 57-year-old man with cirrhosis was hospitalized with decreasing liver function, increasing ascites, and acutely worsening hypertension and renal function. Because of the higher risk of nephrogenic systemic fibrosis (NSF), NCE-MRA of the renal arteries was requested (Figure 22-5 A-B). Another patient, a 52-year-old man with a history of renal transplant and right serum creatinine and rising blood pressure was referred for MRA to evaluate the transplant renal artery anastomosis (Figure 22-5 C).

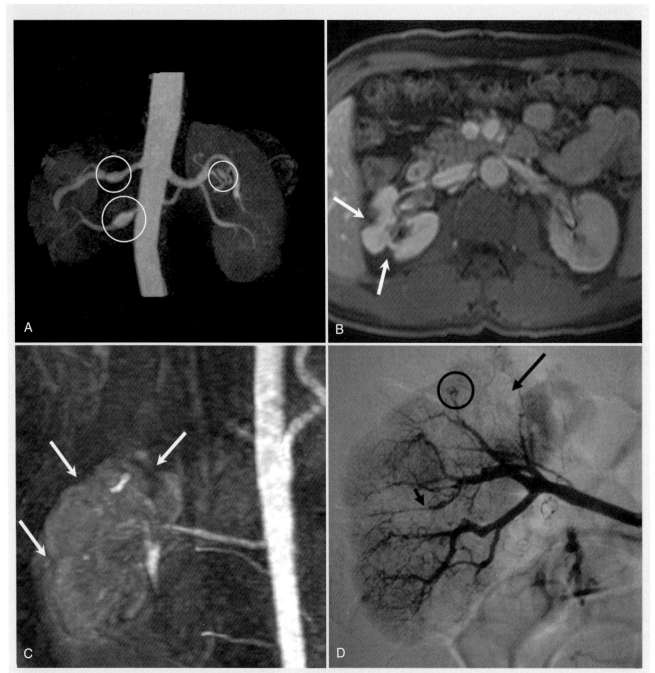

■ **Figure 22-3 A,** MIP image from CE-MRA shows fusiform aneurysms of both right renal arteries and a saccular aneurysm of a segmental branch of the left renal artery (*circles*). The absence of findings suggestive of atherosclerotic disease in the aorta suggests that these aneurysms are related to fibromuscular dysplasia. **B,** Axial postcontrast T1-weighted fast spoiled gradient echo with fat saturation image reveals two wedge-shaped cortical defects in the right kidney (*arrows*), indicating renal infarcts. **C,** MIP image of the right renal artery from CE-MRA does not show any renal artery aneurysms. However, there are several wedge-shaped cortical perfusion defects (*arrows*). **D,** DSA image from a right renal artery injection in the same patient shows several small arcuate artery aneurysms (*circle*), typical of polyarteritis nodosa. In addition, there are areas of hypoperfusion (*long arrow*) and abrupt tapering of the arcuate renal arteries (*short arrow*).

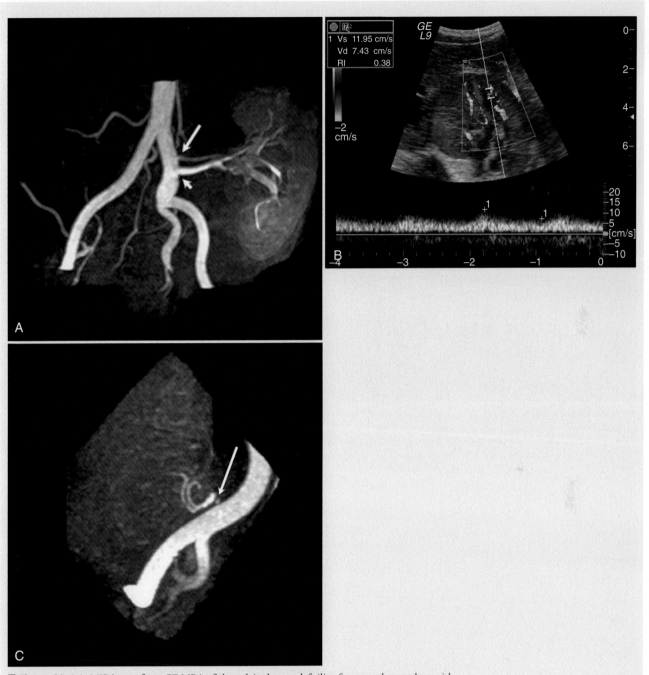

■ **Figure 22-4 A,** MIP image from CE-MRA of the pelvis shows a left iliac fossa renal transplant with normal transplant arteries. Both main (*short arrow*) and accessory (*long arrow*) donor arteries have been transplanted to the left common iliac artery. Both transplant renal artery anastomoses are widely patent. **B,** Duplex ultrasound of an arcuate artery in the mid transplant kidney demonstrates a tardus parvus waveform, suggesting a stenosis in the main transplant renal artery. **C,** MIP image from CE-MRA of the pelvis shows a right iliac fossa renal transplant with a focal severe stenosis (*arrow*) with poststenotic dilatation at the anastomosis of the transplant renal artery and the right external iliac artery.

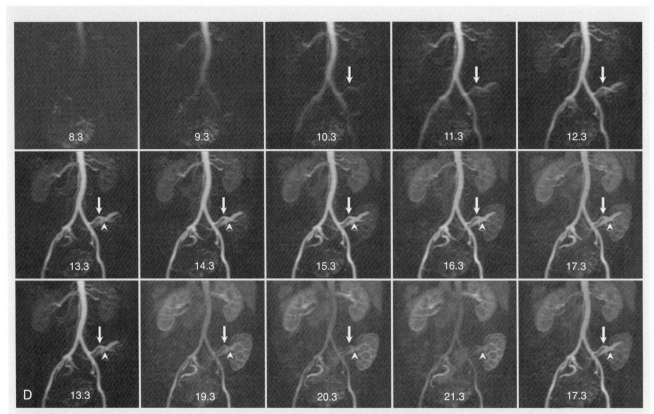

■ **Figure 22-4, cont'd D,** MIP image from a time-resolved CE-MRA study shows a normal transplant renal artery (*arrows*) and very early, abnormal contrast opacification of the transplant renal vein (*arrowheads*), indicative of a transplant renal arteriovenous fistula (AVF). The cause of the AVF is presumably iatrogenic, as a result of prior percutaneous biopsies. The numbers on each of the images correspond to the time frame of the image (in seconds).

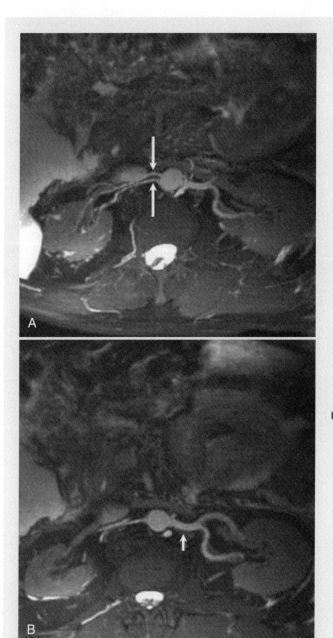

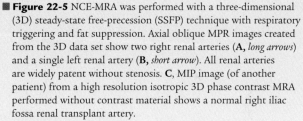

■ **Figure 22-5** NCE-MRA was performed with a three-dimensional (3D) steady-state free-precession (SSFP) technique with respiratory triggering and fat suppression. Axial oblique MPR images created from the 3D data set show two right renal arteries (**A,** *long arrows*) and a single left renal artery (**B,** *short arrow*). All renal arteries are widely patent without stenosis. **C**, MIP image (of another patient) from a high resolution isotropic 3D phase contrast MRA performed without contrast material shows a normal right iliac fossa renal transplant artery.

Comments

Primary indications for NCE-MRA include women who are pregnant and patients at an increased risk of NSF, because of the teratogenic effects of gadolinium and the reported association between gadolinium-based contrast agents and NSF, respectively. A variety of NCE-MRA techniques are available, including time-of-flight (TOF), phase contrast (PC), and balanced steady-state free precession (SSFP) techniques. Respiratory motion limited the utility of traditional TOF and PC techniques for abdominal, including renal, MRA. However, newer, rapid breath-hold SSFP and free-breathing respiratory gated PC and SSFP techniques have been developed and compared with CE-MRA for the evaluation of the renal arteries. Initial results indicate a high sensitivity and specificity for detecting renal artery stenosis $\geq 50\%$ when compared with CE-MRA. In addition, the use of PC-based techniques allow for one to assess the hemodynamic significance of stenoses.

SUGGESTED READING

Browne RF, Riordan EO, Roberts JA, et al: Renal artery aneurysms: diagnosis and surveillance with 3D contrast-enhanced magnetic resonance angiography. Eur Radiol 2004;14:1807-1812.

Chan YL, Leung CB, Yu SC, et al: Comparison of non-breath-hold high resolution gadolinium-enhanced MRA with digital subtraction angiography in the evaluation of allograft renal artery stenosis. Clin Radiol 2001;56:127-132.

Fain SB, King BF, Breen JF, et al: High-Spatial-Resolution Contrast enhanced MR Angiography of the Renal Arteries: A Prospective Comparison with Digital Subtraction Angiography. Radiology 2001;218:481-490.

Herborn CU, Watkins DM, Runge VM, et al: Renal arteries: Comparison of steady-state free precession MR angiography and contrast-enhanced MR angiography. Radiology 2006;239:263-268.

Jain R, Sawhney S: Contrast-enhanced MR angiography (CE-MRA) in the evaluation of vascular complications of renal transplantation. Clin Radiol 2005;60:1171-1181.

Lum DP, Johnson KM, Paul RK, et al: Transstenotic pressure gradients: Measurement in swine—retrospectively ECG-gated 3D phase-contrast MR angiography versus endovascular pressure-sensing guidewires. Radiology 2007;245:751-760.

Maki JH, Wilson GJ, Eubank WB, et al: Navigator-gated MR angiography of the renal arteries: A potential screening tool for renal artery stenosis. AJR Am J Roentgenol 2007;188:W540-W546.

Safian RD, Textor SC: Renal-artery stenosis. N Engl J Med 2001;344:431-442.

Slovut DP, Olin JW: Fibromuscular dysplasia. N Engl J Med 2004;350:1862-1871.

Vasbinder GB, Nelemans PJ, Kessels AG, et al: Diagnostic tests for renal artery stenosis in patients suspected of having renovascular hypertension: A meta-analysis. Ann Intern Med 2001;135:401-411.

Willoteaux S, Faivre-Pierret M, Moranne O, et al: Fibromuscular dysplasia of the main renal arteries: Comparison of contrast-enhanced MR angiography with digital subtraction angiography. Radiology 2006;241:922-929.

Wyttenbach R, Braghetti A, Wyss M, et al: Renal artery assessment with nonenhanced steady-state free precession versus contrast-enhanced MR angiography. Radiology 2007;245:186-195.

Chapter 23

Coronary Arteries and Bypass Grafts

Hajime Sakuma and Yasutaka Ichikawa

KEY POINTS

- Free-breathing 3D coronary MR angiography allows for visualization of all major coronary arteries without administration of contrast medium or radiation exposure to the patient.

- Acquisition of free-breathing whole heart coronary MR angiography requires imaging time of 5 to 20 minutes.

- Whole heart coronary MR angiography permits noninvasive detection of significant coronary artery disease, with a sensitivity of greater than 80% and specificity of greater than 90% in single center studies.

- Coronary MR angiography provides noninvasive detection and size measurement of coronary artery aneurysms in patients with Kawasaki disease.

- Coronary MR angiography is well suited for assessing coronary artery disease in patients with renal failure, because no contrast administration is required.

- Coronary MR angiography is useful in evaluating stenosis of the coronary arterial lumen in patients with heavy coronary calcification.

- 32-channel cardiac coils can provide substantial reduction of imaging time of whole heart coronary MR angiography with higher study success rate.

- High-resolution 3D coronary MRA images can be obtained with 3-Tesla MR imagers if images are acquired after contrast.

- Phase contrast cine MR imaging is useful for the functional assessment of the stenoses in coronary artery bypass grafts.

CORONARY MR ANGIOGRAPHY

Catheter X-ray coronary angiography has been used as the gold standard for identifying significant luminal narrowing of the coronary arteries. However, a considerable number of patients undergoing elective catheter coronary angiography are found to have no significant coronary arterial disease. Consequently there is a strong need for a noninvasive test that can reliably delineate narrowing of the coronary arteries. Contrast enhanced multislice CT is now widely used as a noninvasive method that can provide reliable exclusion of the coronary artery disease. From a patient's point of view, however, coronary MR angiography is more preferable to coronary CT angiography in screening coronary artery disease, because it does not expose the patient to radiation or necessitates a rapid injection of iodinated contrast material.

Noninvasive imaging of the coronary artery with MR angiography is technically challenging, because of small size of the vessel, complex motion caused by cardiac contraction and respiration, and substantially slower data acquisition speed by CMR as compared with multislice CT. In recent years image quality, volume coverage, and acquisition speed of 3D coronary MR angiography were substantially improved, permitting the acquisition of high-quality 3D MR angiograms encompassing the entire coronary arteries within a reasonably short imaging time.

Free-breathing 3D coronary MR angiography acquired with respiratory and electrocardiographic gating is currently the most commonly used MR approach for the assessment of coronary arteries in patients with heart disease. Respiratory gating is achieved by using a navigator echo method that measures the position of the right lung-diaphragm interface by using the MR signal. Electrocardiographic gating is also used to acquire image data during the rest period of the coronary artery in the cardiac cycle. Steady-state free precession sequences permit acquisition of 3D coronary angiograms that encompasses the entire heart with high blood contrast. By using a "whole heart coronary MR angiography" approach, one can visualize all three major coronary arteries without administration of contrast medium or radiation exposure to the patient (Figures 23-1 and 23-2). Imaging time of whole heart coronary MR angiography ranged between 5 to 20 minutes.

Detection of Coronary Artery Disease with MR Angiography

Whole heart coronary MR angiography has been shown to be useful for the detection of significant coronary artery disease, with the sensitivity and specificity similar to those by 16-slice multislice CT in recent studies (Table 23-1, Figures 23-3 and 23-4). Coronary MR angiography may be useful for the diagnosis of:

- Coronary artery anomalies
- Coronary artery aneurysm in patients with Kawasaki disease
- Coronary arterial stenoses in patients with renal failure.
- Coronary arterial stenoses in patients with heavy calcification.
- Screening coronary artery disease in asymptomatic subjects and those with low likelihood of coronary artery disease.

Non–contrast-enhanced coronary MR angiography is well suited for assessing coronary artery disease in patients with renal failure, because no contrast administration is required. Coronary MR angiography is also useful in the visualization of coronary arterial lumen in patients with heavy coronary calcification (Figure 23-5). Coronary MR angiography might be used in screening coronary artery disease in asymptomatic subjects and those with low likelihood of coronary artery disease, because MR does not expose the subjects to ionizing radiation, which is associated with certain risks of radiation induced cancer. Coronary MR angiography provides noninvasive detection and size measurement of coronary artery aneurysms in patients with Kawasaki disease (Figure 23-6).

TABLE 23-1 Sensitivity and Specificity of Whole-Heart Coronary MR Angiography and CT Angiography in Detecting Patients with Significant Coronary Artery Disease

MODALITY	SENSITIVITY	SPECIFICITY	STUDY
Whole-heart coronary	78%	96%	Sakuma H: J Am Coll Cardiol 2006;48:1946.
MR angiography	78%	91%	Jahnke C: Eur Heart J 2005;26:2313.
Multislice CT	76%	95%	16-slice CT (n = 826, metaanalysis) Hamon M: J Am Coll Cardiol 2006;48:1896.
	87%	96%	40–64-slice CT (n = 536, metaanalysis) Hamon M: J Am Coll Cardiol 2006;48:1896.

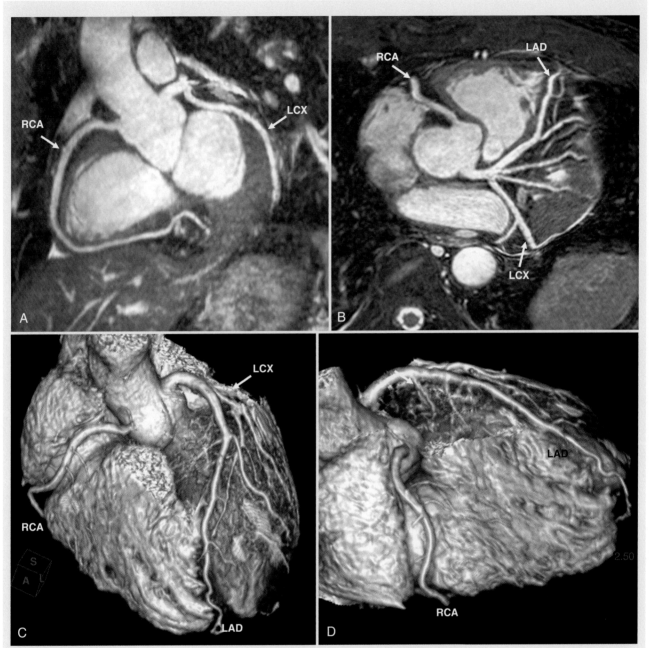

■ **Figure 23-1** Free-breathing, whole heart coronary MR angiography in a 42-year-old man with normal coronary artery. Non–contrast-enhanced three-dimensional MRA images were acquired with a 1.5T MR imager by using a steady-state free precession sequence, navigator echo gating, TR/TE of 4.6/2.3 msec, fat saturation and T2 preparation. **A,** Curved multi-planar reformatted image clearly depicts the right coronary artery (RCA) and left circumflex (LCX) arteries. **B,** Oblique axial curved multi-planar reformatted image visualizes the left main coronary artery, left anterior descending (LAD) artery, and proximal RCA and LCX arteries. Free-breathing, whole heart coronary MR angiography in a 42-year-old man with normal coronary arteries. **C,** Left anterior oblique volume rendered image. **D,** Right lateral volume rendered image. Whole heart coronary MR angiography can provide visualization of major coronary arteries without administration of contrast medium or exposing the subject to ionizing radiation.

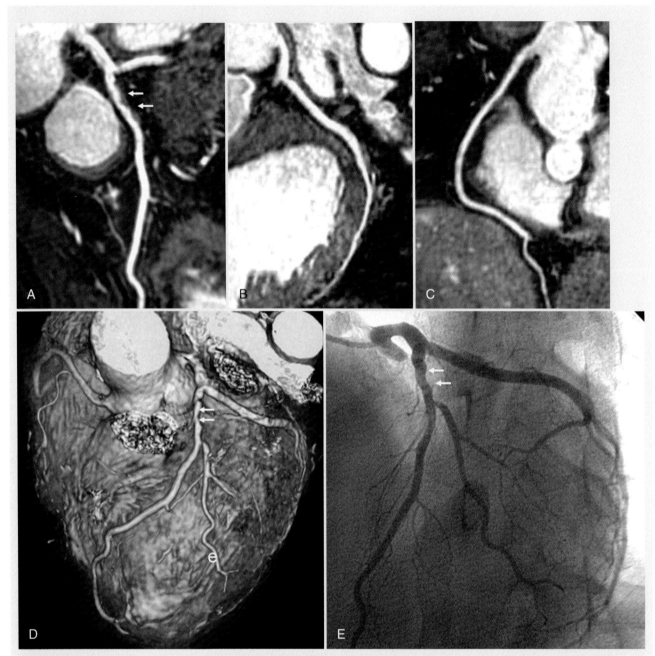

■ **Figure 23-2** Whole heart coronary MR angiograms in a 61-year-old man with suspected coronary artery disease. **A,** Curved multi-planar reformatted (MPR) image of the left anterior descending (LAD) artery. **B,** Curved MPR image of the left circumflex artery (LCX). **C,** Curved MPR image of the right coronary artery (RCA). **D,** Volume rendered image of whole heart coronary MR angiograms. **E,** Catheter coronary angiography. Mild luminal narrowing by atherosclerotic plaque is observed in the proximal part of LAD artery on curved MPR image (**A,** *arrows*) and volume rendered image (**D,** *arrows*). No coronary artery disease was found in LCX (**B**) or RCA (**C**). Catheter coronary angiography (**E**) shows a mild stenosis (less than 50% of the luminal diameter) in the proximal LAD artery.

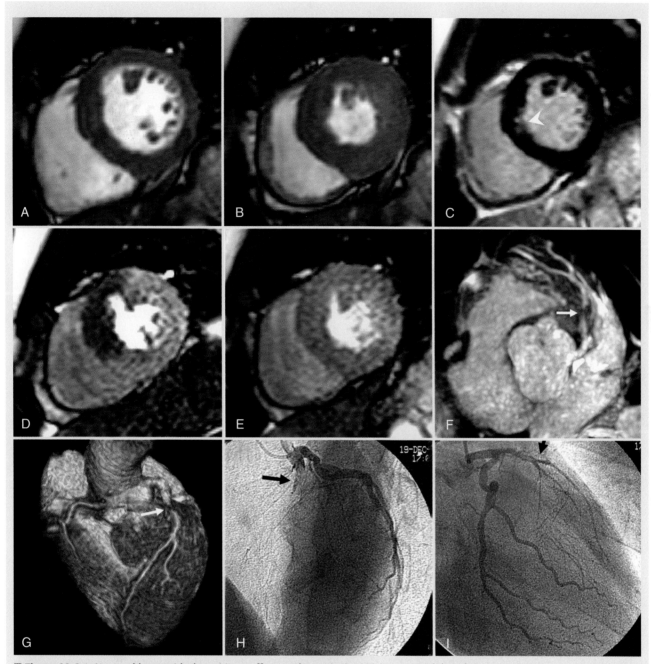

■ **Figure 23-3** A 61-year-old man with chest pain on effort. **A,** Short axis cine MR image at end-diastole.
B, Short axis cine MR images at end-systole. **C,** Late gadolinium enhanced MR image. **D,** Stress
myocardial perfusion CMR. **E,** Rest myocardial perfusion CMR. LV wall motion was normal on cine MR
images (**A, B**). On late gadolinium enhanced CMR, small subendocardial infarction was noted in the
septum (**C,** *arrowhead*). Stress myocardial perfusion CMR revealed severe ischemia in the anteroseptal
wall, which corresponded to the LAD territories (**D**). Rest perfusion CMR was normal (**E**). A 61-year-
old man with chest pain on effort. Free-breathing whole heart coronary MR angiography was acquired
after late gadolinium enhanced CMR. **F,** Thin SLAB maximal intensity projection image of whole heart
coronary MR angiography. **G,** Volume rendered image of whole heart coronary MR angiography.
H, Left anterior oblique view of catheter coronary angiography. **I,** Right anterior oblique view of
catheter coronary angiography. Occlusion or severe stenosis in the proximal LAD artery was indicated
on whole heart coronary MR angiography (**F** and **G,** *white arrows*). Distal part of the LAD artery was
patent on MR angiography. Occlusion of LAD artery was observed on catheter coronary angiogram
(**H, I,** *black arrows*).

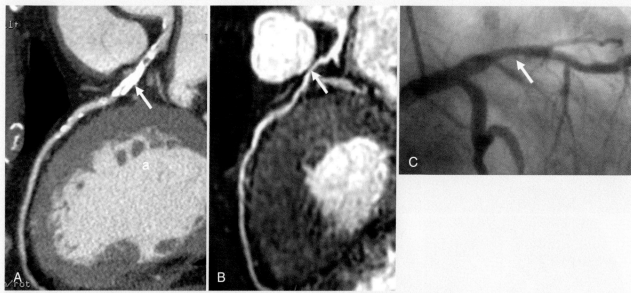

■ **Figure 23-4** A 81-year-old patient with chest pain on effort. **A,** Curved multi-planar reformatted image of whole heart coronary MR angiography revealed diffuse narrowing in the proximal left anterior descending (LAD) artery. Atherosclerotic plaque was also noted along the LAD lumen as an area with intermediate signal intensity (*white arrows*) compared with the epicardial fat on MR angiogram. **B,** Selective coronary angiography demonstrated diffuse narrowing in the proximal LAD artery (*black arrows*).

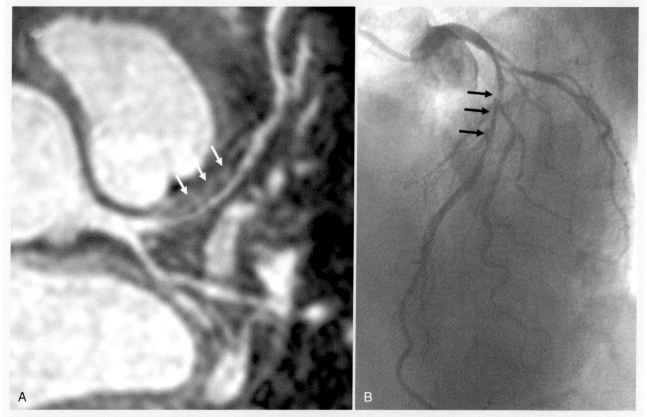

■ **Figure 23-5** A 71-year-old man with chest pain. **A,** Curved multi-planar reformatted image of 64-slice computed tomography (CT) angiography showed heavy calcification of atherosclerotic plaque in the proximal part of left anterior descending (LAD) artery (*arrows*). Lumen of the heavily calcified coronary artery could not be evaluated on CT angiography. Whole heart coronary MR angiography was subsequently performed. **B,** Curved multi-planar reconstruction of whole heart coronary MR angiography showed significant luminal narrowing in the resoximal LAD artery that could not be assessed by multislice CT angiography. **C,** Catheter coronary angiogram confirmed 50% stenosis in the proximal LAD.

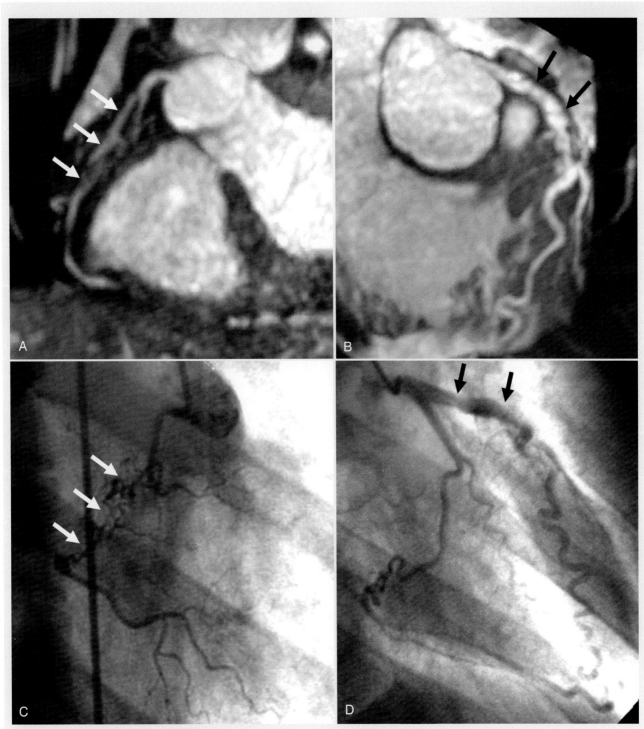

■ **Figure 23-6** A 24-year-old man with a history of Kawasaki disease. **A,** Thin SLAB maximal intensity projection image of the right coronary artery (RCA) reconstructed from whole heart coronary MR angiography showed aneurysm with thrombus (*white arrows*). **B,** Thin SLAB maximal intensity projection image of the left anterior descending (LAD) artery revealed aneurysmal dilatation of LAD artery (*black arrows*). **C,** Catheter coronary angiography of RCA. **D,** Catheter coronary angiography of left coronary artery. RCA was occluded and right ventricular branch of RCA was visualized via small collateral vessels (**C**). Aneurysmal dilatation of LAD artery was observed on catheter coronary angiography (**D,** *black arrows*).

Recent Advances in Coronary MR Angiography

Limitations of the current free-breathing whole heart coronary MR angiography include lengthy imaging time (5 to 20 minutes) and failure of respiratory gated data acquisition in patients who demonstrated an unstable breathing pattern or drift of the diaphragm position during scan. Imaging speed is very important not only to obtain higher patient throughput but also to improve study success rate, as reduced scan time leads to low likelihood of failure in respiratory gated acquisition. Thirty-two-channel cardiac coils permit use of a higher parallel imaging acceleration factor (SENSE factor ≥4) as compared with the acceleration factor by ordinary cardiac coils (SENSE factor 2), which allows for substantial reduction of imaging time of whole heart coronary MR angiography (several minutes to 10 minutes) with higher study success rate (Figure 23-7).

There is an increasing interest in coronary MR imaging using a 3-Tesla MR imager, because signal-to-noise ratio increases approximately linearly with field strength. Because of high radiofrequency power deposition at 3 Tesla that limits maximal flip angle in steady-state free-precession sequence, image quality of non–contrast-enhanced whole heart coronary MRA is not as good as anticipated. However, excellent whole heart coronary MR angiograms can be obtained with a 3-Tesla MR imager, by acquiring 3D coronary MRA images with a Turbo-filed echo sequence following late gadolinium-enhanced CMR (Figures 23-8 and 23-9).

CMR OF CORONARY ARTERY BYPASS GRAFT

The assessment of occlusion and stenosis of coronary artery bypass grafts is required postoperatively in many circumstances. Patency or occlusion of coronary artery bypass graft can be assessed either by using cine MR imaging, contrast-enhanced 3D MR angiography and non–contrast-enhanced whole heart MR angiography (Figure 23-10). In addition to the detection of graft occlusion, noninvasive identification of graft stenoses is important in evaluating patients who present chest pain after bypass graft surgery. Free-breathing 3D MR angiography enables the assessment of vein graft stenoses with a fair diagnostic accuracy. Phase contrast cine MR imaging provides flow quantification in the coronary artery bypass graft, and can be used as a method for functional evaluation of the graft (Figures 23-11 and 23-12). Reduced blood flow volume in the coronary artery bypass graft indicates significant stenosis of the graft conduit or impaired run-off. Comparison between diastolic and systolic flow peaks in blood flow curve in the cardiac cycle is also useful in assessing graft function. In normal coronary arteries and coronary artery bypass grafts without stenosis, diastolic flow peak is typically higher than systolic flow peak, with a diastolic-to-systolic flow ratio of greater than 1.0. However, the diastolic-to-systolic flow ratio is decreased in the coronary artery bypass graft with significant stenosis.

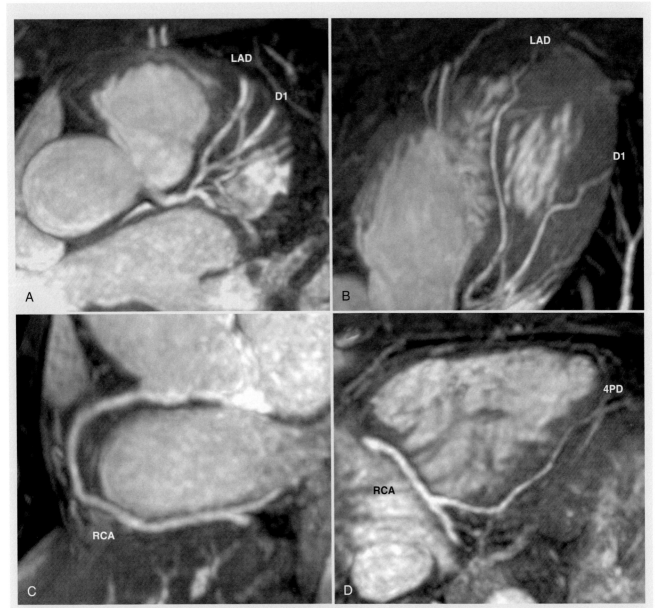

■ **Figure 23-7** Free-breathing whole heart coronary MR angiography acquired with 32-channel cardiac coils and 1.5 Tesla MR imager in a subject with normal coronary artery. **A,** Thin SLAB maximal intensity projection image of left main coronary artery, left anterior descending artery (LAD), and the first diagonal branch (D1). **B,** Thin SLAB maximal intensity projection image of LAD artery and D1. **C,** Thin SLAB maximal intensity projection image of right coronary artery (RCA). **D,** Thin SLAB maximal intensity projection image of distal RCA and posterior descending artery (4PD). High parallel imaging factor (SENSE factor of 4) was employed to reduce imaging time. Acquisition of whole heart coronary MRA was completed within 3 minutes. Distal parts of LAD, D1, and 4PD were well visualized. No significant coronary artery disease was found in this case.

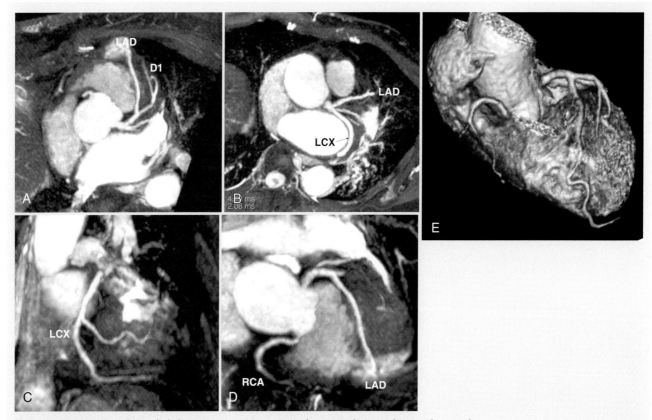

■ **Figure 23-8** Free-breathing whole heart coronary MR angiography at 3 Tesla in a subject with normal coronary artery. **A,** Thin SLAB maximal intensity projection image of left main coronary artery, left anterior descending artery (LAD), and the first diagonal branch (D1). **B,** Thin SLAB maximal intensity projection image of LAD artery and left circumflex artery (LCX). **C,** Thin SLAB maximal intensity projection image of LCX. **D,** Thin SLAB maximal intensity projection image of LAD and right coronary artery (RCA). **E,** Volume rendered images of whole heart coronary MRA. MR angiographic images were acquired with a 3D turbo field-echo (TFE) sequence after obtaining late gadolinium enhanced MR images. Improved signal to noise ratio achieved by 3 Tesla MR imager resulted in excellent visualization of LCX (**B**) and its marginal branch (**C**). Imaging time was approximately 8 minutes by using 6-channel cardiac coils and parallel imaging factor (SENSE) of 2.

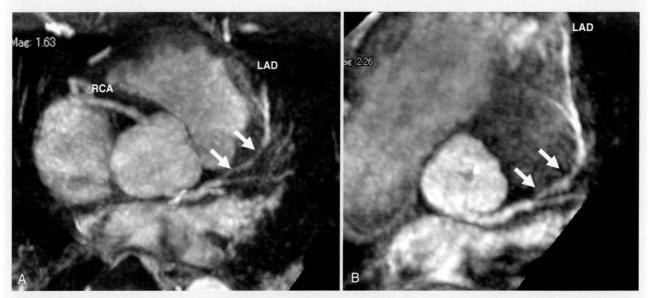

■ **Figure 23-9** A 70-year-old woman with chest pain on effort. Free-breathing whole heart coronary MR angiography were acquired following late–gadolinium-enhanced CMR by using a 3 Tesla MR imager and 6-channel cardiac coils. **A,** Thin SLAB maximal intensity projection image of left main coronary artery, left anterior descending artery (LAD), and right coronary artery (RCA). **B,** Thin SLAB maximal intensity projection image of LAD artery. Stenosis in the proximal LAD was noted on 3 Tesla coronary MR angiogram.

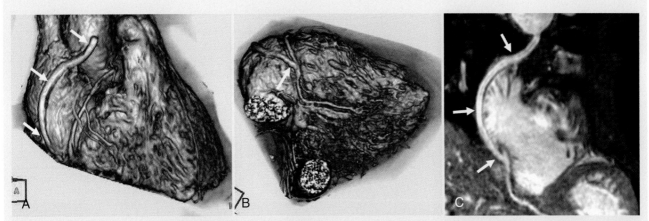

■ **Figure 23-10** Noninvasive visualization of coronary artery bypass graft by whole heart coronary MR angiography in a 58-year-old patient. **A,** Volume rendered image of saphenous vein graft (SVG, *white arrows*) from ascending aorta to the distal part of right coronary artery (RCA). **B,** Volume rendered image of distal anastomosis of the SVG graft to RCA. **C,** Curved multiplanar reformatted image of whole heart coronary MRA clearly demonstrated the SVG graft patency. No stenosis was found at distal anastomosis between SVG graft and distal RCA (**C**).

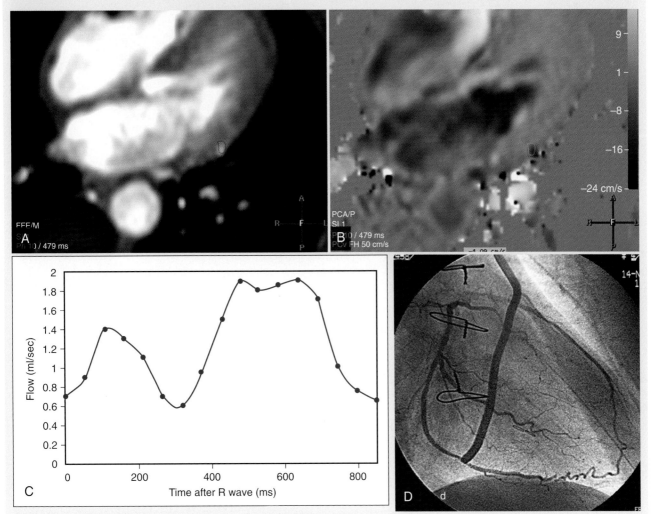

■ **Figure 23-11** A 73-year-old man after coronary artery bypass grafting. Saphenous vein graft (SVG) from ascending aorta was connected to the left circumflex artery (LCX). Phase contrast cine MR images were acquired during a single-breath-hold time by using VENC value of ± 50 cm/sec. **A,** Magnitude image of phase contrast cine CMR. **B,** Phase difference (velocity) image of phase contrast cine CMR. **C,** Time-velocity curve of SVG measured by phase contrast cine CMR. Diastolic peak was higher than systolic peak on flow volume versus time after R-wave curve. Calculated SVG flow volume was 77 ml/min, suggesting sufficient SVG flow. **D,** On selective angiography of SVG graft, no significant stenosis was found in the SVG graft or at distal anastomosis site.

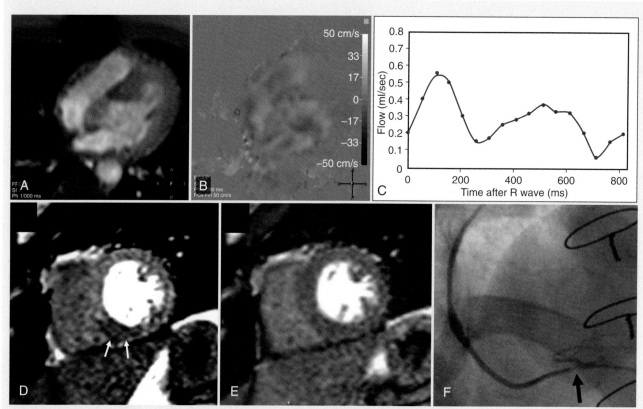

■ **Figure 23-12** A 50-year-old man after coronary artery bypass grafting. Saphenous vein graft (SVG) from ascending aorta was connected to the distal right coronary artery (RCA). Phase contrast cine MR images were acquired during a single-breath-hold time by using VENC value of ± 50 cm/sec. **A,** Magnitude image of phase contrast cine CMR. **B,** Phase difference (velocity) image of phase contrast cine CMR. **C,** Time-velocity curve of SVG measured by phase contrast cine CMR. Diastolic peak was higher than diastolic peak on flow volume versus time after R-wave curve, indicating impaired graft function. Calculated SVG flow volume was 21 ml/min, which confirmed reduced SVG flow. **D,** Stress myocardial perfusion CMR. **E,** Rest myocardial perfusion CMR. Stress myocardial perfusion CMR revealed ischemia in the inferior wall, which corresponded to impaired graft flow to RCA territory (*white arrows*). Rest perfusion CMR was normal (**E**). **F,** Selective angiography of SVG graft demonstrated significant stenosis in the SVG graft near the distal anastomosis site (*black arrow*).

SUGGESTED READING

Coronary MR Angiography Techniques

Jahnke C, Paetsch I, Schnackenburg B, et al: Coronary MR angiography with steady-state free precession: Individually adapted breath-hold technique versus free-breathing technique. Radiology 2004;232:669-676.

Plein S, Jones TR, Ridgway JP, Sivananthan MU: Three-dimensional coronary MR angiography performed with subject-specific cardiac acquisition windows and motion-adapted respiratory gating. Am J Roentgenol 2003;180:505-512.

Sakuma H, Ichikawa Y, Suzawa N, et al: Assessment of coronary arteries with total study time of less than 30 minutes by using whole-heart coronary MR angiography. Radiology 2005;237:316-321.

Spuentrup E, Katoh M, Buecker A, et al: Free-breathing 3D steady-state free precession coronary MR angiography with radial k-space sampling: Comparison with cartesian k-space sampling and cartesian gradient-echo coronary MR angiography—pilot study. Radiology 2004;231:581-586.

Weber OM, Martin AJ, Higgins CB: Whole-heart steady-state free precession coronary artery magnetic resonance angiography. Magn Reson Med 2003;50:1223-1228.

Coronary MR Angiography for Coronary Artery Disease

Jahnke C, Paetsch I, Nehrke K, et al: Rapid and complete coronary arterial tree visualization with magnetic resonance imaging: Feasibility and diagnostic performance. Eur Heart J 2005;26:2313-2319.

Kefer J, Coche E, Legros G, et al: Head-to-head comparison of three-dimensional navigator-gated magnetic resonance imaging and 16-slice computed tomography to detect coronary artery stenosis in patients. J Am Coll Cardiol 2005;46:92-100.

Kim WY, Danias PG, Stuber M, et al: Coronary magnetic resonance angiography for the detection of coronary stenoses. N Eng J Med 2001;345:1863-1869.

Sakuma H, Ichikawa Y, Chino S, et al: Detection of coronary artery stenosis with whole heart coronary magnetic resonance angiography. J Am Coll Cardiol 2006;48:1946-1950.

Coronary MR Angiography in Kawasaki Disease

Greil GF, Stuber M, Botnar RM, et al: Coronary magnetic resonance angiography in adolescents and young adults with Kawasaki disease. Circulation 2002;105:908-911.

Mavrogeni S, Papadopoulos G, Douskou M, et al: Magnetic resonance angiography is equivalent to X-ray coronary angiography for the evaluation of coronary arteries in Kawasaki disease. J Am Coll Cardiol 2004;43:649-652.

Recent advances in Coronary MR Angiography

Gharib AM, Herzka DA, Ustun AO, et al: Coronary MR angiography at 3T during diastole and systole. J Magn Reson Imaging 2007;26:921-926.

Gharib AM, Ho VB, Rosing DR, et al: Coronary artery anomalies and variants: Technical feasibility of assessment with coronary MR angiography at 3 T. Radiology 2008;247:220-227.

Nehrke K, Börnert P, Mazurkewitz P, et al: Free-breathing whole-heart coronary MR angiography on a clinical scanner in four minutes. J Magn Reson Imaging 2006;23:752-756

CMR of Coronary Artery Bypass Graft

Bedaux WL, Hofman MB, Vyt SL, et al: Assessment of coronary artery bypass graft disease using cardiovascular magnetic resonance determination of flow reserve. J Am Coll Cardiol 2002;40:1848-1855.

Ishida N, Sakuma H, Cruz BP, et al: MR flow measurement in the internal mammary artery-to-coronary artery bypass graft: Comparison with graft stenosis at radiographic angiography. Radiology 2001;220:441-447.

Langerak SE, Vliegen HW, de Roos A, et al: Detection of vein graft disease using high-resolution magnetic resonance angiography. Circulation 2002;105:328-333.

Salm LP, Langerak SE, Vliegen HW, et al: Blood flow in coronary artery bypass vein grafts: Volume versus velocity at cardiovascular MR imaging. Radiology 2004;232:915-920.

Chapter 24

Coronary Anomalies

Shahriar Heidary and Michael V. McConnell

KEY POINTS

- Define the most common and clinically significant coronary anomalies.

- Define common types of coronary fistulae.

- Define which coronary anomalies are low versus high risk.

- Outline the advantages of cardiovascular magnetic resonance (CMR) imaging over conventional X-ray angiography.

- Understand treatment options for common coronary anomalies.

Coronary anomalies are a rare group of congenital disorders with an incidence of approximately 0.6 percent of births. These can broadly be defined as anomalies of origin and course, termination, or intrinsic anatomy (Table 24-1). Patients may be asymptomatic or present with angina, palpitations, or exertional syncope. Although most have a benign course, these conditions can cause sudden cardiac death and myocardial infarction—especially in young adults and athletes. Diagnosis is highly dependent on cardiac imaging. Traditionally, X-ray coronary angiography was used to make the diagnosis. Currently CMR has emerged as a noninvasive method for defining the origin of coronary arteries and their three-dimensional proximal course, without radiation exposure or contrast administration. This makes CMR an ideal choice for young adults with suspected coronary anomaly. Treatment highly depends on the type of anomaly. For those associated with an interarterial course and/or myocardial ischemia, surgical correction is warranted.

TABLE 24-1 Types of Coronary Anomalies

Anomalies of origin and course: high risk

    Anomalous location of coronary ostium outside the aortic root (e.g., pulmonary artery, aortic arch)

    Anomalous origin of the coronary ostium from the contralateral coronary sinus

        Interarterial (Preaortic)

            LCA arising from right sinus

            RCA arising from left sinus

Anomalies of origin and course: low risk

    Separate origin of the LAD and LCx

    Anomalous location of the coronary ostium from the proper aortic sinus of Valsalva (e.g., high, low, commissural)

    Anomalous origin of the coronary ostium from the contralateral coronary sinus

        Retro-aortic

            LCA arising from right sinus

            LCA arising from noncoronary sinus

            LCx arising from right sinus

        Prepulmonary

            LCA arising from right sinus

Anomalies of termination

    Coronary fistulae from coronary arteries to:

        Pulmonary Artery or Vein

        Ventricles or Atria

        SVC or Coronary Sinus

Anomalies of intrinsic anatomy

        Coronary ectasia or hypoplasia

        Coronary aneurysms

        Subendocardial course (myocardial bridge)

Adapted from Angelini P: Coronary artery anomalies: An entity in search of an identity. Circulation 2007;115:1296-1305.

ANOMALIES OF ORIGIN AND COURSE: HIGH RISK

Case 1 Left Coronary Artery from the Right Coronary Sinus with an Interarterial Course

A 13-year-old boy presented with exertional syncope. CMR was ordered to assess for coronary anomaly. Based on the high-risk anatomy, the patient underwent successful surgery with reimplantation of the LM to the correct sinus (Figure 24-1).

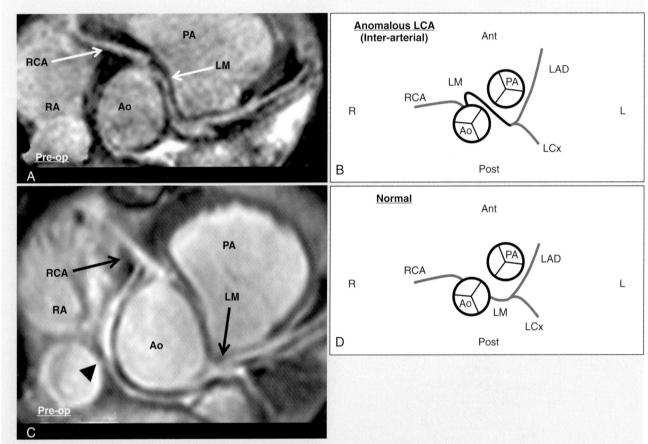

■ **Figure 24-1 A,** Three-dimensional (3D) coronary magnetic resonance angiography (MRA) showing the left main (LM) arising from the right coronary sinus and taking an interarterial (preaortic) course between the aorta (Ao) and the pulmonary artery (PA). A multiplanar reformatting (MPR) method is used to display the 3D MRA image in a single plane. *(Courtesy of G. Greil and R. Botnar.)* **B,** Schematic diagram of the coronary anatomy in panel **A,** showing adjacent origins of the LM and the RCA from the right coronary sinus and the interarterial LM course. **C,** 3D coronary MRA post reimplantation surgery. The LM now arises from the left coronary sinus and follows a normal course. Note the curvilinear structure along the right side of the aorta *(arrowhead)* is postop pericardial fluid. *(Courtesy of G. Greil and R. Botnar.)* **D,** Schematic diagram of normal coronary anatomy, consistent with the patient's postoperative state.

Case 2   Anomalous Left Coronary Artery from the Pulmonary Artery (ALCAPA)

An 18-year-old man presented initially with exertional chest tightness and fatigue while playing basketball. A chest X-ray showed cardiomegaly, and an ECG showed nonspecific ST-T wave abnormalities. A transthoracic echocardiogram revealed moderate LV enlargement, a left ventricle ejection fraction (LVEF) of 35% with global hypokinesis, moderate to severe MR, and severe pulmonary HTN estimated at 100 mm Hg. An exercise myocardial perfusion stress test showed an infarct with severe peri-infarct ischemia in the distal anterior and inferolateral walls at 15 METs of exercise. X-ray coronary angiography revealed an anomalous left coronary artery (LCA) originating from the pulmonary artery (PA) and a large right coronary artery (RCA) providing collaterals to the LCA. He was referred for CMR to better delineate the coronary anomaly and to assess myocardial scar (Figure 24-2). Based on the findings on CMR, he was referred for cardiac surgery where a LIMA graft to the LAD was placed as well as an annuloplasty ring to the mitral valve. His symptoms improved after surgery.

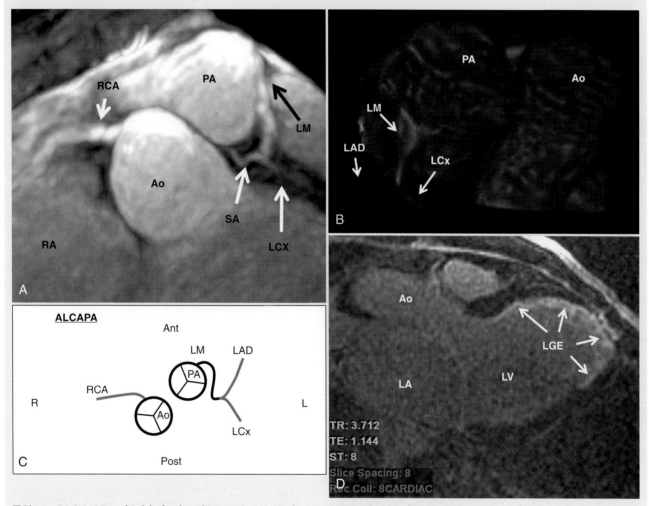

■ **Figure 24-2 A,** 3D multi-slab, free-breathing, navigator-gated coronary MRA showing the LM arising from the PA. The LCX and a small branch toward the SA node are noted in this view, as well as the normal origin of the RCA. Images reformatted as thin maximum intensity projection (MIP). **B,** A volume-rendered 3D coronary MRA image showing the LM arising from the PA and branching into the LAD and LCx. **C,** Schematic diagram of the LM arising from the pulmonary artery. **D,** Postcontrast 3-chamber Inversion Recovery cardiac MR image showing late gadolinium enhancement (LGE) in the LAD territory. The anterior septum and distal posterior wall have subendocardial scar whereas the apex has transmural scar.

ANOMALIES OF ORIGIN AND COURSE: LOW RISK

Case 3 Left Main from Noncoronary Sinus with Retro-Aortic Course

A 21-year-old woman with a past medical history of an aberrant right subclavian artery presented with a nonproductive cough and weight loss for 3 months. A chest X-ray showed a right upper lobe infiltrate suspicious for tuberculosis. After failing standard TB therapy, she was referred for bronchoscopy, which revealed an endobronchial lesion that was later resected. Pathology confirmed an abscess and inflammation secondary to tuberculosis. During the months after her surgery, she continued to have persistent sinus tachycardia, which was associated with intermittent chest pain, palpitations, and dyspnea on exertion. Transthoracic echocardiogram revealed normal RV size and function, normal LV size with moderately reduced LV systolic function, and global hypokinesis. There were no significant valvular abnormalities. She was referred for CMR to further evaluate causes of her cardiomyopathy (Figure 24-3).

Further postcontrast late gadolinium enhancement (LGE) images did not show evidence of scar or fibrosis. This low-risk anomaly was not thought to be causing the patient's symptoms and does not require surgical therapy. She was diagnosed with tachycardia-induced cardiomyopathy and improved with heart failure therapy.

Case 4 Left Main from Right Coronary Sinus with Retro-Aortic Course

A 58-year-old woman with a past medical history of a ventricular septal defect (VSD) and an anomalous LCA presented with intermittent nonexertional chest heaviness over the past year. Her VSD was diagnosed in childhood because she had a murmur, and the anomalous coronary was suspected during a cardiac catheterization while evaluating the VSD. Numerous perfusion scans revealed a normal LV ejection fraction and no evidence of ischemia. She was referred for CMR to determine whether the coronary anomaly was contributing to her symptoms (Figure 24-4).

Because the LCA did not have an interarterial course, it was felt that the patient was not at risk for ischemia from this anomaly. She was diagnosed with atypical chest pain and treated conservatively.

Case 5 Left Coronary Artery from the Right Coronary Sinus with a Prepulmonary Course

A 48-year-old man was hospitalized with chest pain. An ECG showed early repolarization in the precordial leads and 1 mm ST depression inferiorly. X-ray coronary angiography showed an anomalous LM from the right coronary sinus. There was an abrupt termination of the LCx, but as it was a small vessel it was initially managed conservatively. His chest pain resolved over the next 24 hours, but the cardiac enzymes continued to rise despite medical management. He was brought back to the catheterization laboratory and a stent was placed in the LCx. An outpatient CMR was ordered to assess the course of the anomalous LM (Figure 24-5).

The anterior (prepulmonic) course of the LM is a low-risk anomaly and therefore was not intervened on.

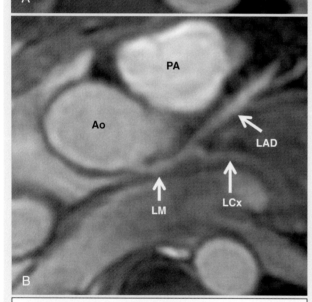

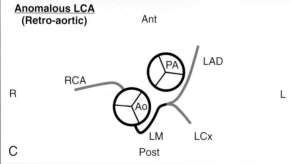

■ **Figure 24-3 A,** 3D multi-slab, free-breathing coronary MRA
depicting the RCA arising from the right sinus and LM arising
from the posterior noncoronary (NC) sinus and coursing
posterior to the Ao [Thin MIP image]. **B,** Additional 3D
coronary MRA image showing the retro-aortic LM bifurcating
into the LAD and LCx. **C,** Schematic diagram of this patient's
low-risk anomalous LM anatomy.

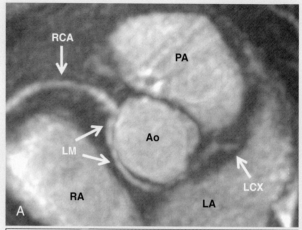

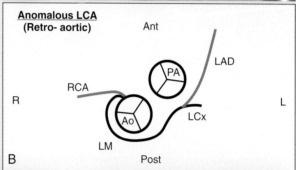

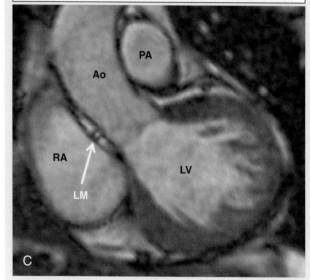

■ **Figure 24-4 A,** 3D coronary MRA showing the LCA arising
from a common origin off the right coronary sinus without
an interarterial course [Thin MIP image]. The long retro-aortic
LM is shown bifurcating into the LAD and LCx. **B,** Schematic
diagram of the coronary anatomy in panel **A. C,** A 2D steady-
state free-precession (SSFP) image further confirmed the retro-
aortic LM (*arrow*) seen in cross-section between the Ao and the
right atrium (RA).

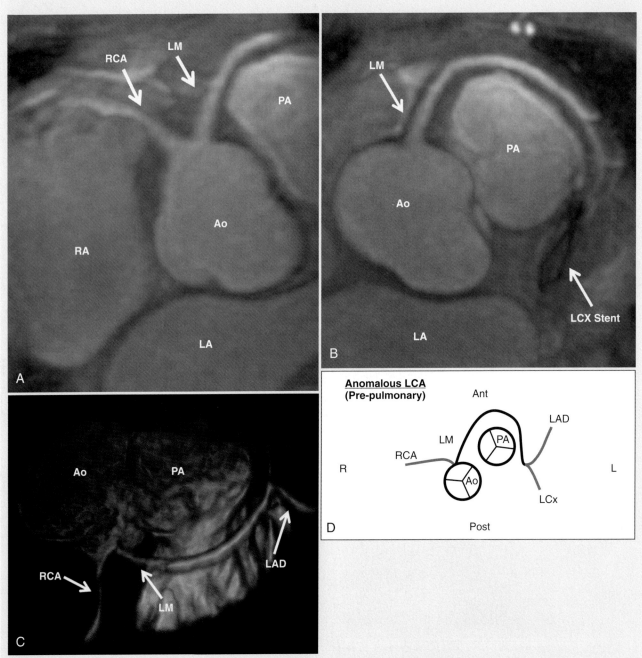

■ **Figure 24-5 A,** 3D coronary MRA showing the patient's LM and RCA arising via separate origins from the right coronary sinus [Thin MIP image]. The proximal LM course is anterior to the PA. **B,** Additional image showing the full prepulmonic course of the anomalous LM, as well as the area of signal loss caused by the LCx stent. **C,** Volume-rendered coronary MRA image showing both the prepulmonic LM and the RCA arising from the right coronary sinus. **D,** Schematic diagram showing this patient's anomalous coronary anatomy.

ANOMALIES OF TERMINATION

Case 6   **Coronary Artery Fistula from the Right Coronary Artery to the Pulmonary Artery**

A 23-year-old man presented with dull chest pain for several months. This nonradiating pain occurred at rest and with exertion, lasting several minutes. He also had mild dyspnea with swimming, as well as occasional palpitations but no syncope. He was referred for CMR to evaluate for a coronary anomaly.

He then underwent a nuclear perfusion scan to evaluate for "coronary steal" from the small fistula, which was negative for ischemia (Figure 24-6). It was therefore determined that the fistula was not the cause of his chest pain and he was treated conservatively.

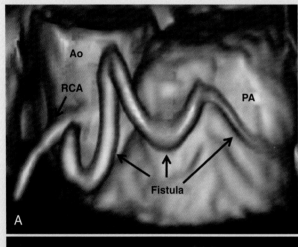

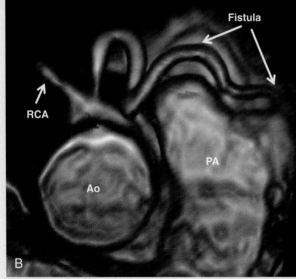

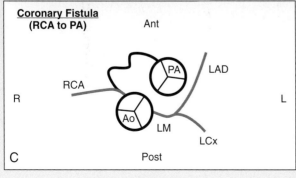

■ **Figure 24-6 A,** Volume-rendered 3D coronary MRA showing the patient's RCA arising from the right coronary sinus of the Ao and giving rise to a fistula coursing anteriorly and connecting to the PA. **B,** Additional volume-rendered image showing the RCA and fistula in relation to the Ao and PA. **C,** Schematic diagram depicting normal origin and course of the RCA and LM but with a fistula connecting the RCA to the PA.

Case 7   Coronary-Cameral Fistula

A 47-year-old man diagnosed in childhood with a congenital arteriovenous fistula. A CMR was obtained to have a new baseline assessment and allow noninvasive follow-up (Figure 24-7).

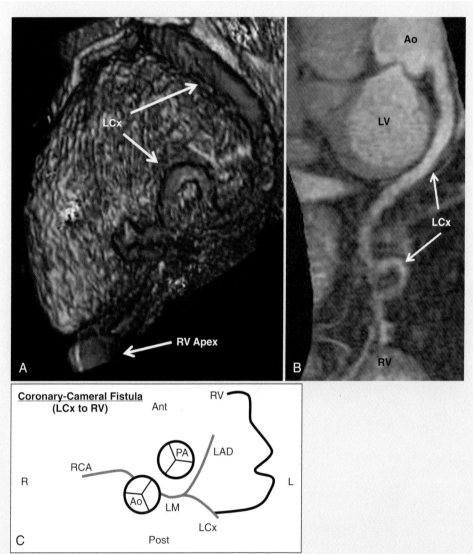

■ **Figure 24-7 A,** Volume-rendered image from a 3D free-breathing, navigator-gated, whole-heart coronary MRA sequence at 3T. There is a dilated and tortuous LCx that communicates distally with the right ventricle at the apex. *(Courtesy of A. Gharib and R. Pettigrew.)* **B,** Curved multi-planar reformatted (MPR) image laying out the tortuous LCx-to-RV fistula. **C,** Schematic diagram of a LCx-to-RV coronary-cameral fistula.

SUMMARY

Coronary anomalies are rare but can cause significant morbidity and mortality. CMR noninvasively and accurately detects anomalies and defines their 3D anatomical course. CMR's lack of invasiveness, ionizing radiation, and contrast administration for this application give it advantages over x-ray or CT angiography. Treatment for high-risk coronary artery anomalies is done to prevent myocardial ischemia or sudden cardiac death. The standard approach is surgical intervention through coronary artery bypass grafting (CABG), reimplantation, or unroofing (marsupialization) of the anomalous coronary vessel.

Coronary artery fistulae can be communications with other vessels (i.e., arteriovenous malformations) or with cardiac chambers (i.e., coronary-cameral fistulae). Both of these anomalies can be congenital or potentially acquired from cardiac procedures (e.g., coronary angiography, CABG, endomyocardial biopsy, cardiac ablation). Most often the fistulae are small and drain into right-sided chambers causing asymptomatic left to right shunts. However, sequelae of larger fistulae can include myocardial ischemia and infarction, congestive heart failure, endocarditis, pulmonary hypertension, aneurysm formation, and rupture. Treatment of these significant fistulae can be achieved through surgical ligation or percutaneous embolization.

SUGGESTED READING

Angelini P: Coronary artery anomalies: An entity in search of an identity. Circulation 2007;115:1296-1305.

Angelini P, Velasco JA, Flamm S: Coronary Anomalies: Incidence, pathophysiology, and clinical relevance. Circulation 2002;105(20):2449-2454.

Angelini P, Walmsley RP, Libreros A, Ott DA: Symptomatic anomalous origination of left coronary artery from the opposite sinus of Valsalva: Clinical presentations, diagnosis, and surgical repair. Tex Heart Inst J 2006;33:171-179.

Cheng T: Prevalence and relevance of coronary anomalies. Cathet Cardiovasc Diagn 1997;42:276-277.

Corrado D, Thiene G, Cocco P, Frescura C: Non-atherosclerotic coronary artery disease and sudden death in young. Br Heart J 1992;68:601-607.

Friedman AH, Fogel MA, Stephens P, et al: Identification, imaging, functional assessment, and management of congenital coronary artery abnormalities in children. Cardiol Young 2007;17(Suppl 2):56-67.

Gharib AM, Ho VB, Rosing DR, et al: Coronary artery anomalies and variants: Technical feasibility of assessment with coronary MR angiography at 3 T. Radiology 2008;247(1):220-227.

Kang WC, Chung WJ, Choi CH, et al: A rare case of anomalous left coronary artery from the pulmonary artery (ALCAPA) presenting congestive heart failure in an adult. Int J Cardiol 2007;115:e63-e67.

Kragel A, Roberts WC: Anomalous origin of either the right or left main coronary artery from the aorta with subsequent coursing between aorta and pulmonary trunk: Analysis of 32 necropsy cases. Am J Cardiol 1988;62:771-777.

Maron B, Shirani J, Poliac LC, et al: Sudden death in young competitive athletes: Clinical, demographic, and pathological profiles. JAMA 1996; 276:3:199-204.

McConnell MV, Ganz P, Selwyn A, et al: Identification of anomalous coronary arteries and their anatomic course by magnetic resonance coronary angiography. Circulation 1995;92(11):3158-3162.

McConnell MV, Stuber M, Manning W: Clinical role of coronary magnetic resonance angiography in the diagnosis of anomalous coronary arteries. J Cardiovasc Magn Reson 2000; 2(3):217-224.

Post J, van Rossum A, Bronzwaer J, et al: Magnetic resonance angiography of anomalous coronary arteries: A new gold standard for delineating the proximal course? Circulation 1995;92(11):3163-3171.

Stuber M, Botnar RM, Danias PG, et al: Double-oblique free-breathing high resolution three-dimensional coronary magnetic resonance angiography. J Am Coll Cardiol 1999;34(2):524-531.

Taylor A, Thorne S, Rubens M, et al: Coronary artery imaging in grown up congenital heart disease: Complementary role of magnetic resonance and x-ray coronary angiography. Circulation 2000; 101(14):1670-1678.

Yamanaka O, Hobbs R: Coronary artery anomalies in 126.595 patients undergoing coronary arteriography. Cathet Cardiov Diagnosis 1990;21:28-40.

Chapter 25

Carotid Atherosclerotic Disease

Chun Yuan, Baocheng Chu, Niranjan Balu, Marina Ferguson, and Thomas S. Hatsukami

KEY POINTS

- Multiple contrast weighted imaging sequences (including bright- and black-blood techniques) are needed for accurate assessment of the luminal surface condition and plaque composition.

- MRI is able to visualize carotid atherosclerosis at different stages and quantify atherosclerotic plaque burden.

- Assessment of luminal narrowing alone may underestimate atherosclerotic plaque burden and the stage of disease.

- Gadolinium contrast enhancement is beneficial for identification and quantification of the fibrous cap, lipid-rich necrotic core, and vessel wall inflammatory status.

- The common carotid artery bifurcation provides an internal fiducial marker for coregistration in serial MRI studies.

- Key plaque features identified by MRI, such as intraplaque hemorrhage and fibrous cap status, are associated with more rapid plaque progression and subsequent ischemic events.

Stroke is a leading cause of long-term disability and is the third most common cause of mortality in many countries. Carotid atherosclerosis is one of the causes of stroke. As a means to prevent cerebrovascular events, carotid endarterectomy has been advocated in patients with high-grade carotid stenosis. However, there is increasing evidence that luminal narrowing may be a poor predictor of carotid plaque vulnerability. The Asymptomatic Carotid Atherosclerosis Study noted that carotid endarterectomy was associated with a reduction in absolute risk for ipsilateral stroke of only 5.9% at 5 years, compared with medical management. If we assume that the projected risk reduction is equally distributed over the course of 5-year follow-up, only one stroke per year would be prevented for every 85 patients undergoing successful endarterectomy.

As such, additional criteria have been sought to better identify patients most at risk of complications from carotid disease. Based on analysis of histologic findings in carotid endarterectomy specimens, fibrous cap rupture, intraplaque hemorrhage, large necrotic cores with thin overlying fibrous caps, plaque neovasculature and inflammatory cell infiltration have been hypothesized to be features of the high-risk, vulnerable plaque.

Although histopathology studies have identified plaque features associated with *prior* ischemic events, it is not possible to determine risk for *future* events based on findings in excised tissue. Until recently progress toward prospectively testing the "vulnerable plaque hypothesis" has been hampered by the inability to accurately and reproducibly identify the crucial plaque features theorized to represent the high-risk lesion in vivo.

Cardiovascular magnetic resonance (CMR) imaging has been extensively validated by multiple investigators as an accurate and reproducible method to characterize human carotid atherosclerosis. Furthermore, CMR is ideally suited for serial studies of plaque progression and regression as it is noninvasive and does not involve ionizing radiation.

The case reports and the list of suggested reading that follow were selected to illustrate this chapter's important points:

Case 1   Assessment of Lumen and Vessel Wall Area

Figure 25-1 shows application of black-blood technique for identification of luminal and outer wall boundaries of carotid arteries.

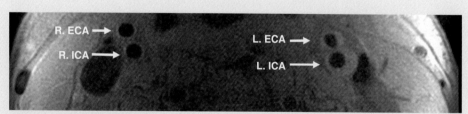

■ **Figure 25-1** Appearance of a diseased left internal carotid artery (ICA) with eccentric plaque on T1-weighted CMR (spatial resolution 0.62 × 0.62 mm, pixel size 0.31 × 0.31 mm). The right carotid artery is normal. Note that the lumen area of the diseased left internal carotid artery is similar to that of the normal right ICA. Thus, measurement of luminal stenosis by conventional angiography would underestimate carotid plaque burden in this individual. The expansion seen in the outer boundary of the left ICA is consistent with the phenomenon of compensatory expansive remodelling, originally described by Glagov. ECA, external carotid artery; ICA, internal carotid artery; R, right; L, left.

Case 2   **Appearance of the Lipid-Rich Necrotic Core**

A 58-year-old man with a history of hypercholesterolemia presented with right upper extremity weakness of four weeks' duration. Duplex ultrasonography discovered a 50% to 79% stenosis in the left internal carotid artery and 1% to 15% stenosis in the right carotid artery. The patient underwent a carotid CMR examination before endarterectomy, which revealed the presence of a large lipid-rich necrotic core in the left carotid artery (Figure 25-2).

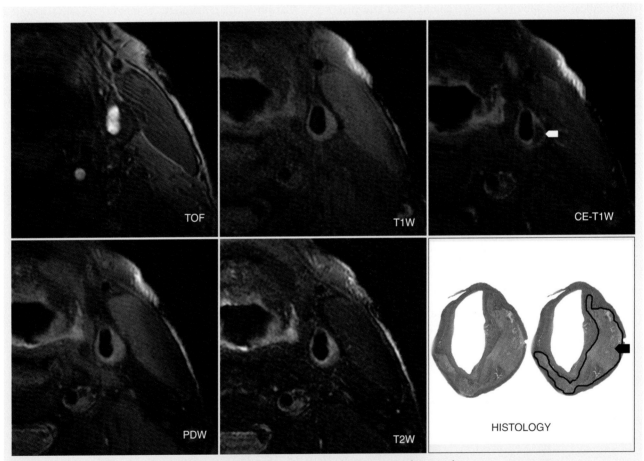

■ **Figure 25-2** Precontrast T1-weighted MR image (T1W) demonstrating a large eccentric plaque in the common carotid artery. Postcontrast T1-weighted image (CE-T1W) demonstrates enhancement of the fibrous cap and less enhancement of the underlying core. The signal pattern (isointense on TOF, iso- to hyperintense on T1W, and less gadolinium-contrast enhancement on CE T1W) is consistent with presence of a lipid-rich necrotic core. The matched histologic cross section confirms the presence and size of the lipid-rich necrotic core. Note that the addition of gadolinium-contrast enhancement facilitates the delineation of the border of the lipid-rich necrotic core. TOF, time-of-flight—bright blood; with the rest all black-blood techniques; T1W, T1-weighted; CE T1W, contrast-enhanced T1-weighted; PDW, proton density-weighted; T2W, T2-weighted.

Case 3   **Identification of the Fibrous Cap and Necrotic Core with Contrast-Enhanced CMR**

A 57-year-old man described multiple episodes consistent with left amaurosis fugax over a period of 5 weeks. Duplex ultrasonography discovered a 80% to 99% left midinternal carotid artery stenosis. A carotid CMR was performed before endarter-ectomy, which showed a large lipid-rich necrotic core in the left common carotid artery. Use of the contrast-enhanced T1-weighted sequence improved the delinea-tion of lipid-rich necrotic core as well as the overlying fibrous cap (Figure 25-3).

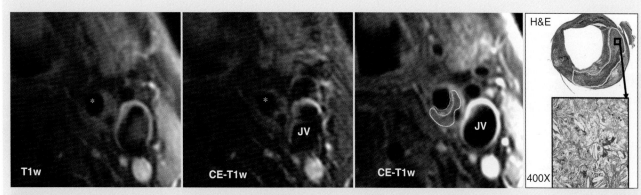

■ **Figure 25-3** Precontrast T1-weighted MR image (T1WI) demonstrating a large eccentric plaque in the common carotid artery (*, lumen of common carotid artery; JV, jugular vein). Postcontrast T1-weighted image (T1WI) demonstrates enhancement of the fibrous cap and less enhancement of the underlying necrotic core. Contours measuring the size of the fibrous cap (*green*) and necrotic core (*yellow*) areas are shown on the Post T1WI on the right. Matched histology from the excised specimen confirmed the corresponding location and size of the fibrous cap (*green*) and necrotic core (*yellow*). The magnified box is a high-power view of the lipid-rich necrotic core containing cholesterol clefts. In a comparison of 108 cross-sectional locations from 21 arteries, quantitative measurements of fibrous cap (FC) length, FC area, and necrotic core (NC) area were collected from matched contrast-enhanced MR images and histology sections. Blinded comparison of corresponding CMR and histology slices showed good correlation for length ($r = 0.73$, $p < 0.001$) and area ($r = 0.80$, $p < 0.001$) of the intact FC. The mean percent necrotic core areas (NC area divided by the wall area) measured by contrast-enhanced CMR and histology were 30.1% and 32.7%, respectively, and were strongly correlated across locations (i = 0.87, $p < 0.001$). *(From Cai J, Hatsukami TS, Ferguson MS, et al: In vivo quantitative measurement of intact fibrous cap and lipid-rich necrotic core size in atherosclerotic carotid plaque: Comparison of high-resolution, contrast-enhanced magnetic resonance imaging and histology. Circulation 2005;112:3437-3444, with permission.)*

Case 4   Intraplaque Hemorrhage

A 69-year-old asymptomatic man with a history of hyperlipidemia, type II diabetes mellitus, and hypertension was seen in follow-up evaluation status post left carotid endarterectomy. A duplex scan discovered an 80% to 99% stenosis in the contralateral, right internal carotid artery. CMR was performed before right carotid endarterectomy and revealed the presence of intraplaque hemorrhage (Figure 25-4).

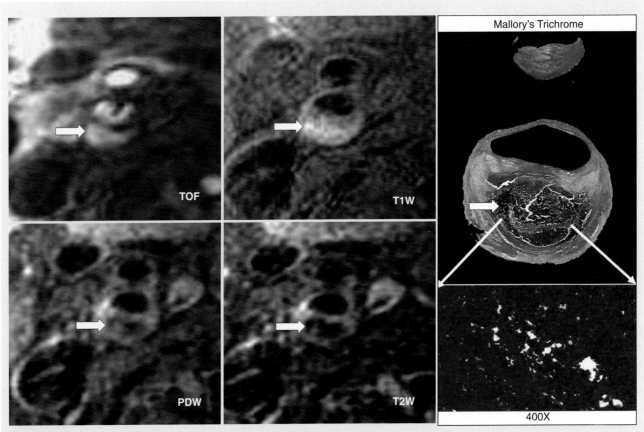

■ **Figure 25-4** High-spatial-resolution, multiple contrast-weighted MRI demonstrates the presence of intraplaque hemorrhage (*arrows*). Intraplaque hemorrhage is identified by the presence of hyperintense signals on TOF and T1W, and variable signal intensities on PDW and T2W, depending on the age of the hemorrhage. Presence of intraplaque hemorrhage was confirmed on the matched histologic cross-section (Mallory's trichrome stain).

Case 5	**Vessel Wall Inflammatory Status: Dynamic Contrast-Enhanced CMR**

As shown in case 3, post–contrast-enhanced T1W imaging demonstrates differential enhancement of plaque tissues in advanced carotid atherosclerosis. Strong enhancement generally suggests the presence of a highly permeable vascular supply and loose extracellular matrix for contrast agent uptake (Figure 25-5). Because neovasculature and increased endothelial permeability are both associated with plaque inflammation, gadolinium enhancement of the vessel wall has been hypothesized to be an indirect marker of vascular wall inflammation. To probe this hypothesis further using quantitative analyses, dynamic contrast-enhanced CMR has been used to measure the actual rate of uptake—characterized by the transfer constant K^{trans}—and compared these measurements to histologic measurements of plaque composition and inflammation. The parameter K^{trans} is well known in oncology, where it has been used to characterize tumor blood supply and permeability. In a recently published study K^{trans} was measured in 27 patients scheduled to undergo carotid endarterectomy. The excised specimens were then histologically analyzed to measure neovasculature and macrophage content. Measurements of K^{trans} correlated significantly with macrophage content ($r = 0.75$, $p < 0.001$) and neovasculature content ($r = 0.71$, $p < 0.001$).

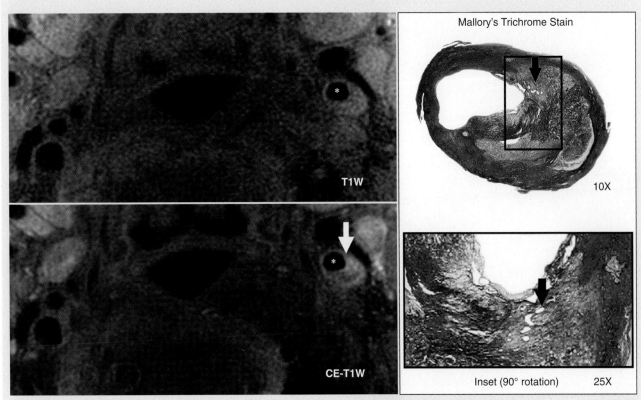

■ **Figure 25-5** Pre- and post–contrast-enhanced CMR sections are on the left. Matched histology shows a region with neovasculature, loose extracellular matrix and macrophage infiltration (*arrow*). Note the enhancement seen on the post–contrast-enhanced CMR (*arrow*) corresponding to the area of neovasculature on histology. The asterisk is located in the common carotid artery lumen. (*From Yuan C, et al. Contrast-enhanced high resolution MRI for atherosclerotic carotid artery tissue characterization. J Magn Reson Imaging 2002;15:62-67, with permission.*)

Case 6   Development of a New Fibrous Cap Rupture and Penetrating Ulcer into Carotid Atherosclerotic Plaque Detected by Serial CMR

Serial carotid CMR scans from a 67-year-old woman who was asymptomatic with regard to her carotid disease but described a history of myocardial infarction on four previous occasions (Figure 25-6). Baseline CMR showed an atherosclerotic plaque with intraplaque hemorrhage in the right internal carotid artery. An intact fibrous cap was present. A follow-up CMR obtained 10 months later identified fibrous cap rupture and an ulcer penetrating into the plaque in the right internal carotid artery. Contrast-enhanced CMR and conventional carotid angiography confirmed the presence of the fibrous cap rupture and ulcer.

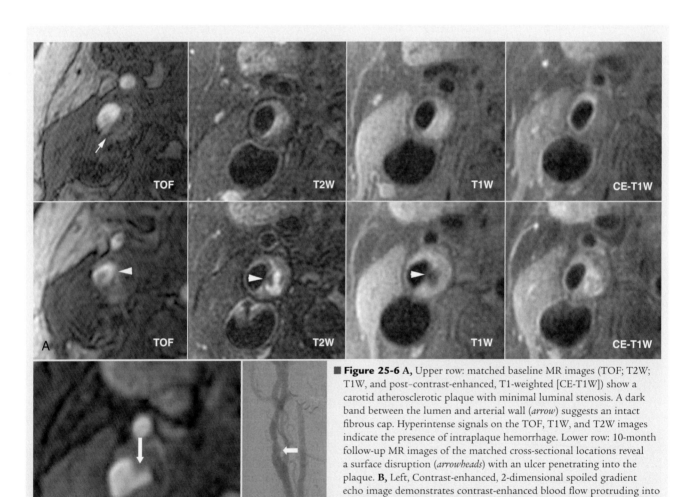

■ **Figure 25-6 A,** Upper row: matched baseline MR images (TOF; T2W; T1W, and post–contrast-enhanced, T1-weighted [CE-T1W]) show a carotid atherosclerotic plaque with minimal luminal stenosis. A dark band between the lumen and arterial wall (*arrow*) suggests an intact fibrous cap. Hyperintense signals on the TOF, T1W, and T2W images indicate the presence of intraplaque hemorrhage. Lower row: 10-month follow-up MR images of the matched cross-sectional locations reveal a surface disruption (*arrowheads*) with an ulcer penetrating into the plaque. **B,** Left, Contrast-enhanced, 2-dimensional spoiled gradient echo image demonstrates contrast-enhanced blood flow protruding into the plaque, suggesting rupture and ulcer (*open arrow*). Right, Carotid angiogram reveals an approximately 5-mm ulcer projecting from the right internal carotid artery (20 mm distal to the bifurcation). This ulcer corresponds in location to the ulceration seen on the MR image. (*From Chu B, Yuan C, Takaya N, et al. Images in cardiovascular medicine. Serial high-spatial-resolution, multi-sequence magnetic resonance imaging studies identify fibrous cap rupture and penetrating ulcer into carotid atherosclerotic plaque. Circulation 2006;113:e660-e661, with permission.*)

| Case 7 | **Carotid Plaque Features Associated with Rapid Progression and Subsequent Ischemic Events** |

Kolodgie and colleagues hypothesized that intraplaque hemorrhage is a potent atherogenic stimulus and results in more rapid increase in necrotic core and plaque size during follow-up. This hypothesis was tested in a case-control study of 29 subjects with 50% to 79% stenosis participating in a prospective natural history study of asymptomatic carotid disease. The volumes of wall, lumen, necrotic core, and intraplaque hemorrhage were measured at baseline and after 18 months. The percent change in wall and lipid-rich necrotic core volume was significantly greater among subjects with intraplaque hemorrhage at baseline, compared with those without hemorrhage (percent change in wall volume 6.8% versus –0.15%, respectively; $p = 0.009$; percent change in lipid-rich necrotic core volume (28.4% versus –5.2%; $p = 0.001$). Lumen volume decreased by 8.5% in the hemorrhage group, and increased by 1.5% in the control group over 18 months ($p = 0.014$) (Figure 25-7A). Furthermore, those with intraplaque hemorrhage at baseline were much more likely to have new plaque hemorrhages at 18 months compared with controls (43% versus 0%; $p = 0.006$). In a prospective CMR study to test the hypothesis that specific carotid plaque features are associated with a higher risk of subsequent ipsilateral transient ischemic attack (TIA) or stroke, 154 participants underwent a baseline carotid CMR examination and were called every 3 months to identify symptoms of new-onset TIA or stroke. Twelve cerebrovascular events that were judged to be carotid-related occurred during a mean follow-up period of 38.2 months. Cox regression analysis demonstrated significant associations between ischemic events and presence of a thin or ruptured fibrous cap (hazard ratio, 17.0; $p < 0.001$), intraplaque hemorrhage (hazard ratio, 5.2; $p = 0.005$), and larger mean necrotic core area (hazard ratio for 10 mm^2 increase, 1.6; $p = 0.01$) in the carotid plaque. Figures 25-7B and 25-7C show Kaplan-Meier survival estimates for ipsilateral event-free-survival among patients with and without intraplaque hemorrhage and thin/ruptured fibrous cap, respectively.

In a recent review of 260 carotid CMR examinations performed in asymptomatic subjects, the prevalence of arteries with intraplaque hemorrhage or fibrous cap rupture was assessed across a range of luminal stenoses. The findings shown in Figure 25-7D indicate that up to a third of subjects with asymptomatic 50% to 79% stenosis have evidence of plaque disruption or intraplaque hemorrhage. Surprisingly, disruption or hemorrhage was noted in approximately 10% of asymptomatic individuals with only 16% to 49% carotid stenosis.

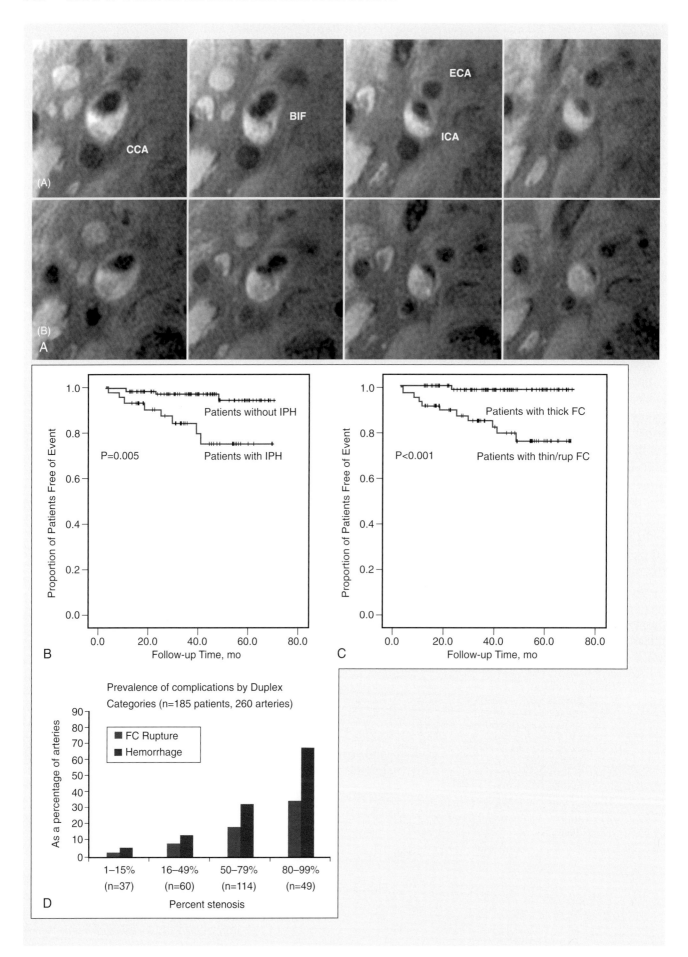

■ **Figure 25-7 A,** T1-weighted images of progression of atherosclerosis associated with intraplaque hemorrhage in the right carotid artery. Each column presents matched cross-sectional locations in carotid artery from baseline CMR (**A**) and CMR obtained 18 months later (**B**). Lumen area was decreased, and wall area was increased in each location on the second examination. CCA, common carotid artery; BIF, common carotid bifurcation; ICA, internal carotid artery; ECA, external carotid artery. *(From Takaya N, Yuan C, Chu B, et al: Presence of intraplaque hemorrhage stimulates progression of carotid atherosclerotic plaques. Circulation 2005;23:2768-2775, with permission).* **B,** Kaplan-Meier survival estimates of the proportion of subjects remaining free of ipsilateral TIA or stroke with (lower curve) and without (upper curve) IPH. IPH, intraplaque hemorrhage. **C,** Kaplan-Meier survival estimates of the proportion of subjects remaining free of ipsilateral TIA or stroke with (lower curve) and without (upper curve) thin/ruptured fibrous cap. FC, fibrous cap. *(From Takaya N, Yuan C, Chu B, et al: Association between carotid plaque characteristics and subsequent ischemic cerebrovascular events: A prospective assessment with MRI-initial results. Stroke 2006;37:818-823, with permission.)* **D,** Prevalence of CMR-identified fibrous cap (FC) rupture and intraplaque hemorrhage by degree of stenosis in carotid plaques (n = 260) of asymptomatic volunteers. The degree of stenosis was determined by duplex ultrasound. *(From Saam T, Underhill HR, Chu B, et al: Prevalence of AHA Type VI carotid atherosclerotic lesions identified by MRI for different levels of stenosis as measured by duplex ultrasound. J Am Coll Cardiol 2008;51:1014-1021, with permission.)*

SUGGESTED READING

Pathology of Carotid Atherosclerosis

Bassiouny HS, Sakaguchi Y, Mikucki SA, et al: Juxtalumenal location of plaque necrosis and neoformation in symptomatic carotid stenosis. J Vasc Surg 1997;26:585-594.

Redgrave JN, Lovett JK, Gallagher PJ, Rothwell PM. Histological assessment of 526 symptomatic carotid plaques in relation to the nature and timing of ischemic symptoms: The Oxford plaque study. Circulation 2006;113:2320-2328.

Virmani R, Burke A, Ladich E, Kolodgie FD. Pathology of carotid artery atherosclerotic disease. In: Gillard J, Graves M, Hatsukami T, Yuan C (eds): Carotid Disease: The Role of Imaging in Diagnosis and Management. Cambridge, Cambridge University Press, 2007, 1-21.

CMR Technique and Validation

Cai J, Hatsukami TS, Ferguson MS, et al: In vivo quantitative measurement of intact fibrous cap and lipid-rich necrotic core size in atherosclerotic carotid plaque: Comparison of high-resolution, contrast-enhanced magnetic resonance imaging and histology. Circulation 2005;112:3437-3444.

Cai J, Hatsukami TS, Ferguson MS, et al: Classification of human carotid atherosclerotic lesions with in vivo multicontrast magnetic resonance imaging. Circulation 2002;106:1368-1373.

Cappendijk VC, Cleutjens KB, Kessels AG, et al: Assessment of human atherosclerotic carotid plaque components with multisequence MR imaging: initial experience. Radiology 2005;234:487-492.

Fayad ZA, Fuster V. Characterization of atherosclerotic plaques by magnetic resonance imaging. Ann N Y Acad Sci 2000;902:173-186.

Kampschulte A, Ferguson MS, Kerwin WS, et al: Differentiation of intraplaque versus juxtaluminal hemorrhage/thrombus in advanced human carotid atherosclerotic lesions by in vivo magnetic resonance imaging. Circulation 2004;110:3239-3244.

Kerwin WS, O'Brien K D, Ferguson MS, et al: Inflammation in carotid atherosclerotic plaque: A dynamic contrast-enhanced MR imaging study. Radiology 2006;241:459-468.

Moody AR, Murphy RE, Morgan PS, et al: Characterization of complicated carotid plaque with magnetic resonance direct thrombus imaging in patients with cerebral ischemia. Circulation 2003;107:3047-3052.

Trivedi RA, U-King-Im JM, et al: MRI-derived measurements of fibrous-cap and lipid-core thickness: The potential for identifying vulnerable carotid plaques in vivo. Neuroradiology 2004;46:738-743.

Wasserman BA, Smith WI, Trout HH 3rd, et al: Carotid artery atherosclerosis: In vivo morphologic characterization with gadolinium-enhanced double-oblique MR imaging initial results. Radiology 2002;223:566-573.

Application of CMR in Prospective Studies

Corti R, Fuster V, Fayad ZA, et al: Effects of aggressive versus conventional lipid-lowering therapy by simvastatin on human atherosclerotic lesions: A prospective, randomized, double-blind trial with high-resolution magnetic resonance imaging. J Am Coll Cardiol 2005;46:106-112.

Saam T, Underhill HR, Chu B, et al: Prevalence of AHA Type VI carotid atherosclerotic lesions identified by MRI for different levels of stenosis as measured by duplex ultrasound. J Am Coll Cardiol 2008;51:1014-1021.

Takaya N, Yuan C, Chu B, et al: Presence of intraplaque hemorrhage stimulates progression of carotid atherosclerotic plaques. Circulation 2005;23:2768-2775.

Takaya N, Yuan C, Chu B, et al: Association between carotid plaque characteristics and subsequent ischemic cerebrovascular events: A prospective assessment with MRI-initial results. Stroke 2006;37:818-823.

Underhill HR, Yuan C, Zhao XQ, et al: Effect of rosuvastatin therapy on carotid plaque morphology and composition in moderately hypercholesterolemic patients: A high-resolution magnetic resonance imaging trial. Am Heart J 2008;155:584.e1-e8.

Wasserman BA, Sharrett AR, Lai S, et al: Risk factor associations with the presence of a lipid core in carotid plaque of asymptomatic individuals using high-resolution MRI: The multi-ethnic study of atherosclerosis (MESA). Stroke 2008;39:329-335.

Wasserman BA, Wityk RJ, Trout HH 3rd, Virmani R. Low-grade carotid stenosis: Looking beyond the lumen with MRI. Stroke 2005;36:2504-2513.

Chapter 26

Plaque and Wall Assessment

Alistair C. Lindsay, Justin M. Lee, Ilias Kylintireas, Matthew D. Robson, and Robin P. Choudhury

KEY POINTS

- Vascular magnetic resonance imaging is noninvasive, does not involve ionizing radiation, and can provide extensive coverage of large arteries with high accuracy and reproducibility.

- As such, it can be used to characterize the composition of atherosclerotic plaques including information on lipid content, fibrous cap integrity, and plaque hemorrhage or thrombosis.

- In addition to providing information on vascular structure, MR imaging is also capable of assessing vascular function as part of an integrated examination.

- Such measurements of vascular function include arterial pulse wave velocity, aortic compliance and distensibility, and flow-mediated dilatation. Good agreement between ultrasound and MR measurements of these parameters has been proven.

- To date vascular magnetic resonance imaging has mainly been used to asses changes in atherosclerotic plaque structure in response to lipid-lowering therapies.

- Potential future clinical applications of this technology are continuing to emerge. Furthermore, MR imaging has the potential to capitalize on molecular techniques that may shed new insights into plaque biology.

The walls of large arteries display a spectrum of structural and functional abnormalities in the context of atherogenesis and are, therefore, an attractive target for investigation of this disease process. Paradoxically, atherosclerotic plaque burden has been estimated conventionally by means of invasive X-ray arteriography of the vessel lumen. More recently both carotid ultrasound and intravascular coronary ultrasound have been used to interrogate the arterial wall directly. However, these methods of plaque and wall imaging are also limited. For instance, ultrasound cannot reliably provide detail on plaque composition and morphology unless used invasively (intravascular ultrasound) and is confined to imaging limited segments of arteries, which are accessible to the imaging probe.

By comparison, MR imaging is noninvasive, does not involve ionizing radiation, and can provide extensive coverage of large arteries with high accuracy and reproducibility. As a result, MR imaging can be used to characterize atherosclerotic plaques in the aorta and the carotid arteries, and to measure the response to therapy at multiple vascular sites. Furthermore, in addition to studying vascular *structure*, MR imaging is capable of assessing vascular *function* as part of an integrated examination.

Even before the development of macroscopic atherosclerotic lesions, loss of normal arterial elasticity can occur and correlates with established cardiovascular risk factors, and even future risk. Therefore noninvasive measures of arterial "stiffness" (Table 26-1) are of potential use in the assessment of cardiovascular disease. To date these have mostly been assessed using peripheral vascular

TABLE 26-1 Definitions of Indices Reflecting Arterial "Stiffness"

TERM	DEFINITION
Compliance	**Absolute** change in vessel area for a given change in pulse pressure.
Distensibility	**Relative** change in a vessel area for a given change in pulse pressure.
Pulse Wave Velocity	**Velocity** of propagation of the physiological pressure pulse wave along an artery.

ultrasound of a superficial artery such as the brachial, but a recent study has demonstrated good agreement between ultrasound and MR measurements of arterial pulse wave velocity (Case 1), compliance and distensibility (Case 2), and flow mediated dilatation (Case 3).

Magnetic resonance imaging is well-suited for serial investigations of both vascular structure and function. These assets have been utilized in studies examining the effect of drug intervention (Case 4). Potential new applications of vascular MR continue to emerge, such as its use for the assessment of carotid plaque in acute stroke (Case 5). Finally, the development of imaging probes to allow imaging of atherosclerosis at molecular, cellular, and functional levels has the potential to revolutionize current assessment of vascular disease (Case 6).

Case 1 **Measurement of Flow in the Aortic Arch (Pulse Wave Velocity)**

Measurement of pulse wave velocity (PWV) between two sites on the arterial tree can give an indication of arterial stiffness (Figure 26-1). As the arterial wall undergoes compositional change, with or without thickening, compliance may be reduced, and the speed of a transmitted arterial pulse wave is increased. This may be accompanied by an increase in systolic blood pressure, pulse pressure widening, and augmentation of late systolic blood pressure. Aortic PWV independently predicts cardiovascular events in the general population, and in patients with diabetes. Furthermore, a reduction in aortic PWV has been linked to a decreased relative risk for all-cause mortality in patients with end-stage renal failure.

Aortic PWV can be estimated by measuring the velocity of the pulse wave transit from the carotid artery to the femoral artery using ultrasound; however, this technique is limited by several technical factors, such as transducer placement and beam angle. Phase-contrast or velocity-encoded MR allows simultaneous quantification of blood volume through accurately defined and reproducible image planes. To avoid artefact, patient motion must be minimized and the slices must not be positioned near large arterial branches.

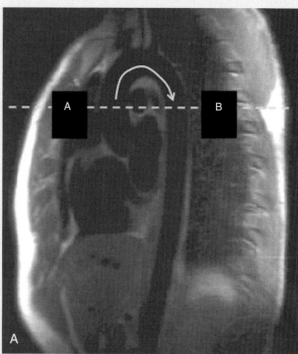

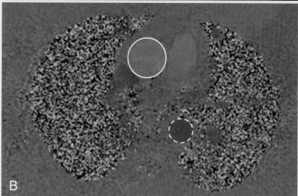

Figure 26-1 A, A sagittal pilot image of the aorta is used to select the transverse plane through the aorta (*dotted line*) at the level of the right pulmonary artery for an ECG-gated spoiled gradient echo sequence with velocity-encoding for phase contrast during free breathing. **B,** Still image of the ascending and proximal descending aorta with velocity encoding. Note that in this example flow in the ascending aorta is bright (*dotted line*), whereas flow in the opposite direction in the descending aorta is dark (*solid line*). **C,** From the phase contrast images a phase velocity map can be constructed and the mean velocity across each vessel area plotted as a function of time (*dotted lines*, below). PWV can then be calculated by dividing the distance between the two levels by the transit time of the flow wave—estimated from the points of maximum change in velocity (acceleration, *solid lines*, below). The distance between the two measurement points is obtained by tracing the centerline of the aortic arch.

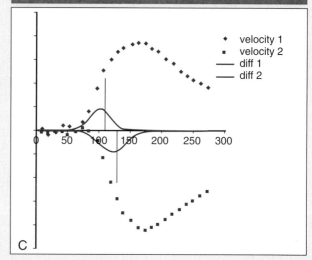

Case 2   Assessment of Arterial Distensibility

Aortic distensibility is defined as the relative change in volume or cross-sectional area for a given change in arterial pressure. The elasticity (and hence the distensibility) of the large arteries is greater proximally because of the higher elastin to collagen ratio in their walls; as a result distensibility is greater in the proximal than the descending aorta. As the elastic fibers of the arteries degenerate with age and in disease, a corresponding increase in arterial stiffness takes place. MR imaging allows careful matching of slice positioning, ensuring that reproducible measurements of aortic distensibility at the same location can be taken (Figure 26-2). Distensibility is reduced in patients with ischemic heart disease and hypertension, and is most accurately calculated when used with central, rather than peripheral, blood pressure measurements. MR imaging can be used to estimate aortic, carotid, and peripheral vascular distensibility noninvasively and with superior reproducibility to ultrasound. Furthermore, in patients with newly diagnosed coronary artery disease initiation of medical therapy, including a statin has been associated with a marked early improvement in aortic distensibility.

Case 3   Measurement of Flow-Mediated Dilatation

Distinct from changes in vessel elasticity (above), a decline in *endothelial function* may also occur long before the appearance of structural atherosclerotic disease. Previously measured invasively, more recently ultrasonographic methods measuring flow mediated dilatation (FMD) have been used to analyze the reactivity of superficial, medium-sized arteries (Figure 26-3). In a typical protocol, the brachial artery is scanned dynamically in three conditions: (1) at baseline; (2) endothelial-dependent vasodilatation during reactive hyperemia induced by suprasystolic pressure inflation of a blood pressure cuff for five minutes distally, on the forearm; and (3) after administration of sublingual nitroglycerin (GTN), which causes maximal (endothelium-independent) vasodilatation. In each state, the diameter of the artery is measured at peak dilatation, and expressed as the percentage change from baseline. In this way FMD has demonstrated a strong link between vascular risk factors and endothelial function in both adults and children. Using magnetic resonance imaging of the brachial artery with measurement of FMD, Wiesmann et al. demonstrated impaired endothelial dysfunction in smokers compared with nonsmoking controls. Similarly, an improvement in endothelial function has been shown in response to low-dose folate supplementation.

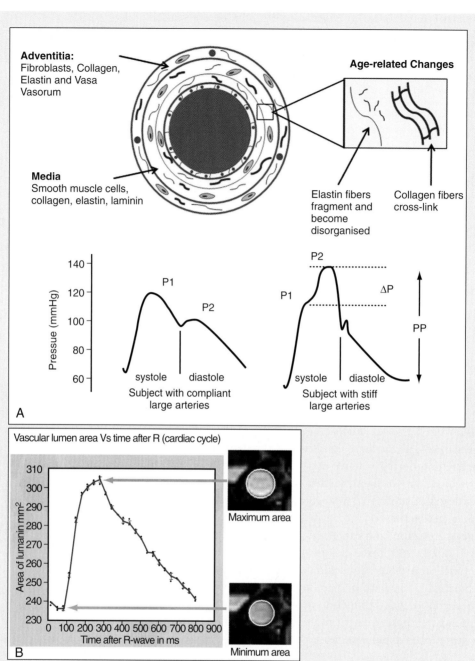

Adventitia:
Fibroblasts, Collagen, Elastin and Vasa Vasorum

Age-related Changes

Media
Smooth muscle cells, collagen, elastin, laminin

Elastin fibers fragment and become disorganised

Collagen fibers cross-link

P1

P2

P2

P1

ΔP

PP

systole   diastole
Subject with compliant large arteries

systole   diastole
Subject with stiff large arteries

Pressue (mmHg)

A

Vascular lumen area Vs time after R (cardiac cycle)

Area of lumanin mm²

Time after R-wave in ms

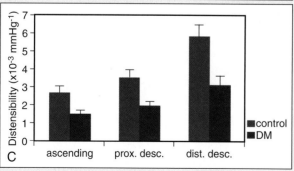

Maximum area

Minimum area

B

Distensibility (x10⁻³ mmHg⁻¹)

ascending   prox. desc.   dist. desc.

■control
■DM

C

■ **Figure 26-2 A,** (Top) Structure of the arterial wall. With aging (inset) the elastic lamellae of the media undergo fragmentation and thinning, accompanied by the increasing deposition and cross-linking of collagen, which is 100 to 1000 times stiffer than elastin. *(Adapted from Adams JC: Molecular organization of cell-matrix contacts: Essential multiprotein assemblies in cell and tissue function. Expert Rev Mol Med 2002;4:1-24, with permission.)* (Bottom) Pulse pressure amplification in a young healthy subject with compliant arteries (left), when compared with a more elderly patient with "stiffer" arteries. Reflected pressure waves (P2) arrive back earlier as the arteries stiffen, leading to an augmentation of systolic blood pressure and a drop in diastolic blood pressure. *(Adapted from Oliver JJ, Webb DJ: Noninvasive assessment of arterial stiffness and risk of atherosclerotic events. Arterioscler Thromb Vasc Biol 2003;23:554-566, with permission.)* **B,** Images of the ascending aorta during diastole and systole. After slice selection from initial sagittal pilot images, ECG-gated steady-state free-precession (SSFP) cine acquisitions of the aorta are taken during breath-hold in both the planes shown above. From these images, maximum and minimum aortic cross-sectional areas over the cardiac cycle are determined using semi-automated edge detection software. Distensibility is then calculated by the dividing the relative change in vessel area by the pulse pressure. **C,** Using the techniques outlined above, lower aortic distensibility has been demonstrated in all of (1) ascending, (2) proximal descending, and (3) distal descending aorta in diabetic patients compared with matched controls. *(Adapted from Lee JM, Shirodaria C, Jackson CE, et al: Multi-modal magnetic resonance imaging quantifies atherosclerosis and vascular dysfunction in patients with type 2 diabetes mellitus. Diab Vasc Dis Res 2007;4:44-48, with permission.)*

Case 4   **Assessment of the Vascular Response to Statin Therapy**

Treatment with HMG CoA reductase inhibitors (statins) has been shown to reduce cardiovascular events by 25% to 30%. Although reductions in clinical events have been shown as little as four weeks after initiation of treatment, conventional imaging modalities, such as carotid ultrasound intima media thickness (CIMT) and intravascular ultrasound (IVUS) have previously been used to examine the effect of a drug on atherosclerotic disease only after much longer periods of time. The early clinical benefits of statins may not reflect purely structural changes in arteries but may also be caused by the pleiotropic effects of the drugs including its effect on improving endothelial function. As described previously, MR imaging can provide insights into some of these parameters through multimodal assessment of the response to statin therapy (Figure 26-4).

Corti et al. were among the first to demonstrate a reduction in carotid and aortic atherosclerosis using serial MR imaging after 12 months of statin treatment. Subsequently the same group demonstrated that more intensive lipid lowering, to LDL-cholesterol less than 100 mg/dl, was associated with a larger decrease in plaque size also over 12 months. More recently, Lee et al. used MR imaging to demonstrate, in the carotid arteries and aorta, reduction in the plaque index (normalized vessel wall area) as early as 3 months after statin initiation. Within the same patients, early changes in atherosclerosis (3 months) were significantly correlated with later change at 12 months.

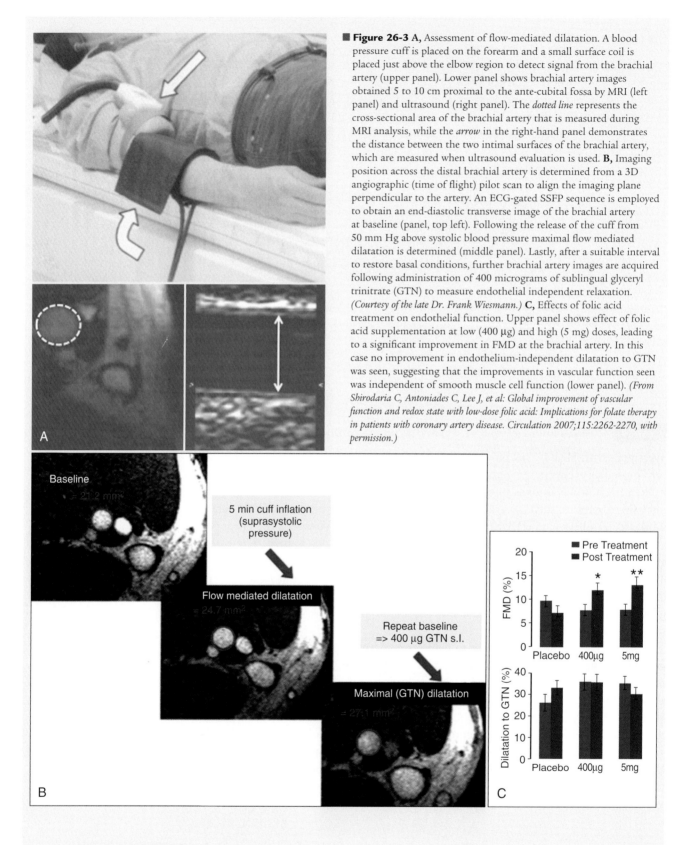

■ **Figure 26-3 A,** Assessment of flow-mediated dilatation. A blood pressure cuff is placed on the forearm and a small surface coil is placed just above the elbow region to detect signal from the brachial artery (upper panel). Lower panel shows brachial artery images obtained 5 to 10 cm proximal to the ante-cubital fossa by MRI (left panel) and ultrasound (right panel). The *dotted line* represents the cross-sectional area of the brachial artery that is measured during MRI analysis, while the *arrow* in the right-hand panel demonstrates the distance between the two intimal surfaces of the brachial artery, which are measured when ultrasound evaluation is used. **B,** Imaging position across the distal brachial artery is determined from a 3D angiographic (time of flight) pilot scan to align the imaging plane perpendicular to the artery. An ECG-gated SSFP sequence is employed to obtain an end-diastolic transverse image of the brachial artery at baseline (panel, top left). Following the release of the cuff from 50 mm Hg above systolic blood pressure maximal flow mediated dilatation is determined (middle panel). Lastly, after a suitable interval to restore basal conditions, further brachial artery images are acquired following administration of 400 micrograms of sublingual glyceryl trinitrate (GTN) to measure endothelial independent relaxation. *(Courtesy of the late Dr. Frank Wiesmann.)* **C,** Effects of folic acid treatment on endothelial function. Upper panel shows effect of folic acid supplementation at low (400 µg) and high (5 mg) doses, leading to a significant improvement in FMD at the brachial artery. In this case no improvement in endothelium-independent dilatation to GTN was seen, suggesting that the improvements in vascular function seen was independent of smooth muscle cell function (lower panel). *(From Shirodaria C, Antoniades C, Lee J, et al: Global improvement of vascular function and redox state with low-dose folic acid: Implications for folate therapy in patients with coronary artery disease. Circulation 2007;115:2262-2270, with permission.)*

Case 5   Stroke

Following a minor stroke or transient ischemic attack (TIA), there is a substantial risk of further stroke, which is especially high early after the initial event. This risk is especially high where a TIA or minor stroke is caused by carotid artery disease (approximately 40% of cases). Although the degree of carotid arterial stenosis and the presence of ulceration, as identified by contrast X-ray arteriography, can to some extent predict which patients are at high risk, angiographic techniques are fundamentally limited in their ability to assess plaque composition and micro-anatomy. Therefore improved imaging methods are required to optimize risk stratification poststroke. Using MR imaging contrast generated by T1-weighted, T2-weighted, and proton-density weighted images with or without gadolinium enhancement, it is possible to determine plaque anatomy, composition, and the integrity of the fibrous cap (Figure 26-5). As a result, potential new imaging targets can be investigated including the integrity of the fibrous cap and the presence of plaque hemorrhage or thrombosis.

For the former, Hatsukami et al. used high-resolution MR imaging with a 3D time-of-flight (TOF) protocol to distinguish intact, thick fibrous cap, from thin, and ruptured, cap. Subsequently, Yuan et al. and Wassermann et al. used gadolinium-based, contrast-enhanced MR imaging (CEMRI) to distinguish fibrous cap from necrotic core on T1-weighted images—the former enhancing approximately three times as much after contrast injection. Although MR imaging is also capable of distinguishing intraplaque hemorrhage from juxtaluminal thrombosis, the correlation between these findings and clinical symptoms is less well defined. Detailed plaque imaging, when combined with angiographic technique and diffusion-weighted imaging (DWI) of the brain, may allow MR imaging to characterize the pathophysiology of stroke, noninvasively. Although not yet validated in clinical trials, magnetic resonance vascular imaging is likely to be increasingly used in the acute setting.

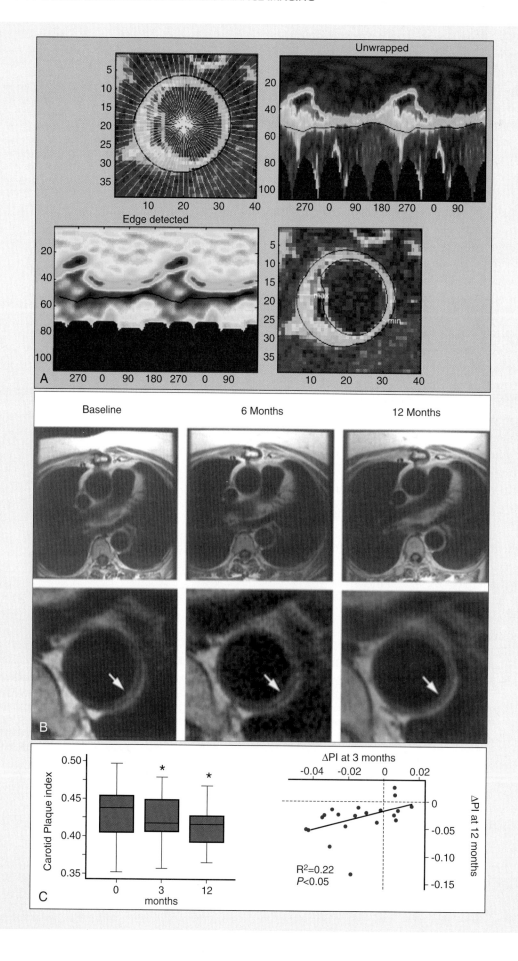

■ **Figure 26-4 A,** Serial time point studies in which images are obtained at multiple levels in a number of arteries generates large data sets. For image segmentation, we and others have developed semi-automated software that uses arterial images imported into a mathematical analysis package. In the example given here, the *difference* in signal between adjoining voxels is then translated into a color-coded image to allow objective definition of the vessel wall boundaries. Outer (top left and right) and inner (bottom left) wall boundaries are first manually defined on these images. From this accurate wall area and plaque volume can be measured, and the outlines or "masks" can be stored for future analysis and comparison (bottom right). **B,** Serial T2-weighted images of a patient treated with simvastatin for 1 year, showing the descending aorta at baseline (before treatment), 6 months, and 12 months follow-up. Upper panel shows mediastinal images with coronary blood vessel pattern confirming precise matching. Close-up of the ascending aorta (lower panel) indicates maximal atherosclerotic plaque size. *(Adapted from Corti R, Fayad ZA, Fuster V, et al: Effects of lipid-lowering by simvastatin on human atherosclerotic lesions: A longitudinal study by high-resolution, noninvasive magnetic resonance imaging. Circulation 2001;104:249-252, with permission.)* **C,** Graph demonstrating reduction in aortic wall (plaque) area in response to statin treatment, here normalized to vessel area and expressed as plaque index (left). Significant reductions are observed between baseline and 3 months and 12 months treatment. Scatter plot demonstrates that change in plaque index at three months was significantly correlated to the change measured at 12 months (Right). *(Adapted from Lee JM, Wiesmann F, Shirodaria C, et al: Early changes in arterial structure and function following statin initiation: Quantification by magnetic resonance imaging. Atherosclerosis 2008;197:951-958, with permission.)*

Case 6 **Molecular and Cellular Imaging of the Vessel Wall**

Features that may predict erosion or rupture of an atherosclerotic plaque leading to thrombotic complications may include the presence of a thin fibrous cap overlying a large necrotic lipid core, an abundance of inflammatory cells such as macrophages, and the presence of intraplaque or juxtaluminal thrombosis. The ability to identify any or all of these components could be of great clinical utility in diagnosing the vulnerable or high-risk plaque.

To date MR imaging agents have principally been based on either superparamagnetic particles of iron oxide (SPIO) or paramagnetic gadolinium chelates. SPIO induce areas of signal loss on T2*-weighted MR images. Both human and animal studies of atherosclerosis have shown that these particles are taken up by macrophages in inflamed plaques (Figure 26-6). Ultrasmall particles of iron oxide (USPIO) reduced average signal by 24% in a study of human subjects with significant carotid disease who underwent carotid endarterectomy. Gadolinium is a less effective relaxation enhancer and must be delivered at higher concentrations to get sufficient contrast. For this reason, it is loaded into larger-sized particles such as immunomicelles or perfluorocarbon nanoparticles, and such agents have been used to image thrombosis, angiogenesis, and plaque macrophages in vivo.

Contrast agents such as these have begun to describe a new field of molecular and cellular MR imaging that allows characterization of the vessel wall. In the future these technologies aim to supersede our reliance on contrast lumenography as the predominant method of atherosclerotic disease assessment.

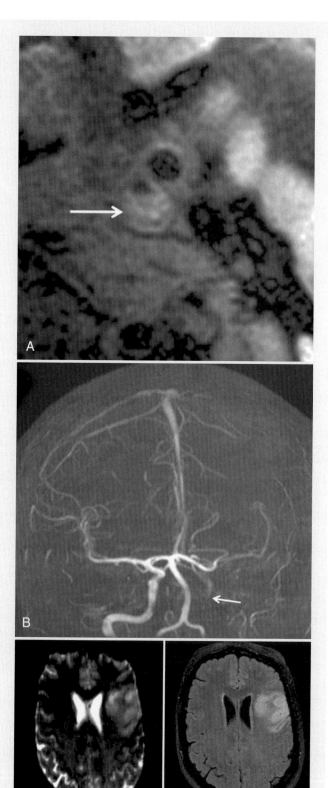

■ **Figure 26-5 A,** T1-weighted image of the left carotid artery of a 47-year-old female presenting with acute expressive dysphasia. A 90% occlusion of the left internal carotid artery is seen (*arrow*); marked heterogeneity of the plaque can be seen. **B,** Magnetic resonance angiogram of the same patient showing interruption of flow through the left common carotid artery (*arrow*) when compared with the contralateral side. Flow in the distal circle internal of artery can be seen as a result of backfilling from the circle of Willis. **C,** Diffusion weighted imaging of the brain (left) reveals a large area of acute ischemia and infarction in the left middle cerebral artery territory, which is confirmed by subsequent FLAIR imaging of the matched slice.

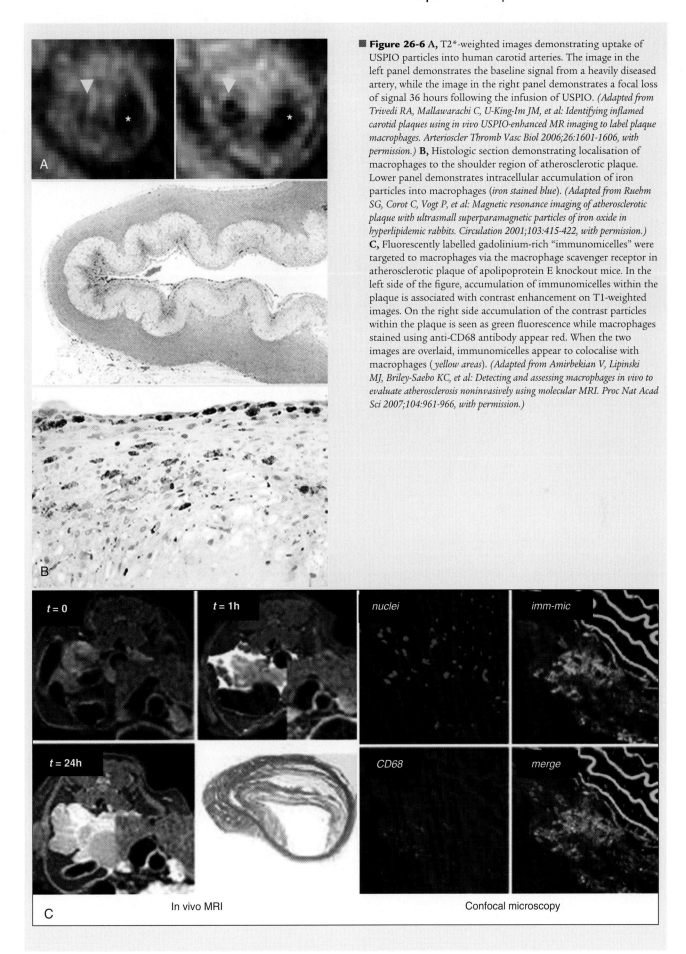

■ **Figure 26-6 A,** T2*-weighted images demonstrating uptake of USPIO particles into human carotid arteries. The image in the left panel demonstrates the baseline signal from a heavily diseased artery, while the image in the right panel demonstrates a focal loss of signal 36 hours following the infusion of USPIO. *(Adapted from Trivedi RA, Mallawarachi C, U-King-Im JM, et al: Identifying inflamed carotid plaques using in vivo USPIO-enhanced MR imaging to label plaque macrophages. Arterioscler Thromb Vasc Biol 2006;26:1601-1606, with permission.)* **B,** Histologic section demonstrating localisation of macrophages to the shoulder region of atherosclerotic plaque. Lower panel demonstrates intracellular accumulation of iron particles into macrophages *(iron stained blue). (Adapted from Ruehm SG, Corot C, Vogt P, et al: Magnetic resonance imaging of atherosclerotic plaque with ultrasmall superparamagnetic particles of iron oxide in hyperlipidemic rabbits. Circulation 2001;103:415-422, with permission.)* **C,** Fluorescently labelled gadolinium-rich "immunomicelles" were targeted to macrophages via the macrophage scavenger receptor in atherosclerotic plaque of apolipoprotein E knockout mice. In the left side of the figure, accumulation of immunomicelles within the plaque is associated with contrast enhancement on T1-weighted images. On the right side accumulation of the contrast particles within the plaque is seen as green fluorescence while macrophages stained using anti-CD68 antibody appear red. When the two images are overlaid, immunomicelles appear to colocalise with macrophages *(yellow areas). (Adapted from Amirbekian V, Lipinski MJ, Briley-Saebo KC, et al: Detecting and assessing macrophages in vivo to evaluate atherosclerosis noninvasively using molecular MRI. Proc Nat Acad Sci 2007;104:961-966, with permission.)*

SUGGESTED READING

Plaque Imaging

Corti R, Fayad ZA, Fuster V, et al: Effects of lipid-lowering by simvastatin on human atherosclerotic lesions: A longitudinal study by high-resolution, noninvasive magnetic resonance imaging. Circulation 2001;104:249-252.

Corti R, Fuster V, Fayad ZA, et al: Effects of aggressive versus conventional lipid-lowering therapy by simvastatin on human atherosclerotic lesions: A prospective, randomized, double-blind trial with high-resolution magnetic resonance imaging. J Am Coll Cardiol 2005; 46:106.

Kramer CM, Cerilli LA, Hagspiel K, et al: Magnetic resonance imaging identifies the fibrous cap in atherosclerotic abdominal aortic aneurysm. Circulation 2004;109:1016-1021.

Lee JMS, Wiesmann F, Shirodaria S, et al: Early changes in arterial structure and function following statin initiation: Quantification by magnetic resonance imaging. Atherosclerosis 2008 197:951-958.

Saam T, Ferguson MS, Yarnykh VL, et al: Quantitative evaluation of carotid plaque composition by in vivo MRI. Arterioscler Thromb Vasc Biol 2005;25:234-239.

Yuan C, Kerwin WS, Ferguson MS, et al: Contrast-enhanced high resolution MRI for atherosclerotic carotid artery tissue characterization. J Magn Reson Imaging 2002;15:62-67.

Yuan C, Zhang SX, Polissar NL, et al: Identification of fibrous cap rupture with magnetic resonance imaging is highly associated with recent transient ischemic attack or stroke. Circulation 2002;105:181-185.

Vascular Function

Cohn JN: Arterial stiffness, vascular disease, and risk of cardiovascular events. Circulation 2006;113:601-603.

Lee JM, Shirodaria C, Jackson CE, et al: Multi-modal magnetic resonance imaging quantifies atherosclerosis and vascular dysfunction in patients with type 2 diabetes mellitus. Diab Vasc Dis Res 2007;4: 44-48.

Leeson CP, Robinson M, Francis JM, et al: Cardiovascular magnetic resonance imaging for non-invasive assessment of vascular function: Validation against ultrasound. J Cardiovasc Magn Reson 2006;8: 381-387.

Mattace-Raso FU, van der Cammen TJ, Hofman A, et al: Arterial stiffness and risk of coronary heart disease and stroke: The Rotterdam Study. Circulation 2006;113:657-663.

Metafratzi ZM, Efremidis SC, Skopelitou AS, De Roos A: The clinical significance of aortic compliance and its assessment with magnetic resonance imaging. J Cardiovasc Magn Reson 2002;4:481-491.

Oliver JJ, Webb DJ: Noninvasive assessment of arterial stiffness and risk of atherosclerotic events. Arterioscler Thromb Vasc Biol 2003;23:554-566.

Wiesmann F, Petersen SE, Leeson PM, et al: Global impairment of brachial, carotid, and aortic vascular function in young smokers: Direct quantification by high-resolution magnetic resonance imaging. J Am Coll Cardiol 2004;44:2056-2064.

Molecular Imaging

Choudhury RP, Fuster V, Fayad ZA: Molecular, cellular and functional imaging of atherothrombosis. Nat Rev Drug Discov 2004;3:913-925.

Index